The Assessment and Treatment of Addiction

The Assessment and Treatment of Addiction

Best Practices and New Frontiers

Edited by:

ITAI DANOVITCH, MD, MBA, DFASAM, FAPA
Chairman
Associate Clinical Professor
Department of Psychiatry and Behavioral Neurosciences
Cedars Sinai Medical Center
Los Angeles, CA, United States

LARISSA J. MOONEY, MD
Associate Clinical Professor
Department of Psychiatry and Biobehavioral Sciences
University of California, Los Angeles
Los Angeles, CA, United States

Chief, Greater Los Angeles VA Substance Use Disorders Section
Los Angeles, CA, United States

ELSEVIER

ELSEVIER

3251 Riverport Lane
St. Louis, Missouri 63043

Publisher: Patrick Manley
Acquisition Editor: Lauren Boyle
Editorial Project Manager: Jennifer Horigan
Production Project Manager: Poulouse Joseph
Cover Designer: Alan Studholme

Typeset by TNQ Technologies

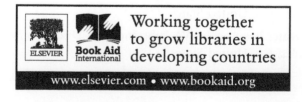

List of Contributors

Itai Danovitch, MD, MBA, DFASAM, FAPA
Chairman
Associate Clinical Professor
Department of Psychiatry and Behavioral
  Neurosciences
Cedars Sinai Medical Center
Los Angeles, CA, United States

Larissa J. Mooney, MD
Associate Clinical Professor
Department of Psychiatry and Biobehavioral Sciences
University of California
Los Angeles, CA, United States
Chief
Greater Los Angeles VA Substance Use Disorders
  Section
Los Angeles, CA, USA,

Jonathan M. Wai, MD
Addiction Psychiatry Fellow
Division on Substance Use Disorders
Columbia University Department of Psychiatry
New York, NY, United States

David A. Wiss, MS, RDN
Doctoral Student
Fielding School of Public Health, Community
  Health Sciences
University of California, Los Angeles
Los Angeles, CA, United States
Registered Dietitian Nutritionist
Nutrition in Recovery
Los Angeles, CA, United States

Tony P. George, MD, FRC
Professor of Psychiatry
Department of Psychiatry
University of Toronto
Toronto, ON, Canada

Kristen Schmidt, MD, MAPH
Addiction Psychiatry Fellow
Psychiatry and Biobehavioral Sciences
University of California
Los Angeles, CA, United States

Elie G. Aoun, MD
General, Addictions and Forensic Psychiatrist
Forensic Psychiatry Research Fellow
Columbia University
New York, NY, United States

Alan J. Budney, PhD
Professor
Center for Technology and Behavioral Health
Geisel School of Medicine, Dartmouth College
Hanover, NH, United States

Andrew Saxon, MD
Director, Center of Excellence in Substance Abuse
  Treatment and Education
Mental Health
VA Puget Sound Health Care System
Seattle, WA, United States
Professor
Psychiatry and Behavioral Sciences
University of Washington
Seattle, WA, United States

David A. Gorelick, MD, PhD, DLFAPA
Professor
Department of Psychiatry
University of Maryland School of Medicine
Baltimore, MD, United States

Lara A. Ray, PhD
Professor
Department of Psychology
University of California, Los Angeles
Los Angeles, CA, United States

Keith G. Heinzerling, MD, MPH
Associate Professor in Residence
Department of Family Medicine
UCLA
Los Angeles, CA, United States

Suzette Glasner, PhD
Associate Professor
Department of Psychiatry and School of Nursing
UCLA
Los Angeles, CA, United States

Tess K. Drazdowski, PhD
Postdoctoral Scholar, UCLA
Integrated Substance Abuse Programs (ISAP)
Department of Psychiatry and Biobehavioral Sciences
Los Angeles, CA, United States

Seth Ammerman, MD, FAAP, FSAHM, DABAM
Clinical Professor
Division of Adolescent Medicine
Department of Pediatrics
Stanford University/Lucile Packard Children's
    Hospital Stanford
Palo Alto, CA, United States

Anna Lembke, MD
Associate Professor of Psychiatry in Addiction Medicine
    and courtesy faculty appointment in Pain Medicine
Medical Director
Addiction Medicine Chief
Addiction Medicine Dual Diagnosis Clinic
Program Director
Addiction Medicine Fellowship
Stanford University School of Medicine
Stanford, CA, United States

Ismene Petrakis, MD
Professor
Department of Psychiatry
Yale University School of Medicine
West Haven, CT, United States

Dolores Vojvoda, MD
Assistant Professor of Psychiatry
Department of Psychiatry
Yale University School of Medicine
New Haven, CT, United States

Director, PTSD/Anxiety Firm
Department of Psychiatry
VA Connecticut Healthcare System
West Haven, CT, United States

Mark S. Gold, MD
Professor and Chairman
Department of Psychiatry
University of Florida
Gainesville, FL, United States

A. Benjamin Srivastava, MD
Resident Physician
Department of Psychiatry
Washington University School of Medicine
Saint Louis, MO, United States

John F. Kelly, PhD
Elizabeth R. Spallin Associate Professor of Psychiatry
    in Addiction Medicine, Harvard Medical School
Department of Psychiatry
Harvard Medical School
Boston, MA, United States

Director, Recovery Research Institute
Massachusetts General Hospital
Boston, MA, United States

David Mee-Lee, MD
President
Owner
DML Training and Consulting
Davis, CA, United States

Jeffrey Becker, MD, ABIHM
Psychiatrist
CA, United States

Frances R. Levin, MD
Kennedy-Leavy Professor of Psychiatry
Columbia University Irving Medical Center
Director
Division on Substance Use Disorders
New York State Psychiatric Institute
New York, NY, United States

Diana Martinez, MD
Professor of Psychiatry at Columbia University Irving
    Medical Center
Division on Substance Use Disorders
Columbia University Department of Psychiatry
New York, NY, United States

Darby Lowe, BSc
Addictions Division, CAMH
Department of Psychiatry
University of Toronto
Toronto, ON, Canada

Alexandria S. Coles, BA
Addictions Division, CAMH
Department of Psychiatry
University of Toronto
Toronto, ON, Canada

Karolina Kozak, MSc
Addictions Division, CAMH
Department of Psychiatry
University of Toronto
Toronto, ON, Canada

Jacob T. Borodovsky, PhD
Health & Behavior Research Center
Washington University School of Medicine
St. Louis, MO, United States

Lisa A. Marsch, PhD
Professor
Center for Technology and Behavioral Health
    Geisel School of Medicine, Dartmouth College
Hanover, NH, United States

Sarah E. Lord, PhD
Professor
Center for Technology and Behavioral Health
    Geisel School of Medicine, Dartmouth College
Hanover, NH, United States

Emily Hartwell, MA
Department of Psychology
University of California, Los Angeles
Los Angeles, CA, United States

Rejoyce Green, BA
Department of Psychology
University of California, Los Angeles
Los Angeles, CA, United States

Alexandra Venegas, BS
Department of Psychology
University of California, Los Angeles
Los Angeles, CA, United States

Managing Challenges in the Assessment and Treatment of Addiction

Larissa J. Mooney and Itai Danovitch

Scientific research has characterized addiction as a disease of the brain marked by significant clinical and social impairment caused by loss of control over substance use. The underpinnings of addiction span biological, psychological, environmental, and social factors. Typical of other chronic diseases, recovery from substance use disorders (SUDs) often includes episodes of relapse to some level of substance use, which may warrant more careful monitoring, improved adherence to treatment, or a change in treatment approach to facilitate symptom remission. The best outcomes of treatment for many SUDs are generally obtained by a long-term, comprehensive, individualized approach integrating pharmacotherapy and behavioral interventions to manage symptoms and promote recovery.

In the United States, substance-related overdose deaths are at an all-time high and are now the leading cause of death among individuals under age 50 years. The sharpest rise in recent years has been largely driven by a sharp rise in use of opioids and sedative hypnotics. Despite this public health crisis, only approximately 10% of individuals with SUDs who need treatment receive it. Thus, there is an urgent need to increase the availability of evidence-based screening, diagnosis, and treatment of SUDs. Innovative intervention strategies and more accessible treatment programs should be expanded and available in nonspecialty healthcare settings such as primary care and mental health clinics. Health systems and networks need to implement service delivery models that improve coordination, integration, and quality of care.

The focus of this book is on the assessment and treatment of SUDs, traditionally referred to as "addiction" and still used in current clinical practice and research, including in the most recent version of the *Diagnostic and Statistical Manual (DSM-5)*. The book is organized into three broad sections that cover emerging findings, established practices, and novel approaches for addressing SUDs. The specific content covered within each section was selected with attention to the predicaments and concerns that healthcare providers and patients regularly face. Thus, the topics covered range from patient-level interventions to systems issues, such as measuring quality. Some chapters provide an overview of evidence-based treatment approaches for SUDs, such as recent developments in pharmacological and behavioral treatment options for the major categories of SUDs, as well as the needs of special populations, such as adolescents and older adults. Other chapters cover neurobiology, nutrition, trauma, chronic pain, and psychoneuroendocrinology phenomena that have implications for treatment and clinical management. Finally, several chapters address novel concepts and emerging areas of research in the field that will become the basis for future approaches to identifying, treating, and managing SUDs.

Our overarching goal is to equip healthcare providers, researchers, administrators, and policymakers with information required to advance the field and provide quality care to individuals with SUDs. We are grateful for the outstanding work of the contributing authors, each a leader in the field, without which this book would not have been possible.

Contents

CHAPTER 1

Neurochemical Imaging in Addiction: How Science Informs Practice

JONATHAN M. WAI, MD • FRANCES R. LEVIN, MD • DIANA MARTINEZ, MD

OVERVIEW

Substance use disorders are characterized by the Diagnostic and Statistical Manual of Mental Disorders (DSM-5) as "a cluster of cognitive, behavioral, and physiological symptoms indicating that the individual continues using the substance despite significant substance-related problems".[1] The diagnostic criteria are further categorized into the symptom clusters of impaired control over use, compulsivity, harmful consequences, and the physiological symptoms of tolerance and withdrawal. These symptoms may persist despite clear negative consequences due to environmental, psychological, or biological reinforcers of behavior. The uncontrollable substance intake that characterizes addiction is clinically distinct from the occasional use of an addictive drug without loss of control,[2] and current addiction research is focused on characterizing the mechanisms underpinning that distinction. This chapter will review the discoveries of neurochemical imaging studies in human subjects and explore how these findings may translate to treatments for addiction.

NEUROANATOMICAL STRUCTURES

A brief review of the neuroanatomical structures most relevant to addiction will aid in understanding the neurochemical imaging literature. These structures have mostly been identified through research using animal models. The nucleus accumbens is located within the ventral striatum and is most closely associated with the reinforcing properties of substances.[3,4] Projections from the ventral tegmental area to the nucleus accumbens shell are important for regulating motivational salience.[5,6] Rewarding events increase dopaminergic release in the accumbens, which reinforces the behaviors that led to the reward.[7,8] The amygdala also receives dopaminergic input from the ventral tegmental area, as well as other input from the prefrontal cortex, nucleus accumbens, brain stem, and hypothalamus.[9] It is involved in attributing predictors to motivationally salient, or rewarding, events.[10] The prefrontal cortex, particularly the anterior cingulate and ventral orbital cortices, is involved in reward-based decision-making,[11] a process that appears to be strongly influenced by the predictability of a reward.[12,13]

NEUROTRANSMITTERS

Dopamine has a central role in mediating reinforced behavior. The mesolimbic dopamine system, which connects the ventral tegmental area in the midbrain to the nucleus accumbens in the ventral striatum, is specifically involved in the reward and reinforcement value of addictive substances.[14] When dopamine is released from the ventral tegmental area in response to novel salient stimuli, this promotes learning and diverts attention to these events.[15] There are 5 subtypes of dopamine receptors (D1-D5), which are further classified into the D1-like (D1 and D5) and D2-like (D2, D3, D4) families.[16] The D1-like receptors act to increase the second messenger cyclic adenosine monophosphate (cAMP), while the D2-like receptors decrease cAMP.[17] Because of the similar properties of these receptors within their respective families and similar behavior in neuroimaging studies, they will be referred to only as D1 or D2 receptors in this chapter.

Changes in dopaminergic signaling in humans were first identified in cocaine addiction by Volkow et al.,[18] but have now been seen in many other addictions, including alcohol, opioid, tobacco, and methamphetamine use disorder. Recent studies have also found impaired dopamine systems in cannabis use disorder. Low D2 receptor binding has been hypothesized to

The Assessment and Treatment of Addiction. https://doi.org/10.1016/B978-0-323-54856-4.00001-8

represent a vulnerability to the rewarding effect of pharmacologic rewards over naturally occurring reinforcers.[19,20]

NEUROCHEMICAL IMAGING

Positron emission tomography (PET) and single-photon emission computed tomography (SPECT) are imaging modalities that can be used to measure receptor density and changes in neurotransmitters in the human brain. The injection of a radioligand, which is a radioactive molecule that binds to a specific receptor, can be detected with PET or SPECT scanners. Radioligands have been developed for a number of different receptors in the brain, such as D1 and D2 dopamine receptors, μ-opioid receptors, serotonergic receptors, and more.

The outcome measure for these brain imaging studies is called the "binding potential" (BP). BP is a measure of the radioligand–receptor complexes in the brain, and it is defined as the product of receptor density (B_{max}) and the affinity of the radioligand for the receptor $(1/K_D)$[21] such that:

$$BP = \frac{B_{max}}{K_D} = B_{max} * \frac{1}{K_D} = B_{max} * affinity$$

However, it is also important in brain imaging to recognize that while the radioligand binds to the receptor, a small amount will bind to nonspecific proteins in the brain. This is called "nonspecific binding" and it affects the "signal to noise" of the radioligand. The most common method used to account for nonspecific binding is to use a reference region. This is a brain region that does not have the receptor being targeted and contains only the nonspecific binding of the radioligand.[22] This is abbreviated as the BP_{ND} because it uses the nonspecific binding in tissue as a reference region. This is calculated as:

$$BP_{ND} = f_{ND} * \frac{B_{max}}{K_D}$$

In this equation, f_{ND} is the free fraction of drug in the nondisplaceable reference region.[23] For example, when imaging D2 receptors with the radiotracer [11C]raclopride, the cerebellum is often used as the reference region because there are no cerebellar dopamine receptors. Other measures of binding potential are BP_F and BP_P, which use the equilibrium ratios of specifically bound radioligand relative to the free radioligand in tissue or the total radioligand in plasma, respectively. These other measures require more invasive procedures, such as arterial blood monitoring, to estimate the binding potential. While nomenclature can vary, these are the simplest definitions of the binding potential measures.[22]

In addition to measuring receptor binding potential, the stimulant "challenge" method can also be used to study changes in dopamine transmission (see Fig. 1.1). This technique uses a PET radioligand that images the D2 receptor and scans are obtained before and after a stimulant, such as amphetamine or methylphenidate. Since the stimulant increases endogenous dopamine in the brain, there are fewer D2 receptors available to bind to the radioligand. This results in a decrease in BP, with a greater decrease in BP representing increased levels of endogenous dopamine release. This decrease is likely from internalization of the D2 receptors rather than direct competition of dopamine and the radiotracer in the poststimulant scan.[24,25]

Thus, the use of PET imaging can provide the following information on dopamine transmission: (1) baseline binding of the D2 receptor in the human brain;

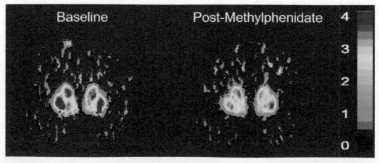

FIG. 1.1 Representative PET scan showing the decrease in D2 receptor binding following a stimulant challenge with methylphenidate 60mg PO. Methylphenidate administration decreases the amount of D2 receptors available to bind to [11C]raclopride by increasing extracellular dopamine. Values for the binding potential are shown in the color bar.

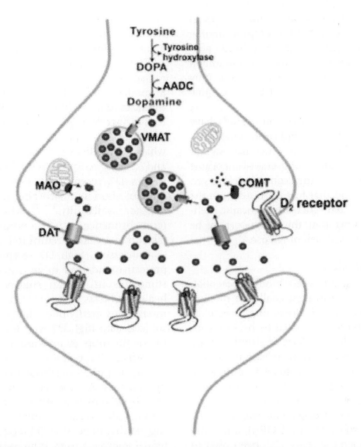

FIG. 1.2 A dopaminergic synapse. DAT = dopamine transporter, MAO = monoamine oxidase, VMAT = vesicular monoamine transporter, COMT = catechol-O-methyltransferase, AADC = aromatic L-amino acid decarboxylase. (Adapted from Ravan S, Martinez D, Slifstein M, Abi-Dargham A. Molecular imaging in alcohol dependence. In: Handbook of Clinical Neurology. Vol 125. Elsevier; 2014:293-311. https://doi.org/10.1016/B978-0-444-62619-6.00018-5.)

and (2) dopamine release from the presynaptic neurons in response to a pharmacologic challenge with a stimulant drug.

COCAINE
Cocaine and Dopamine

Neurochemical imaging has been used to investigate changes in dopamine receptors (D1 and D2) as well as presynaptic dopamine release in cocaine use disorder. With chronic cocaine use, there have been consistent findings of dysfunctional dopamine signaling along multiple parts of the synapse. Fig. 1.2 illustrates the components of the synaptic cleft of a dopamine neuron.

Dopamine Receptors

Numerous PET imaging studies have shown that DSM-IV cocaine dependence is associated with a decrease in D2 receptor binding. Volkow et al.[18] first used [18F]N-methylspiroperidol to show decreased D2 receptor binding potential in the striatum, which has been repeatedly replicated with similar findings.[26–30] This decrease has been correlated with decreased cerebral glucose metabolism in the orbitofrontal cortex and cingulate measured with [18F]fludeoxyglucose,[13] suggesting associated dysregulation of inhibitory control and decision-making leading to compulsive drug taking. When the striatal substructures are differentiated into the caudate, putamen, and ventral striatum, low D2 receptor binding potential is seen across each subdivision.[28,30] These findings have been found to persist after 3 months of abstinence[26] and studies in nonhuman primates suggests that D2 receptor binding may not return to precocaine use levels until after 1 year.[31] Additionally, imaging studies in nonhuman primates have demonstrated that this decrease is only seen in chronic and not short-term cocaine exposure.[31–34]

Changes in the dopamine D1 receptor family have also been implicated in cocaine addiction. One study using [^{11}C]NNC-112 showed no difference in D1 receptor binding in persons with DSM-IV cocaine dependence compared to healthy controls. However, this same study also found that low D1 binding in the ventral striatum predicted increased cocaine self-administration, suggesting that this receptor may be associated with an increased risk of relapse.[35]

Dopamine Transmission

In addition to decreased D2 receptor binding potential, several studies using the stimulant challenge method have found decreased striatal dopamine release in cocaine-dependent subjects compared to healthy controls.[27,36] While the euphoric effects of stimulants are positively associated with dopamine release in healthy controls,[37–41] cocaine-dependent subjects experience less subjectively positive responses to psychostimulants and there is no association between their subjective response and the amount of dopamine release.[27] PET scans with 6-[^{18}F]-flouro-L-DOPA (FDOPA), a radiolabeled precursor to dopamine, have also been used to measure presynaptic dopamine activity. Subjects with DSM-IV cocaine dependence who were abstinent for 11–30 days had decreased FDOPA uptake when compared to healthy controls,[42] suggesting that there is decreased dopamine synthesis during this abstinence period.

Another technique uses alpha-methyl-p-tyrosine (AMPT) to inhibit tyrosine hydroxylase.[43] Tyrosine hydroxylase is an enzyme required for dopamine synthesis and its inhibition results in lowered endogenous dopamine. By performing a PET scan with AMPT induced dopamine depletion after a preliminary [^{11}C]raclopride scan and measuring the difference, studies have shown that endogenous dopamine is reduced in individuals with DSM-IV cocaine dependence.[30]

Clinical Significance

Although the literature is clear that there are widespread dopaminergic deficits in individuals with cocaine use disorder when compared to healthy individuals, the question of the significance of this relationship remains—does low D2 receptor availability represent a vulnerability to cocaine addiction, or is it a result of it? There are limited studies with human subjects that can address this, but animal studies can be used to infer a model where decreased D2 receptor availability increases the likelihood of substance use, which in turn further decreases D2 receptor binding. Social stress in rhesus monkeys leads to decreased D2 receptors, which is predictive of cocaine self-administration,[44] and chronic cocaine self-administration further decreases D2 receptor binding potential.[31] Prolonged, but not short term, cocaine use decreases dopamine receptor availability,[32–34] which recovers with long-term abstinence.[31,45,46] In nonhuman primates, it may take up to a year to return to baseline levels.[31]

Conversely, high D2 receptor availability may be protective and lead to an unpleasant experience with stimulants in human studies.[38,47] In these studies, healthy subjects with low D2 receptor availability rated intravenous methylphenidate as more enjoyable, while subjects with high D2 receptor levels were more likely to rate the drug as unpleasant. This suggests that baseline striatal D2 receptor availability modulates the reinforcing properties of stimulants and thus affects the risk of addiction. Additionally, using an adenovirus vector in rodents to increase the expression of D2 receptors results in reduced cocaine intake.[48] These studies together suggest that increasing D2 receptor availability is a potential approach to treating cocaine use disorder.

Other Dopamine Studies

The dopamine transporter (DAT) is a presynaptic monoamine transporter that mediates dopamine reuptake from the synapse. Cocaine intoxication and addiction are mediated primarily through dopaminergic pathways, with acute effects due to inhibition of dopamine uptake by binding to the DAT.[49] DAT can be imaged with radiotracers [^{123}I]β-CIT for SPECT and [^{11}C]cocaine in PET to measure the density of dopaminergic neurons. Studies show mixed results, with DAT being elevated for up to 6 weeks after cessation of cocaine use,[50–52] but returning to normal levels after early abstinence. These studies suggest that there are likely no long-term changes in DAT as a result of chronic cocaine use and thus little evidence of long-term changes to the density of dopamine neurons. The findings of the PET and SPECT literature studying dopamine in cocaine use disorder are summarized in Table 1.1.

TABLE 1.1
Summary of the Findings of PET and SPECT Literature Studying the Dopaminergic Changes in Cocaine Dependence

Target	COCAINE STUDIES SHOWING CHANGE		
	Decreased	No Difference	Increased
D2 Receptor Binding	Volkow et al.,[18] Volkow et al.,[26] Volkow et al.,[27] Martinez et al.,[28] Martinez et al.,[30] and Martinez et al.[29]		
Dopamine Transmission	Volkow et al.,[27] Martinez et al.,[36] and Martinez et al.[29]		
Endogenous Dopamine	Martinez et al.[30]		
DAT		Volkow et al.[52] and Wang et al.[51]	Malison et al.[50]
Dopamine Synthesis	Wu et al.[42]		

The columns display the studies that show a decrease, increase, or no change of the dopaminergic component in the row.

Other Neurotransmitters

Using [11C]carfentanil as a radiotracer to the μ-opioid receptor, studies have found increased BP in the anterior cingulate, frontal and temporal cortices, caudate, and thalamus in early abstinence, and increased BP in cingulate, frontal cortex, caudate, and thalamus after 4 weeks of abstinence.[53,54] μ-opioid receptor binding also correlates with self-reports of craving for cocaine. Serotonergic dysfunction has also been observed in acutely abstinent chronic cocaine users. Using [123I] β-CIT, Jacobson et al.[55] observed increased serotonin transporter binding in the diencephalon and brainstem. This finding suggests that serotonin levels may be decreased in the synapse during acute abstinence.

Summary

In summary, there are consistent PET findings in subjects with cocaine use disorder showing (1) decreased dopamine D2 receptor availability, (2) decreased presynaptic dopamine release, and (3) reduced endogenous dopamine. These pharmacologic effects of cocaine are seen only after chronic cocaine exposure. Additionally, there are differential changes in the dopamine system depending on the duration of abstinence. It remains unclear if these changes predispose patients to or are result of cocaine use, but there is some evidence that both of these processes occur. Animal studies suggest that correction of the dopaminergic deficit can reduce cocaine use. As will be discussed later on, recent studies developing treatments for cocaine use disorder have capitalized on these findings from brain imaging studies by addressing this neurochemical deficit.

METHAMPHETAMINE

Like cocaine, chronic methamphetamine use has been associated with decreased striatal D2 receptor binding and blunted presynaptic dopamine release.[56–58] However, unlike cocaine, chronic methamphetamine use has been consistently associated with decreased DAT levels. Table 1.2 summarizes the PET findings for DAT in chronic methamphetamine abuse. DAT levels are decreased by 16%–30% in subjects that range in periods of abstinence from days to years,[59–66] most often in the caudate, putamen, and ventral striatum. DAT is most decreased when abstinence periods are shorter, with Volkow et al.[62] finding recovery to normal measures of DAT after 9 months of abstinence. This same study also showed that levels of DAT positively correlated with performance in motor and verbal memory tasks, although this finding was not replicated in other studies.[59,60] Conflicting studies have found decreases in DAT persisting even after at least several years of abstinence.[60,61] As decreased DAT represents a decrease in dopaminergic neurons, these results suggest that chronic methamphetamine use results in neuronal loss. In the serotonin system, widespread decrease of the serotonin transporter has been observed in areas that include the orbitofrontal

TABLE 1.2
Comparison of the Percent Decrease in DAT Binding and Time of Abstinence (in Order of Least to Greatest Decrease in DAT Binding)

Study	Abstinence Period Mean (Range)	Maximal % Decrease of DAT
Johanson et al.[59]	3.4 y (3 m–18 y)	15% (caudate)
McCann et al.[61]	3.3 y (4 m–5 y)	25% (putamen)
McCann et al.[60]	2.4 y (8 m–>10 y)	23% (caudate)
Iyo et al.[66]	9 m[a] (0 m–18 m)	26% (ventral striatum)
Volkow et al.[65]	6 m (0.5 m–36 m)	28% (caudate)
Sekine et al.[63]	5.6 m (7 d–1.5 y)	30% (ventral striatum)
Chou et al.[64]	Days (not specified)	30% (whole striatum)

The percent % is the maximal decrease reported in any striatal brain region. Abstinence period is provided as the time of abstinence prior to the PET scan and is reported as an average and range: y is years, m is months, d is days.
[a] estimated average, actual data not provided.
Adapted from Urban NBL, Martinez D. Neurobiology of addiction. Insight from neurochemical imaging. *Psychiatr Clin North Am.* 2012;35(2): 521–541. https://doi.org/10.1016/j.psc.2012.03.011.

and occipital cortices, midbrain, thalamus, caudate, and cerebellum,[67,68] suggesting damage to and loss of neurons in the serotonergic system in addition to the loss of dopaminergic neurons observed in studies looking at DAT levels. Taken together, these studies show that methamphetamine use disorder is associated with blunted striatal dopamine transmission, which is similar to the findings in cocaine use disorder. However, insofar as DAT serves as a marker for integrity of the dopaminergic neuron, these imaging studies also indicate that chronic methamphetamine use may cause more neuronal injury and have more permanent effects than chronic cocaine use.

ALCOHOL
Dopamine Receptors
The changes in the D2 receptor binding associated with chronic alcohol use are also similar to what has been observed with chronic cocaine use. In subjects with DSM-IV alcohol dependence, D2 striatal binding is decreased by about 10%–20% when compared to healthy controls.[69–73] This reduced binding is seen in multiple regions across the striatum, including the nucleus accumbens. Striatal D2 binding is also inversely associated with increased alcohol craving,[71] which in turn is positively correlated with risk of relapse.[70] Taken together, these studies suggest that persons with alcohol use disorder who have low D2 receptor binding are at an increased risk for relapse compared to persons with alcohol use disorder with normal D2 binding.

Presynaptic Dopamine
Dopamine transmission in alcohol use disorder has been studied using PET and three different radiotracers: (1) [18F]dihydrotetrobenazine (DTBZ) which labels the type 2 vesicular monoamine transporters (VMAT 2); (2) [11C]raclopride before and after a psychostimulant challenge to measure presynaptic dopamine release; and (3) FDOPA to the measure the capacity of presynaptic dopamine synthesis.

Overall, these studies show that alcohol use disorder is associated with a decrease in striatal dopamine storage and release. Studies using [18F]DTBZ to label the presynaptic dopamine vesicles found decreased radioligand uptake in the caudate nucleus and putamen, representing decreased dopamine stores.[74] Using the [11C]raclopride stimulant challenge produces similar findings, showing decreased endogenous dopamine release when comparing persons with DSM-IV alcohol dependence to healthy controls,[75] specifically in the putamen and ventral striatum.[76,77]

Experiments performed with FDOPA have not shown a clear decrease in the uptake of this radiotracer. While increased FDOPA in the left putamen and right caudate[78] has been observed, Heinz et al.[70] found no significant difference in net striatal FDOPA uptake when comparing persons with DSM-IV alcohol dependence to controls. However, this study did find that FDOPA uptake in the ventral striatum was negatively associated with increased alcohol craving, suggesting that decreased dopamine synthesis in persons with alcohol use disorder increases cravings and risk of relapse.

Imaging of the DAT using varied methodology (PET/SPECT/autoradiograph) and radiotracers ([^{123}I]β-CIT, [^{11}C]D-threo-methylphenidate) has yielded mixed results. Most studies show decreased or no change in DAT concentrations in early withdrawal or prolonged sobriety compared to healthy controls,[73,79–83] with only one group finding increased DAT in violent subjects with DSM-III alcoholism using SPECT after 4 weeks of abstinence.[81] These findings suggest that while alcohol withdrawal may result in a transient decrease in DAT binding, there are no long-term changes in DAT availability and thus no changes in dopamine neurons density.

Similar to chronic cocaine use, it remains undetermined whether these changes in dopamine pathways predispose or result from chronic alcohol use. Volkow et al.[72] found D2 receptor binding to be unaffected after 4 months of abstinence. Rominger et al.[84] also did not find a difference in striatal D2 receptor binding in early abstinence, although they did find striatal and thalamic D2 receptor binding to be increased 30% after 1 year of abstinence. Conversely, there is evidence of low D2 binding increasing liability for development of an alcohol use disorder. Healthy nonaddicted family members with alcohol use disorder have higher D2 receptor binding,[85] suggesting that these individuals may be protected by a more robust dopamine signaling pathway. Additionally, similar to what was observed in cocaine studies, using an adenovirus vector to increase D2 receptor expression in rats decreases alcohol self-administration.[86] Table 1.3 summarizes the findings of PET studies looking at dopamine in alcohol use disorder.

GABA

Studies on the GABA$_A$ receptor have mostly used the PET radioligand [^{11}C]flumazenil, or SPECT tracer [^{123}I]iomazenil and have had mixed results. Multiple studies have found decreased GABA$_A$ receptor availability at 1–7 months of abstinence.[87–89] However, increased GABA$_A$ receptor availability for persons with comorbid DSM-IV alcohol and tobacco dependence was observed at 1 week of abstinence, but this normalized to control levels after 4 weeks of abstinence.[90] Other studies found no difference in GABA$_A$ receptor binding in persons with DSM-IV alcohol dependence compared to healthy controls.[91,92] Variations in cohort sizes and differing times of abstinence may account for these discrepancies in findings. Additionally, these findings may be from reduced grey matter volume and not truly reduced receptor density,[93] although one study found decreased GABA receptors even in the absence of grey matter atrophy.[89]

Other Neurotransmitters

Studies have looked at the serotonin transporter and serotonin receptors 1A and 1B with overall mixed results.[94–97] Again, these studies have varied methodologies and patient characteristics, but generally found decreased serotonin transporter, no difference in serotonin 1A receptor, and increased binding to the serotonin 1B receptor in the ventral striatum of persons with DSM-IV alcohol dependence.

The opioid transporter has been investigated with the radiotracer [^{11}C]carfentanil (selective for the μ-opioid receptor), [^{11}C]diprenorphine (a nonselective opioid

TABLE 1.3
Summary of the Dopaminergic Neuroimaging Studies in Alcohol Dependence

Target	ALCOHOL STUDIES SHOWING CHANGE		
	Decreased	No Difference	Increased
D2 receptor binding	Hietala et al.,[69] Volkow et al.,[73] Volkow et al.,[72] Heinz et al.,[70,71] and Martinez et al.[76] Rominger et al.[84] (immediate)	Rominger et al.[84] after short-term follow-up	Rominger et al.[84] (after 1 year of abstinence)
Dopamine Transmission	Martinez et al.[76] and Volkow et al.[77]		
DAT	Tiihonen et al.,[81] Laine et al.,[79,80] immediate, Repo et al.[83]	Volkow et al.,[73] Heinz et al.,[82] Laine et al.[79,80] (at 4 weeks)	Tiihonen et al.[81]
Presynaptic dopamine storage	Gilman et al.[74]		
Dopamine Synthesis		Heinz et al.[70]	Tiihonen et al.[78]

The columns display the studies that show a decrease, increase, or no change in the dopaminergic component of the row. Among the brain regions with changes in dopaminergic targets are the ventral striatum, caudate, putamen, thalamus, hippocampus, and insula.

receptor partial agonist), or [^{11}C]methlynaltrindole (selective for the δ-opioid receptor). These studies have had variable results, showing an increase or decrease in striatal binding.[98–100] Opioid receptor binding has been positively correlated with alcohol craving, significant in the nucleus accumbens and anterior cingulate cortex in early abstinence, and the anterior cingulate cortex in late abstinence.[101] Further evidence of a role of opioid receptors in alcohol use disorder is that treatment with the μ-opioid receptor blocker, naltrexone, reduces cue-induced alcohol cravings,[102] but with only a moderate effect size on drinking reduction and relapse in subjects with DSM-IV alcohol dependence in meta-analyses.[103] However, activation of κ-opioid receptors decreases striatal dopamine release, suggesting that κ-opioid receptor agonism prevents reinforcement.[104]

OTHER SUBSTANCES OF ABUSE

Studies in DSM-IV heroin-dependent subjects found decreased D2 receptor binding and dopamine release; however, neither measure was predictive of heroin self-administration.[105,106] A small study of μ-opioid receptor availably using [^{11}C]carfentanil in persons with DSM-IV heroin dependence on buprenorphine maintenance found an increase in the ventral striatum, inferofrontal cortex, and anterior cingulate.[107] A study with DSM-IV heroin-dependent subjects on methadone maintenance found decreased μ and κ-opioid receptor availability in the thalamus, amygdala, caudate, anterior cingulate, and putamen compared to healthy controls.[108]

In earlier studies, chronic cannabis use had not been associated with decreased D2 receptor binding when compared to healthy controls.[109–111] A study using a stimulant challenge also found no differences in dopamine release in subjects with DSM-IV cannabis dependence, although this study used subjects who reported only mild to moderate cannabis use.[109] However, two recent studies have shown there to be decreased dopamine transmission with cannabis use,[112,113] as well as an inverse association between dopamine release and the severity of cannabis addiction.[112] These discrepancies may be explained by a higher severity of DSM-IV cannabis dependence in the studies with positive findings.

Studies of the cannabinoid CB1 receptor in chronic, heavy cannabis users using the radiotracer [^{18}F]FMPEP-d2 found downregulation of the CB1 receptor in cortical regions, which reverted to normal levels after a month of continuous monitored abstinence.[114] A study with the radiotracer [^{18}F]MK-9470 also found a global decrease in CB1 receptor availability.[115]

SCIENCE INFORMING TREATMENT
Biomarkers for Treatment Prediction

Neurochemical imaging has demonstrated that decreased D2 receptor binding predicts a pleasurable response to psychostimulants in healthy non-addicted controls,[47] which may increase the addictive liability of stimulants for these individuals. Conversely, individuals with a family history of addiction but do not have a substance use disorder have increased D2 receptor binding.[85] Taken together, these results suggest that in healthy nonaddicted people, low D2 receptor binding may serve as a biomarker for increased risk of developing a substance use disorder when exposed to a stimulant. However, since cocaine use itself lowers D2 receptor binding,[31] this measure would be difficult to interpret if a person is already using stimulants.

In addition to abnormalities in D2 receptor binding potential predicting stimulant response, decreased dopamine release in the ventral striatum is predictive of treatment response and stimulant seeking behavior. In studies of persons with DSM-IV cocaine and amphetamine[29,58] dependence, lower D2 receptor binding as well as lower dopamine transmission increased the risk of relapse. In the study by Wang et al.,[58] subgroup analysis of the treatment-seeking subjects who relapsed found no change in D2 availability after the stimulant challenge, representing almost no dopamine release in response to stimulant administration. Conversely, subjects with DSM-IV methamphetamine dependence with D2 receptor availability and dopamine signaling that did not differ from controls were more likely to complete detoxification in this study. In another study by Martinez et al.,[36] subjects with lower dopamine release were more likely to choose cocaine over an equivalent monetary reward. Fig. 1.3 shows a representation of the decreased dopamine signaling as seen with a PET scan using a stimulant challenge. These studies suggest that decreased striatal dopamine function is associated with a poor response to treatment, and increased dopamine signaling predicts a better treatment response.

Dopamine Transmission and Cocaine Use Disorder—Psychostimulant Substitution

The use of psychostimulants to treat cocaine use disorder has been described in case reports dating back to the 1980s.[116,117] The "Self-Medication Hypothesis" proposed by Khantzian asserts that the specific psychoactive properties of substances of abuse appeal to patients with certain psychiatric disturbances.[118] Individuals with symptoms of attention deficit hyperactivity

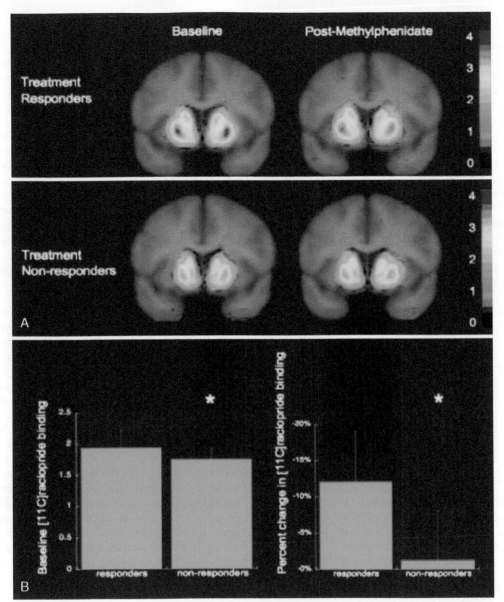

FIG. 1.3 A) Representative PET scans from a cocaine dependent subject who responded to treatment (top) and a treatment non-responder (bottom). The scans shown are at baseline (left) and following 60 mg PO methylphenidate (right). Methylphenidate administration increases extracellular dopamine so that fewer D2 receptors are available to bind to [11C]raclopride. Thus, in treatment responders, methylphenidate administration decreases [11C]raclopride binding, whereas non-responders show little change in [11C] raclopride binding, consistent with high dopamine release in the treatment responder and low dopamine release in the non-responder. The color bar shows the values for binding potential. B) The bar graphs show the changes in [11C]raclopride at baseline and after a stimulant challenge in responders and non-responders. (Adapted from Martinez D, Carpenter KM, Liu F, et al. Imaging dopamine transmission in cocaine dependence: link between neurochemistry and response to treatment. Am J Psychiatry. 2011;168(6):634-641. https://doi. org/10.1176/appi.ajp.2010.10050748.)

disorder (ADHD) or chronic depression were noted to have a preference for cocaine.

The Self-Medication Hypothesis may be applied to treatment trials using stimulants to treat cocaine use disorder. Use of substitution pharmacotherapy has been effective and is common for the treatment of opioid and nicotine use disorders.[119,120] Levin et al.[121] recently demonstrated a dose–response relationship for the use of 60 mg or 80 mg daily of extended-release mixed-amphetamine salts in the treatment of ADHD with comorbid DSM-IV cocaine dependence. Higher medication dosages achieved greater 30% ADHD symptom reduction, higher rates of 3-week continuous abstinence, and an increased odds of a cocaine-negative week when compared to the lower dosing. Both medication treatment arms performed better than placebo. A secondary analysis of this study also found that mixed-amphetamine salts also decreased the weekly proportion of cannabis use.[122]

Treated with higher dosed psychostimulants, cocaine-dependent patients have been found in several studies to have higher abstinence rates compared to lower dosing or placebo.[121,123,124] As patients with cocaine use disorder have deficient dopamine signaling and do not achieve the same dopamine release as healthy controls, they may require higher doses than nonaddicted patients to achieve the desired effect.

Initial studies using methylphenidate at lower doses to treat comorbid ADHD and stimulant use disorder were no more effective than placebo when treating ADHD symptoms[125–128] nor the stimulant use disorder.[125–129] A later study using higher dosages of methylphenidate found that patients taking doses up to 180 mg/day had improved ADHD symptomatology, treatment retention, and more amphetamine-negative urines compared to the placebo group.[130] In general, studies using more robust stimulant dosages have been more effective in decreasing illicit stimulant use.[124,131–133]

While there have been several meta-analyses with equivocal results for the efficacy of stimulant substitution for the treatment of DSM-IV cocaine dependence, the reviewed studies used heterogenous medications with variable activity on dopamine pathways as well as varied methodologies.[134–136] Patient populations were mixed, with several studies recruiting patients with comorbid methadone maintenance,[132,137] and another recruiting only intravenous cocaine users.[138] Analysis of the studies is also complicated by low retention rates, with one study having only 20% of subjects complete.[139] Table 1.4 reviews double-blind randomized controlled trials using a psychostimulant to treat cocaine use disorder. Studies using weaker dopaminergic agents alone, such as modafinil or bupropion, were not included in this table because although they may increase dopamine levels in the synapse, they have very different pharmacokinetic and behavioral properties when compared to classical stimulants.[140]

Studies using methylphenidate[141] or less-potent medications as a cocaine substitution agent may not yield as positive results as amphetamines because of the dysfunction of dopamine transmission among persons with DSM-IV cocaine dependence. Although amphetamines directly cause dopamine release, methylphenidate acts as a reuptake inhibitor to increase dopamine transmission, relying on a more intact dopaminergic system. As seen in PET studies, in some stimulant-dependent patients, 60 mg of oral methylphenidate does not result in any dopamine release at all.[58]

In summary, meta-analyses analyzing substitution treatments for cocaine dependence may have yielded inconclusive results due to (1) patients requiring higher stimulant dosages due to decreased dopamine transmission and (2) lack of sufficient subgroup analyses resulting in the analysis of a heterogenous group with very different phenotypes and treatment. More studies with robust dosing and consistent methods would help to determine the role of stimulant substitution for treating cocaine use disorder.

Adenosine A$_{2A}$ Receptor Antagonists

While dopamine agonists may be used to correct deficits in dopamine transmission, the sustained dopaminergic activity has the theoretical shortcoming of interrupting endogenous dopamine release in response to environmental stimuli. Literature on the efficacy of dopamine agonists for the treatment of addictions is still inconclusive, and there are no studies assessing long-term outcomes. Instead of generating a constant increase of dopaminergic tone using psychostimulants, another approach to dopamine system modulation is to increase the system's ability to react to natural, non-pharmacologic reinforcers. This may be possible by affecting other striatal receptors that regulate the dopamine system.

Adenosine A$_{2A}$ receptors form heteromers with D2 receptors in the striatum.[142,143] Activation of A$_{2A}$ receptors causes allosteric changes in the D2 receptor that decreases its affinity for dopamine.[144–146] A$_{2A}$ antagonism blocks the inhibiting effect of adenosine on the A$_{2A}$ receptor and can act to "boost" the signal

TABLE 1.4
Randomized Double-Blind Placebo-Controlled Trials Using Stimulant Substitution to Treat Cocaine Dependence

Study	Intervention	Methylphenidate Equivalents[a]	Completers[b]	Study Population	Significant Outcomes
POSITIVE RESULTS					
Grabowski et al.[131]	dextroamphetamine SR 15–30 mg/d BID, or 30–60 mg/d, BID, 38 day dose titration with dose doubling	40–80 mg, 80–160 mg	Placebo: 22.9%; 15–30 mg: 40.4%; 30–60 mg: 8.7%	cocaine dependent	Retention best for 15–30 mg group. Cocaine-positive urines were decreased in both treatment groups compared to placebo. The 30–60 mg group also had a greater decrease in cocaine-positive urines compared to the 15–30 group.
Grabowski et al.[132]	dextroamphetamine SR 15–30 mg/d BID, or 30–60 mg/d BID, 38 day dose titration with dose doubling	40–80 mg, 80–160 mg	Placebo: 25%; 15–30 mg: 50%; 30–60 mg: 39.3%	cocaine and opioid dependent	Decreased cocaine use in the 30–60 group compared to placebo, but not 15–30 group.
Levin et al.[121]	mixed amphetamine salts XR 60 mg daily or 80 mg daily, flexible dosing, 1 week placebo lead in	120 mg, 160 mg	Placebo: 67%; 60 mg: 75%; 80 mg: 79%	cocaine dependent with ADHD	Greater 30% ADHD symptom reduction, cocaine negative weeks, and 3-week abstinence in both treatment groups compared to placebo.
Mooney et al.[124]	methamphetamine IR 30 mg/d 6 times a day, or SR 30 mg daily, 5–7 day stabilization phase with dose titration	240 mg	Placebo: 33%; 30 mg IR: 30%; 30 mg SR: 32%	cocaine dependent	Decreased positive urines and decreased craving in the SR group compared to placebo, but not the IR group.
MIXED RESULTS					
Levin et al.[126]	methylphenidate 40–60 mg/d BID, flexible dosing, 2 week induction	40–60 mg	Placebo: 45% Medication: 43%	cocaine dependent with ADHD	No difference in ADHD symptoms or cocaine use, although secondary analysis showed lower probability of cocaine positive urine samples in medication group compared to placebo.

Continued

TABLE 1.4
Randomized Double-Blind Placebo-Controlled Trials Using Stimulant Substitution to Treat Cocaine Dependence—cont'd

Study	Intervention	Methylphenidate Equivalents[a]	Completers[b]	Study Population	Significant Outcomes
NEGATIVE RESULTS					
Dürsteler-MacFarland et al.[137]	methylphenidate 60 mg/d BID, fixed dose without titration	60 mg	Placebo: 81% Medication 60%	cocaine and heroin dependent, on diacetylmorphine maintenance	No difference in cocaine free urines, self-reported cocaine use, or retention.
Grabowski et al.[131]	methylphenidate 45 mg/d BID, 2 week human laboratory stabilization period	45 mg	49%[c]	cocaine dependent	No difference in cocaine use or retention.
Mooney et al.[133]	lisdexamfetamine 70 mg daily, 1 week induction titration	55 mg	Placebo: 71% Medication: 57%	cocaine dependent	No difference in cocaine use. Decreased cocaine craving in treatment group.
Schmitz et al.[139]	modafinil 400 mg/d TID, dextroamphetamine SR 60 mg/d TID, or modafinil 200 mg/d TID plus D-amphetamine 30 mg/d TID, 5-day run-up titration	160 mg	20%[c]	cocaine dependent	Increased cocaine use in the combination group compared to placebo, no difference in others.
Schubiner et al.[129]	methylphenidate IR 30–90 mg/d TID (mean 26.25 mg), pemoline (stopped), 1-week titration, flexible dosing	30–90 mg	Placebo: 58% Medication: 45%	cocaine dependent with ADHD	Improved ADHD symptoms compared to placebo, no changes in cocaine measures.
Shearer et al.[138]	dextroamphetamine IR 20–60 mg daily (mean 41 mg), 1 week dose titration starting at 20 mg, flexible dosing	52.5–160 mg	Placebo: 36% Medication: 38%	intravenous cocaine dependent (24 commorbid opioid dependent)	No significant difference between treatment groups.

a Methylphenidate equivalents are approximate and were converted from the stimulant dose based on the recommended dosage ranges and authors' experience with the medications.
b Differences in retention rates not significant unless noted in outcomes.
c Exact retention rates of groups not published, but groups did not significantly differ.

of D2 receptors in response to endogenous dopamine. This increase in dopamine tone may help to reacclimate patients to rewarding nonpharmacologic environmental stimuli. This increase in dopamine transmission may also improve response to behavioral treatments, similar to what has been observed in PET studies.[29,58]

A[2A] antagonists (istradefylline, preladent, tozadenant)[144,147–150] are already being used in clinical trials for Parkinson's disease, but are not yet available for human investigations to treat substance use disorders. However, tozadenant (as compound SYN115) was administered to cocaine-dependent subjects while performing a working memory task and resulted in greater activation of striatal regions on fMRI when compared to placebo, suggesting enhanced dopaminergic function.[144]

κ-Opioid Receptor Antagonists

The κ-opioid receptor binds to the endogenous ligand, dynorphin, and acts to decrease dopamine release.[151] Nonselective opioid antagonists have already shown some efficacy in treating addiction. Naltrexone, a nonselective opioid receptor antagonist, is approved for treatment of alcohol use disorder, and buprenorphine, a nonselective partial opioid receptor agonist, reduces alcohol craving. Selective κ-opioid receptor antagonists have been shown to have antidepressant, anxiolytic effects and also alleviate symptoms of nicotine and cocaine use disorder in animal models.[152,153]

The first human safety study of a κ-opioid receptor antagonist, JDTic was stopped due to the emergence of unsustained ventricular tachycardia in two subjects at similar times after dosing.[154] κ-Opioid receptor antagonists are known to have cardiovascular effects that are protective in rats, such as reduced arrhythmias[155] and positive inotropy.[156] However, it remains unclear if cardiovascular side effects in humans are from the particular agent studied or κ-opioid receptor antagonists as a class. JDTic may affect the heart by activating the stress kinase c-Jun N-terminal kinase (JNK), which has broad cellular effects.[157]

Nonselective opioid receptor antagonists such as naltrexone and buprenorphine do not have cardiac side effects, nor does the κ-opioid receptor antagonist LY2456302, which does not affect JNK and does not have any cardiac side effects.[158] LY2456302 has recently been shown to be safe for further studies in humans[159] and is under investigation as a potential drug for the treatment of depression and addiction.

SUMMARY

The neurochemical imaging literature suggests that individuals may be predisposed by both genetic and environmental factors to addiction, and chronic substance use can further cause neurotransmitter signaling changes that exacerbate preexisting variations in reward pathways. This has implications for risk of addiction, but also for the likelihood of response to certain treatments. Despite the different mechanisms of action of drugs of abuse, all addictive substances have action on the dopamine system. Pharmacologic treatments that have actions directly or indirectly on dopamine transmission have the potential to treat various addictions.

REFERENCES

1. American Psychiatric Association. *Diagnostic and Statistical Manual of Mental Disorders*. American Psychiatric Association; 2013. https://doi.org/10.1176/appi.books.9780890425596.
2. Koob GF, Volkow ND. Neurocircuitry of addiction. *Neuropsychopharmacology*. 2009;35(10):217–238. https://doi.org/10.1038/npp.2009.110.
3. Di Chiara G, Imperato A. Drugs abused by humans preferentially increase synaptic dopamine concentrations in the mesolimbic system of freely moving rats. *Proc Natl Acad Sci USA*. 1988;85(14):5274–5278. https://doi.org/10.1073/pnas.85.14.5274.
4. Wise RA. Neurobiology of addiction. *Curr Opin Neurobiol*. 1996. https://doi.org/10.1016/S0959-4388(96)80079-1.
5. Bassareo V, Di Chiara G. Differential responsiveness of dopamine transmission to food-stimuli in nucleus accumbens shell/core compartments. *Neuroscience*. 1999;89(3):637–641. https://doi.org/10.1016/S0306-4522(98)00583-1.
6. Sellings LH, Clarke PB. Segregation of amphetamine reward and locomotor stimulation between nucleus accumbens medial shell and core. *J Neurosci*. 2003;23(15):6295–6303. https://www.ncbi.nlm.nih.gov/pubmed/12867514.
7. Ito R, Dalley JW, Howes SR, Robbins TW, Everitt BJ. Dissociation in conditioned dopamine release in the nucleus accumbens core and shell in response to cocaine cues and during cocaine-seeking behavior in rats. *J Neurosci*. 2000;20(19):7489–7495. http://www.ncbi.nlm.nih.gov/pubmed/11007908.
8. Cheng JJ, de Bruin JPC, Feenstra MGP. Dopamine efflux in nucleus accumbens shell and core in response to appetitive classical conditioning. *Eur J Neurosci*. 2003;18(5):1306–1314. https://doi.org/10.1046/j.1460-9568.2003.02849.x.
9. Georges F, Aston-Jones G. Potent regulation of midbrain dopamine neurons by the bed nucleus of the stria terminalis. *J Neurosci*. 2001;21(16):RC160. http://www.ncbi.nlm.nih.gov/pubmed/11473131.

10. Everitt BJ, Cardinal RN, Parkinson JA, Robbins TW. Appetitive behavior: impact of amygdala-dependent mechanisms of emotional learning. *Ann NY Acad Sci.* 2003;985:233–250. http://www.ncbi.nlm.nih.gov/pubmed/12724162.

11. Bush G, Vogt BA, Holmes J, et al. Dorsal anterior cingulate cortex: a role in reward-based decision making. *Proc Natl Acad Sci USA.* 2002;99(1):523–528. https://doi.org/10.1073/pnas.012470999.

12. Berns GS, McClure SM, Pagnoni G, Montague PR. Predictability modulates human brain response to reward. *J Neurosci.* 2001;21(8):2793–2798. http://www.ncbi.nlm.nih.gov/pubmed/11306631.

13. Volkow ND, Wang G-J, Ma Y, et al. Expectation enhances the regional brain metabolic and the reinforcing effects of stimulants in cocaine abusers. *J Neurosci.* 2003;23(36):11461–11468. https://doi.org/23/36/11461.

14. Gilpin NW, Koob GF. Neurobiology of alcohol dependence: focus on motivational mechanisms. *Alcohol Res Health.* 2008;31(3):185–195. http://www.ncbi.nlm.nih.gov/pubmed/19881886.

15. Kalivas PW, Volkow ND. The neural basis of addiction: a pathology of motivation and choice. *Am J Psychiatry.* 2005;162(8):1403–1413. https://doi.org/10.1176/appi.ajp.162.8.1403.

16. Hou H, Tian M, Zhang H. Positron emission tomography molecular imaging of dopaminergic system in drug addiction. *Anat Rec Adv Integr Anat Evol Biol.* 2012;295(5):722–733. https://doi.org/10.1002/ar.22457.

17. Sibley DR, Monsma FJ. Molecular biology of dopamine receptors. *Trends Pharmacol Sci.* 1992;13(2):61–69. https://doi.org/10.1016/0165-6147(92)90025-2.

18. Volkow ND, Fowler JS, Wolf AP, et al. Effects of chronic cocaine abuse on postsynaptic dopamine receptors. *Am J Psychiatry.* 1990;147(6):719–724. https://doi.org/10.1176/ajp.147.6.719.

19. Volkow ND, Fowler JS, Wang G-J, Goldstein RZ. Role of dopamine, the frontal cortex and memory circuits in drug addiction: insight from imaging studies. *Neurobiol Learn Mem.* 2002;78(3):610–624. https://doi.org/10.1006/nlme.2002.4099.

20. Melis M, Spiga S, Diana M. The dopamine hypothesis of drug addiction: hypodopaminergic state. In: *International Review of Neurobiology.* Vol. 63. 2005:101–154. https://doi.org/10.1016/S0074-7742(05)63005-X.

21. Mintun MA, Raichle ME, Kilbourn MR, Wooten GF, Welch MJ. A quantitative model for the in vivo assessment of drug binding sites with positron emission tomography. *Ann Neurol.* 1984;15(3):217–227. https://doi.org/10.1002/ana.410150302.

22. Innis RB, Cunningham VJ, Delforge J, et al. Consensus nomenclature for in vivo imaging of reversibly binding radioligands. *J Cereb Blood Flow Metab.* 2007;279600493:1533–1539. https://doi.org/10.1038/sj.jcbfm.9600493.

23. Slifstein M, Laruelle M. Models and methods for derivation of in vivo neuroreceptor parameters with PET and SPECT reversible radiotracers. *Nucl Med Biol.* 2001;28(5):595–608. https://doi.org/10.1016/S0969-8051(01)00214-1.

24. Laruelle M. Imaging synaptic neurotransmission with *in vivo* binding competition techniques: a critical review. *J Cereb Blood Flow Metab.* 2000;20(3):423–451. https://doi.org/10.1097/00004647-200003000-00001.

25. Skinbjerg M, Liow J-S, Seneca N, et al. D2 dopamine receptor internalization prolongs the decrease of radioligand binding after amphetamine: a PET study in a receptor internalization-deficient mouse model. *Neuroimage.* 2010;50(4):1402–1407. https://doi.org/10.1016/j.neuroimage.2010.01.055.

26. Volkow ND, Fowler JS, Wang G-J, et al. Decreased dopamine D2 receptor availability is associated with reduced frontal metabolism in cocaine abusers. *Synapse.* 1993;14(2):169–177. https://doi.org/10.1002/syn.890140210.

27. Volkow ND, Wang G-J, Fowler JS, et al. Decreased striatal dopaminergic responsiveness in detoxified cocaine-dependent subjects. *Nature.* 1997;386(6627):830–833. https://doi.org/10.1038/386830a0.

28. Martinez D, Broft A, Foltin RW, et al. Cocaine dependence and D2 receptor availability in the functional subdivisions of the striatum: relationship with cocaine-seeking behavior. *Neuropsychopharmacology.* 2004;29(6):1190–1202. https://doi.org/10.1038/sj.npp.1300420.

29. Martinez D, Carpenter KM, Liu F, et al. Imaging dopamine transmission in cocaine dependence: link between neurochemistry and response to treatment. *Am J Psychiatry.* 2011;168(6):634–641. https://doi.org/10.1176/appi.ajp.2010.10050748.

30. Martinez D, Greene K, Broft A, et al. Lower level of endogenous dopamine in patients with cocaine dependence: findings from PET Imaging of D_2/D_3 receptors following acute dopamine depletion. *Am J Psychiatry.* 2009;166(10):1170–1177. https://doi.org/10.1176/appi.ajp.2009.08121801.

31. Nader MA, Morgan D, Gage HD, et al. PET imaging of dopamine D2 receptors during chronic cocaine self-administration in monkeys. *Nat Neurosci.* 2006;9(8):1050–1056. https://doi.org/10.1038/nn1737.

32. Farfel GM, Kleven MS, Woolverton WL, Seiden LS, Perry BD. Effects of repeated injections of cocaine on catecholamine receptor binding sites, dopamine transporter binding sites and behavior in rhesus monkey. *Brain Res.* 1992;578(1–2):235–243. https://doi.org/10.1016/0006-8993(92)90252-5.

33. Moore RJ, Vinsant SL, Nader MA, Porrino LJ, Friedman DP. Effect of cocaine self-administration on dopamine D2 receptors in rhesus monkeys. *Synapse.* 1998;30(1):88–96. https://doi.org/10.1002/(SICI)1098-2396(199809)30:1<88::AID-SYN11>3.0.CO;2-L.

34. Nader M, Daunais JB, Moore T, et al. Effects of cocaine self-administration on striatal dopamine systems in rhesus monkeys initial and chronic exposure. *Neuropsychopharmacology.* 2002;27(1):35–46. https://doi.org/10.1016/S0893-133X(01)00427-4.

35. Martinez D, Slifstein M, Narendran R, et al. Dopamine D1 receptors in cocaine dependence measured with PET and the choice to self-administer cocaine. *Neuropsychopharmacology.* 2009;34(7):1774–1782. https://doi.org/10.1038/npp.2008.235.

36. Martinez D, Narendran R, Foltin RW, et al. Amphetamine-induced dopamine release: markedly blunted in cocaine dependence and predictive of the choice to self-administer cocaine. *Am J Psychiatry*. 2007;164(4): 622–629. https://doi.org/10.1176/ajp.2007.164.4.622.

37. Volkow ND, Wang G-J, Telang F, et al. Cocaine cues and dopamine in dorsal striatum: mechanism of craving in cocaine addiction. *J Neurosci*. 2006;26(24):6583–6588. https://doi.org/10.1523/JNEUROSCI.1544-06.2006.

38. Volkow ND, Wang GJ, Fowler JS, et al. Prediction of reinforcing responses to psychostimulants in humans by brain dopamine D2 receptor levels. *Am J Psychiatry*. 1999;156(9):1440–1443. https://doi.org/10.1176/ajp.156.9.1440.

39. Drevets WC, Gautier C, Price JC, et al. Amphetamine-induced dopamine release in human ventral striatum correlates with euphoria. *Biol Psychiatry*. 2001;49(2):81–96. https://doi.org/10.1016/S0006-3223(00)01038-6.

40. Abi-Dargham A, Kegeles LS, Martinez D, Innis RB, Laruelle M. Dopamine mediation of positive reinforcing effects of amphetamine in stimulant naïve healthy volunteers: results from a large cohort. *Eur Neuropsychopharmacol*. 2003;13(6):459–468. https://doi.org/10.1016/j.euroneuro.2003.08.007.

41. Martinez D, Slifstein M, Broft A, et al. Imaging human mesolimbic dopamine transmission with positron emission tomography. Part II: amphetamine-induced dopamine release in the functional subdivisions of the striatum. *J Cereb Blood Flow Metab*. 2003;23(3): 285–300. https://doi.org/10.1097/01.WCB.0000048520.34839.1A.

42. Wu J, Bell K, Najafi A, et al. Decreasing striatal 6-FDOPA uptake with increasing duration of cocaine withdrawal. *Neuropsychopharmacology*. 1997;17(6):402–409. https://doi.org/10.1016/S0893-133X(97)00089-4.

43. Laruelle MDM, D'Souza CD, Baldwin RM, et al. Imaging D2 receptor occupancy by endogenous dopamine in humans. *Neuropsychopharmacology*. 1997;17(3):162–174. https://doi.org/10.1016/S0893-133X(97)00043-2.

44. Morgan D, Grant KA, Gage HD, et al. Social dominance in monkeys: dopamine D2 receptors and cocaine self-administration. *Nat Neurosci*. 2002;5(2):169–174. https://doi.org/10.1038/nn798.

45. Maggos C, Tsukada H, Kakiuchi T, et al. Sustained withdrawal allows normalization of in vivo [^{11}C]N-Methylspiperone dopamine D2 receptor binding after chronic Binge cocaine a positron emission tomography study in rats. *Neuropsychopharmacology*. 1998;19(2): 146–153. https://doi.org/10.1016/S0893-133X(98)00009-8.

46. Beveridge TJR, Smith HR, Nader MA, Porrino LJ. Abstinence from chronic cocaine self-administration alters striatal dopamine systems in rhesus monkeys. *Neuropsychopharmacology*. 2009;34(5):1162–1171. https://doi.org/10.1038/npp.2008.135.

47. Volkow ND, Wang G-J, Fowler JS, et al. Brain DA D2 receptors predict reinforcing effects of stimulants in humans: replication study. *Synapse*. 2002;46(2):79–82. https://doi.org/10.1002/syn.10137.

48. Thanos PK, Michaelides M, Umegaki H, Volkow ND. D2R DNA transfer into the nucleus accumbens attenuates cocaine self-administration in rats. *Synapse*. 2008;62(7): 481–486. https://doi.org/10.1002/syn.20523.

49. White FJ, Kalivas PW. Neuroadaptations involved in amphetamine and cocaine addiction. *Drug Alcohol Depend*. 1998;51(1–2):141–153. https://doi.org/10.1016/S0376-8716(98)00072-6.

50. Malison RT, Best SE, van Dyck CH, et al. Elevated striatal dopamine transporters during acute cocaine abstinence as measured by [^{123}I] beta-CIT SPECT. *Am J Psychiatry*. 1998;155(6):832–834. https://doi.org/10.1176/ajp.155.6.832.

51. Wang GJ, Volkow ND, Fowler JS, et al. Cocaine abusers do not show loss of dopamine transporters with age. *Life Sci*. 1997;61(11):1059–1065. https://doi.org/10.1016/S0024-3205(97)00614-0.

52. Volkow N, Wang GJ, Fowler JS, et al. Cocaine uptake is decreased in the brain of detoxified cocaine abusers. *Neuropsychopharmacology*. 1996;14(3):159–168. https://doi.org/10.1016/0893-133X(95)00073-M.

53. Zubieta JK, Gorelick DA, Stauffer R, Ravert HT, Dannals RF, Frost JJ. Increased mu opioid receptor binding detected by PET in cocaine-dependent men is associated with cocaine craving. *Nat Med*. 1996; 2(11):1225–1229. https://doi.org/10.1038/nm1196-1225.

54. Gorelick DA, Kim YK, Bencherif B, et al. Imaging brain mu-opioid receptors in abstinent cocaine users: time course and relation to cocaine craving. *Biol Psychiatry*. 2005;57(12):1573–1582. https://doi.org/10.1016/j.biopsych.2005.02.026.

55. Jacobsen LK, Staley JK, Malison RT, et al. Elevated central serotonin transporter binding availability in acutely abstinent cocaine-dependent patients. *Am J Psychiatry*. 2000; 157(7):1134–1140. https://doi.org/10.1176/appi.ajp.157.7.1134.

56. Volkow ND, Chang L, Wang GJ, et al. Low level of brain dopamine D2 receptors in methamphetamine abusers: association with metabolism in the orbitofrontal cortex. *Am J Psychiatry*. 2001;158(12):2015–2021. https://doi.org/10.1176/appi.ajp.158.12.2015.

57. Lee B, London ED, Poldrack RA, et al. Striatal dopamine D2/D3 receptor availability is reduced in methamphetamine dependence and is linked to impulsivity. *J Neurosci*. 2009;29(47):14734–14740. https://doi.org/10.1523/JNEUROSCI.3765-09.2009.

58. Wang GJ, Smith L, Volkow ND, et al. Decreased dopamine activity predicts relapse in methamphetamine abusers. *Mol Psychiatry*. 2012;17(9):918–925. https://doi.org/10.1038/mp.2011.86.

59. Johanson C-E, Frey KA, Lundahl LH, et al. Cognitive function and nigrostriatal markers in abstinent methamphetamine abusers. *Psychopharmacol Berl*. 2006;185(3): 327–338. https://doi.org/10.1007/s00213-006-0330-6.

60. McCann UD, Kuwabara H, Kumar A, et al. Persistent cognitive and dopamine transporter deficits in abstinent methamphetamine users. *Synapse*. 2008;62(2):91–100. https://doi.org/10.1002/syn.20471.

61. McCann UD, Wong DF, Yokoi F, Villemagne V, Dannals RF, Ricaurte GA. Reduced striatal dopamine transporter density in abstinent methamphetamine and methcathinone users: evidence from positron emission tomography studies with [^{11}C]WIN-35,428. *J Neurosci.* 1998;18(20):8417–8422. http://www.ncbi.nlm.nih.gov/pubmed/9763484.

62. Volkow ND, Chang L, Wang GJ, et al. Loss of dopamine transporters in methamphetamine abusers recovers with protracted abstinence. *J Neurosci.* 2001; 21(23):9414–9418. http://www.ncbi.nlm.nih.gov/pubmed/11717374.

63. Sekine Y, Iyo M, Ouchi Y, et al. Methamphetamine-related psychiatric symptoms and reduced brain dopamine transporters studied with PET. *Am J Psychiatry.* 2001;158(8):1206–1214. https://doi.org/10.1176/appi.ajp.158.8.1206.

64. Chou Y-H, Huang W-S, Su T-P, Lu R-B, Wan F-J, Fu Y-K. Dopamine transporters and cognitive function in methamphetamine abuser after a short abstinence: a SPECT study. *Eur Neuropsychopharmacol.* 2007;17(1):46–52. https://doi.org/10.1016/j.euroneuro.2006.05.002.

65. Volkow ND, Chang L, Wang GJ, et al. Association of dopamine transporter reduction with psychomotor impairment in methamphetamine abusers. *Am J Psychiatry.* 2001;158(3):377–382. https://doi.org/10.1176/appi.ajp.158.3.377.

66. Iyo M, Sekine Y, Mori N. Neuromechanism of developing methamphetamine psychosis: a neuroimaging study. *Ann NY Acad Sci.* 2004;1025(1):288–295. https://doi.org/10.1196/annals.1316.036.

67. Sekine Y, Ouchi Y, Takei N, et al. Brain serotonin transporter density and aggression in abstinent methamphetamine abusers. *Arch Gen Psychiatry.* 2006;63(1):90–100. https://doi.org/10.1001/archpsyc.63.1.90.

68. Kish SJ, Fitzmaurice PS, Boileau I, et al. Brain serotonin transporter in human methamphetamine users. *Psychopharmacol Berl.* 2009;202(4):649–661. https://doi.org/10.1007/s00213-008-1346-x.

69. Hietala J, West C, Syvälahti E, et al. Striatal D2 dopamine receptor binding characteristics in vivo in patients with alcohol dependence. *Psychopharmacol Berl.* 1994;116(3):285–290. https://doi.org/10.1007/BF02245330.

70. Heinz A, Siessmeier T, Wrase J, et al. Correlation of alcohol craving with striatal dopamine synthesis capacity and D$_{2/3}$ receptor availability: a combined [^{18}F]DOPA and [^{18}F]DMFP PET study in detoxified alcoholic patients. *Am J Psychiatry.* 2005;162(8):1515–1520. https://doi.org/10.1176/appi.ajp.162.8.1515.

71. Heinz A, Siessmeier T, Wrase J, et al. Correlation between dopamine D(2) receptors in the ventral striatum and central processing of alcohol cues and craving. *Am J Psychiatry.* 2004;161(10):1783–1789. https://doi.org/10.1176/appi.ajp.161.10.1783.

72. Volkow ND, Wang GJ, Maynard L, et al. Effects of alcohol detoxification on dopamine D2 receptors in alcoholics: a preliminary study. *Psychiatry Res – Neuroimaging.* 2002; 116(3):163–172. https://doi.org/10.1016/S0925-4927(02)00087-2.

73. Volkow ND, Wang GJ, Fowler JS, et al. Decreases in dopamine receptors but not in dopamine transporters in alcoholics. *Alcohol Clin Exp Res.* 1996;20(9):1594–1598. https://doi.org/10.1111/j.1530-0277.1996.tb05936.x.

74. Gilman S, Koeppe RA, Adams KM, et al. Decreased striatal monoaminergic terminals in severe chronic alcoholism demonstrated with (+)[^{11}C]Dihydrotetrabenazine and positron emission tomography. *Ann Neurol.* 1998;44(3):326–333. https://doi.org/10.1002/ana.410440307.

75. Martinez D, Narendran R. Imaging neurotransmitter release by drugs of abuse. In: *Current Topics in Behavioral Neurosciences.* Vol. 3. 2010:219–245. https://doi.org/10.1007/7854_2009_34.

76. Martinez D, Gil R, Slifstein M, et al. Alcohol dependence is associated with blunted dopamine transmission in the ventral striatum. *Biol Psychiatry.* 2005;58(10):779–786. https://doi.org/10.1016/j.biopsych.2005.04.044.

77. Volkow ND, Wang G-J, Telang F, et al. Profound decreases in dopamine release in striatum in detoxified alcoholics: possible orbitofrontal involvement. *J Neurosci.* 2007;27(46):12700–12706. https://doi.org/10.1523/JNEUROSCI.3371-07.2007.

78. Tiihonen J, Vilkman H, Räsänen P, et al. Striatal presynaptic dopamine function in type 1 alcoholics measured with positron emission tomography. *Mol Psychiatry.* 1998;3(2):156–161. https://doi.org/10.1038/sj.mp.4000365.

79. Laine TP, Ahonen A, Torniainen P, et al. Dopamine transporters increase in human brain after alcohol withdrawal. *Mol Psychiatry.* 1999;4(2):189–191, 104–105. https://doi.org/10.1038/sj.mp.4000514.

80. Laine TP, Ahonen A, Räsänen P, Tiihonen J. Dopamine transporter availability and depressive symptoms during alcohol withdrawal. *Psychiatry Res.* 1999;90(3):153–157. https://doi.org/10.1016/S0925-4927(99)00019-0.

81. Tiihonen J, Kuikka J, Bergström K, et al. Altered striatal dopamine re-uptake site densities in habitually violent and non-violent alcoholics. *Nat Med.* 1995;1(7):654–657. https://doi.org/10.1038/nm0795-654.

82. Heinz A, Goldman D, Jones DW, et al. Genotype influences in vivo dopamine transporter availability in human striatum. *Neuropsychopharmacology.* 2000;22(2):133–139. https://doi.org/10.1016/S0893-133X(99)00099-8.

83. Repo E, Kuikka JT, Bergström KA, Karhu J, Hiltunen J, Tiihonen J. Dopamine transporter and D2-receptor density in late-onset alcoholism. *Psychopharmacol Berl.* 1999;147(3):314–318. https://doi.org/10.1007/s002130051173.

84. Rominger A, Cumming P, Xiong G, et al. [^{18}F]Fallypride PET measurement of striatal and extrastriatal dopamine D2/3 receptor availability in recently abstinent alcoholics. *Addict Biol.* 2012;17(2):490–503. https://doi.org/10.1111/j.1369-1600.2011.00355.x.

85. Volkow ND, Wang G-J, Begleiter H, et al. High levels of dopamine D2 receptors in unaffected members of alcoholic families: possible protective factors. *Arch Gen Psychiatry.* 2006;63(9):999–1008. https://doi.org/10.1001/archpsyc.63.9.999.

86. Thanos PK, Volkow ND, Freimuth P, et al. Overexpression of dopamine D2 receptors reduces alcohol self-administration. *J Neurochem.* 2001;78(5):1094–1103. https://doi.org/10.1046/j.1471-4159.2001.00492.x.

87. Abi-Dargham A, Krystal JH, Anjilvel S, et al. Alterations of benzodiazepine receptors in type II alcoholic subjects measured with SPECT and [123I]Iomazenil. *Am J Psychiatry.* 1998;155(11):1550–1555. https://doi.org/10.1176/ajp.155.11.1550.

88. Lingford-Hughes AR, Wilson SJ, Cunningham VJ, et al. GABA-benzodiazepine receptor function in alcohol dependence: a combined 11C-flumazenil PET and pharmacodynamic study. *Psychopharmacol Berl.* 2005;180(4):595–606. https://doi.org/10.1007/s00213-005-2271-x.

89. Lingford-Hughes AR, Acton PD, Gacinovic S, et al. Reduced levels of GABA-benzodiazepine receptor in alcohol dependency in the absence of grey matter atrophy. *Br J Psychiatry.* 1998;173:116–122. https://doi.org/10.1192/BJP.173.2.116.

90. Staley JK, Gottschalk C, Petrakis IL, et al. Cortical gamma-aminobutyric acid type A-benzodiazepine receptors in recovery from alcohol dependence: relationship to features of alcohol dependence and cigarette smoking. *Arch Gen Psychiatry.* 2005;62(8):877–888. https://doi.org/10.1001/archpsyc.62.8.877.

91. Litton JE, Neiman J, Pauli S, et al. PET analysis of [11C]flumazenil binding to benzodiazepine receptors in chronic alcohol-dependent men and healthy controls. *Psychiatry Res.* 1993;50(1):1–13. https://doi.org/10.1016/0925-4927(93)90019-E.

92. Lingford-Hughes AR, Acton PD, Gacinovic S, et al. Levels of gamma-aminobutyric acid-benzodiazepine receptors in abstinent, alcohol-dependent women: preliminary findings from an 123I-iomazenil single photon emission tomography study. *Alcohol Clin Exp Res.* 2000;24(9):1449–1455. https://doi.org/10.1097/00000374-200009000-00018.

93. Cosgrove KP, Esterlis I, Mason GF, Bois F, O'Malley SS, Krystal JH. Neuroimaging insights into the role of cortical GABA systems and the influence of nicotine on the recovery from alcohol dependence. *Neuropharmacology.* 2011;60(7–8):1318–1325. https://doi.org/10.1016/j.neuropharm.2011.01.020.

94. Hu J, Henry S, Gallezot JD, et al. Serotonin 1B receptor imaging in alcohol dependence. *Biol Psychiatry.* 2010;67(9):800–803. https://doi.org/10.1016/j.biopsych.2009.12.028.

95. Heinz A, Jones DW, Bissette G, et al. Relationship between cortisol and serotonin metabolites and transporters in alcoholism [correction of alcolholism]. *Pharmacopsychiatry.* 2002;35(4):127–134. https://doi.org/10.1055/s-2002-33197.

96. Szabo Z, Owonikoko T, Peyrot M, et al. Positron emission tomography imaging of the serotonin transporter in subjects with a history of alcoholism. *Biol Psychiatry.* 2004;55(7):766–771. https://doi.org/10.1016/j.biopsych.2003.11.023.

97. Martinez D, Slifstein M, Gil R, et al. Positron emission tomography imaging of the serotonin transporter and 5-HT1A receptor in alcohol dependence. *Biol Psychiatry.* 2009;65(2):175–180. https://doi.org/10.1016/j.biopsych.2008.08.034.

98. Bencherif B, Wand GS, McCaul ME, et al. Mu-opioid receptor binding measured by [11C]carfentanil positron emission tomography is related to craving and mood in alcohol dependence. *Biol Psychiatry.* 2004;55(3):255–262. https://doi.org/10.1016/j.biopsych.2003.07.007.

99. Weerts EM, Wand GS, Kuwabara H, et al. Positron emission tomography imaging of mu- and delta-opioid receptor binding in alcohol-dependent and healthy control subjects. *Alcohol Clin Exp Res.* 2011;35(12):2162–2173. https://doi.org/10.1111/j.1530-0277.2011.01565.x.

100. Heinz A, Reimold M, Wrase J, et al. Correlation of stable elevations in striatal mu-opioid receptor availability in detoxified alcoholic patients with alcohol craving: a positron emission tomography study using carbon 11-labeled carfentanil. *Arch Gen Psychiatry.* 2005;62(1):57–64. https://doi.org/10.1001/archpsyc.62.1.57.

101. Williams TM, Davies SJC, Taylor LG, et al. Brain opioid receptor binding in early abstinence from alcohol dependence and relationship to craving: an [11C]diprenorphine PET study. *Eur Neuropsychopharmacol.* 2009;19(10):740–748. https://doi.org/10.1016/j.euroneuro.2009.06.007.

102. Myrick H, Anton RF, Li X, Henderson S, Randall PK, Voronin K. Effect of naltrexone and ondansetron on alcohol cue-induced activation of the ventral striatum in alcohol-dependent people. *Arch Gen Psychiatry.* 2008;65(4):466–475. https://doi.org/10.1001/archpsyc.65.4.466.

103. Maisel NC, Blodgett JC, Wilbourne PL, Humphreys K, Finney JW. Meta-analysis of naltrexone and acamprosate for treating alcohol use disorders: when are these medications most helpful? *Addiction.* 2012. https://doi.org/10.1111/j.1360-0443.2012.04054.x.

104. Gianoulakis C. Endogenous opioids and addiction to alcohol and other drugs of abuse. *Curr Top Med Chem.* 2009;9(11):999–1015. https://doi.org/10.2174/156802609789630956.

105. Martinez D, Saccone PA, Liu F, et al. Deficits in dopamine D2 receptors and pre-synaptic dopamine in heroin dependence: commonalities and differences with other types of addiction. *Biol Psychiatry.* 2012;1(713):192–198. https://doi.org/10.1016/j.biopsych.2011.08.024.

106. Wang GJ, Volkow ND, Fowler JS, et al. Dopamine D2 receptor availability in opiate-dependent subjects before and after naloxone-precipitated withdrawal. *Neuropsychopharmacology.* 1997. https://doi.org/10.1016/S0893-133X(96)00184-4.

107. Zubieta J, Greenwald MK, Lombardi U, et al. Buprenorphine-induced changes in mu-opioid receptor availability in male heroin-dependent volunteers a preliminary study. *Neuropsychopharmacology.* 2000;23(3):326–334. https://doi.org/10.1016/S0893-133X(00)00110-X.

108. Kling MA, Carson RE, Borg L, et al. Opioid receptor imaging with positron emission tomography and [(^{18})F]cyclofoxy in long-term, methadone-treated former heroin addicts. *J Pharmacol Exp Ther.* 2000;295(3):1070–1076. http://www.ncbi.nlm.nih.gov/pubmed/11082442.

109. Urban NBL, Slifstein M, Thompson JL, et al. Dopamine release in chronic cannabis users: a [^{11}C]Raclopride positron emission tomography study. *Biol Psychiatry.* 2012;71(8): 677–683. https://doi.org/10.1016/j.biopsych.2011.12.018.

110. Sevy S, Smith GS, Ma Y, et al. Cerebral glucose metabolism and D2/D3 receptor availability in young adults with cannabis dependence measured with positron emission tomography. *Psychopharmacol Berl.* 2008;197(4): 549–556. https://doi.org/10.1007/s00213-008-1075-1.

111. Stokes PR, Egerton A, Watson B, et al. History of cannabis use is not associated with alterations in striatal dopamine D_2/D_3 receptor availability. *J Psychopharmacol.* 2012;26(1): 144–149. https://doi.org/10.1177/0269881111414090.

112. Volkow ND, Wang G-J, Telang F, et al. Decreased dopamine brain reactivity in marijuana abusers is associated with negative emotionality and addiction severity. *Proc Natl Acad Sci USA.* 2014;111(30):E3149–E3156. https://doi.org/10.1073/pnas.1411228111.

113. van de Giessen E, Weinstein JJ, Cassidy CM, et al. Deficits in striatal dopamine release in cannabis dependence. *Mol Psychiatry.* 2017;22(1):68–75. https://doi.org/10.1038/mp.2016.21.

114. Hirvonen J, Goodwin RS, Li C-T, et al. Reversible and regionally selective downregulation of brain cannabinoid CB1 receptors in chronic daily cannabis smokers. *Mol Psychiatry.* 2012;17(6):642–649. https://doi.org/10.1038/mp.2011.82.

115. Ceccarini J, Kuepper R, Kemels D, Van Os J, Henquet C, Van Laere K. [^{18}F]MK-9470 PET measurement of cannabinoid CB1 receptor availability in chronic cannabis users. *Addict Biol.* 2015;20(2):357–367. https://doi.org/10.1111/adb.12116.

116. Khantzian EJ, Gawin F, Kleber HD, Riordan CE. Methylphenidate (Ritalin) treatment of cocaine dependence—a preliminary report. *J Subst Abuse Treat.* 1984;1(2):107–112. https://doi.org/10.1016/0740-5472(84)90033-3.

117. Khantzian EJ. *Clinical and Research Reports an Extreme Case of Cocaine Dependence and Marked Improvement with Methylphenidate Treatment*; 1983. http://ajp.psychiatryonline.org/doi/pdf/10.1176/ajp.140.6.784.

118. Khantzian EJ. The self-medication hypothesis of addictive disorders: focus on heroin and cocaine dependence. In: *The Cocaine Crisis.* Boston, MA: Springer US; 1987: 65–74. https://doi.org/10.1007/978-1-4613-1837-8_7.

119. Lancaster T, Stead L, Silagy C, Sowden A. Effectiveness of interventions to help people stop smoking: findings from the Cochrane Library. *BMJ Clin Res Ed.* 2002;325: 881–886. https://doi.org/10.1016/j.mcna.2011.08.003.

120. Mattick RP, Breen C, Kimber J, Davoli M. Buprenorphine Maintenance versus Placebo or Methadone Maintenance for Opioid Dependence. In: Mattick RP, ed. *Cochrane Database of Systematic Reviews.* Chichester, UK: John Wiley & Sons, Ltd.; 2014:CD002207. https://doi.org/10.1002/14651858.CD002207.pub4.

121. Levin FR, Mariani JJ, Specker S, et al. Extended-release mixed amphetamine salts vs placebo for comorbid adult attention-deficit/hyperactivity disorder and cocaine use disorder. *JAMA Psychiatry.* 2015;72(6):593. https://doi.org/10.1001/jamapsychiatry.2015.41.

122. Notzon DP, Mariani JJ, Pavlicova M, et al. Mixed-amphetamine salts increase abstinence from marijuana in patients with Co-occurring attention-deficit/hyperactivity disorder and cocaine dependence HHS public access. *Am J Addict.* 2016;25(8):666–672. https://doi.org/10.1111/ajad.12467.

123. Mariani JJ, Pavlicova M, Bisaga A, Nunes EV, Brooks DJ, Levin FR. Extended-release mixed amphetamine salts and topiramate for cocaine dependence: a randomized controlled trial. *Biol Psychiatry.* 2012. https://doi.org/10.1016/j.biopsych.2012.05.032.

124. Mooney ME, Herin DV, Schmitz JM, et al. Effects of oral methamphetamine on cocaine use: a randomized, double-blind, placebo-controlled trial. *Drug Alcohol Depend.* 2009;101(12):34–41. https://doi.org/10.1016/j.drugalcdep.2008.10.016.

125. Carpentier PJ, de Jong CAJ, Dijkstra BAG, Verbrugge CAG, Krabbe PFM. A controlled trial of methylphenidate in adults with attention deficit/hyperactivity disorder and substance use disorders. *Addiction.* 2005;100(12): 1868–1874. https://doi.org/10.1111/j.1360-0443.2005.01272.x.

126. Levin FR, Evans SM, Brooks DJ, Garawi F. Treatment of cocaine dependent treatment seekers with adult ADHD: double-blind comparison of methylphenidate and placebo. *Drug Alcohol Depend.* 2007. https://doi.org/10.1016/j.drugalcdep.2006.07.004.

127. Levin FR, Evans SM, Brooks DJ, Kalbag AS, Garawi F, Nunes EV. Treatment of methadone-maintained patients with adult ADHD: double-blind comparison of methylphenidate, bupropion and placebo. *Drug Alcohol Depend.* 2006;81(2):137–148. https://doi.org/10.1016/j.drugalcdep.2005.06.012.

128. Konstenius M, Jayaram-Lindström N, Beck O, Franck J. Sustained release methylphenidate for the treatment of ADHD in amphetamine abusers: a pilot study. *Drug Alcohol Depend.* 2010;108(1–2):130–133. https://doi.org/10.1016/j.drugalcdep.2009.11.006.

129. Schubiner H, Saules KK, Arfken CL, et al. Double-blind placebo-controlled trial methylphenidate treat adult ADHD patients with comorbid cocaine dependence. *Exp Clin Psychopharmacol.* 2002. https://doi.org/10.1037/1064-1297.10.3.286.

130. Konstenius M, Jayaram-Lindström N, Guterstam J, Beck O, Philips B, Franck J. Methylphenidate for attention deficit hyperactivity disorder and drug relapse in criminal offenders with substance dependence: a 24-week randomized placebo-controlled trial. *Addiction.* 2014;109(3): 440–449. https://doi.org/10.1111/add.12369.

131. Grabowski J, Rhoades H, Schmitz J, et al. Dextroamphetamine for cocaine-dependence treatment: a double-blind randomized clinical trial. *J Clin Psychopharmacol.* 2001; 21(5):522–526. https://doi.org/10.1097/00004714-200110000-00010.

132. Grabowski J, Rhoades H, Stotts A, et al. Agonist-like or antagonist-like treatment for cocaine dependence with methadone for heroin dependence: two double-blind randomized clinical trials. *Neuropsychopharmacology*. 2004; 29(5):969–981. https://doi.org/10.1038/sj.npp.1300392.

133. Mooney ME, Herin DV, Specker S, et al. Pilot study of the effects of lisdexamfetamine on cocaine use: a randomized, double-blind, placebo-controlled trial. *Drug Alcohol Depend*. 2015;153:94–103. https://doi.org/10.1016/j.drugalcdep.2015.05.042.

134. Castells X, Cunill R, Vidal X, Capellà D. Psychostimulant drugs for cocaine dependence. *Cochrane Database Syst Rev*. 2016;(9). https://doi.org/10.1002/14651858.CD007380.pub4.

135. Carpentier P-J, Levin FR. Pharmacological treatment of ADHD in addicted patients. *Harv Rev Psychiatry*. 2017; 25(2):50–64. https://doi.org/10.1097/HRP.00000000000 00122.

136. Dürsteler K, Berger E-M, Strasser H, et al. Clinical potential of methylphenidate in the treatment of cocaine addiction: a review of the current evidence. *Subst Abuse Rehabil*. 2015;6:61. https://doi.org/10.2147/SAR.S50807.

137. Dürsteler-MacFarland KM, Farronato NS, Strasser J, et al. A randomized, controlled, pilot trial of methylphenidate and cognitive-behavioral group therapy for cocaine dependence in heroin prescription. *J Clin Psychopharmacol*. 2013. https://doi.org/10.1097/JCP.0b013e31 827bfff4.

138. Shearer J, Wodak A, van Beek I, Mattick RP, Lewis J. Pilot randomized double blind placebo-controlled study of dexamphetamine for cocaine dependence. *Addiction*. 2003;98(8):1137–1141. https://doi.org/10.1046/j.1360-0443.2003.00447.x.

139. Schmitz JM, Rathnayaka N, Green CE, et al. Combination of modafinil and d -amphetamine for the treatment of cocaine dependence: a preliminary investigation. *Front Psychiatry*. 2012. https://doi.org/10.3389/fpsyt.2012.00077.

140. Wisor J. Modafinil as a catecholaminergic agent: empirical evidence and unanswered questions. *Front Neurol*. 2013;4:139. https://doi.org/10.3389/fneur.2013.00139.

141. Grabowski J, Roache JD, Schmitz JM, Rhoades H, Creson D, Korszun A. Replacement medication for cocaine dependence: methylphenidate. *J Clin Psychopharmacol*. 1997;17(6):485–488. https://doi.org/10.1097/00004714-199712000-00008.

142. Trifilieff P, Rives M-L, Urizar E, et al. Detection of antigen interactions ex vivo by proximity ligation assay: endogenous dopamine D2-adenosine A2A receptor complexes in the striatum. *Biotechniques*. 2011;51(2):111–118. https://doi.org/10.2144/000113719.

143. Barret O, Hannestad J, Alagille D, et al. Adenosine 2A receptor occupancy by tozadenant and preladenant in rhesus monkeys. *J Nucl Med*. 2014;55(10):1712–1718. https://doi.org/10.2967/jnumed.114.142067.

144. Moeller FG, Steinberg JL, Lane SD, et al. Increased orbitofrontal brain activation after administration of a selective adenosine A2A antagonist in cocaine dependent subjects. *Front Psychiatry*. 2012. https://doi.org/10.3389/fpsyt.2012.00044.

145. Ferré S, Casadó V, Devi LA, et al. G protein-coupled receptor oligomerization revisited: functional and pharmacological perspectives. *Pharmacol Rev*. 2014;66(2):413–434. https://doi.org/10.1124/pr.113.008052.

146. Ferré S, Ciruela F, Quiroz C, et al. Adenosine receptor heteromers and their integrative role in striatal function. *Sci World J*. 2007;7:74–85. https://doi.org/10.1100/tsw.2007.211.

147. Uchida S, Kadowaki-Horita T, Kanda T. Effects of the adenosine A2A receptor antagonist on cognitive dysfunction in Parkinson's disease. *Int Rev Neurobiol*. 2014;119:169–189. https://doi.org/10.1016/B978-0-12-801022-8.00008-8.

148. Hodgson RA, Bedard PJ, Varty GB, et al. Preladenant, a selective A2A receptor antagonist, is active in primate models of movement disorders. *Exp Neurol*. 2010;225(2):384–390. https://doi.org/10.1016/j.expneurol.2010.07.011.

149. Hauser RA, Cantillon M, Pourcher E, et al. Preladenant in patients with Parkinson's disease and motor fluctuations: a phase 2, double-blind, randomised trial. *Lancet Neurol*. 2011;10(3):221–229. https://doi.org/10.1016/S1474-4422(11)70012-6.

150. Hauser RA, Olanow CW, Kieburtz KD, et al. Tozadenant (SYN115) in patients with Parkinson's disease who have motor fluctuations on levodopa: a phase 2b, double-blind, randomised trial. *Lancet Neurol*. 2014;13(8):767–776. https://doi.org/10.1016/S1474-4422(14)70148-6.

151. Bruchas MR, Land BB, Chavkin C. The dynorphin/kappa opioid system as a modulator of stress-induced and pro-addictive behaviors. *Brain Res*. 2010; 1314(1981):44–55. https://doi.org/10.1016/j.brainres.2009.08.062.

152. Carroll FI, Carlezon Jr WA. Development of κ opioid receptor antagonists. *J Med Chem*. 2013;56(6):2178–2195. https://doi.org/10.1021/jm301783x.

153. Carroll FI, Dolle RE. The discovery and development of the N-substituted trans-3,4-dimethyl-4-(3′-hydroxyphenyl)piperidine class of pure opioid receptor antagonists. *ChemMedChem*. 2014;9(8):1638–1654. https://doi.org/10.1002/cmdc.201402142.

154. Buda KJ, Carroll FI, Kosten TR, Swearingen D, Walters BB. A double-blind, placebo-controlled study to evaluate the safety, tolerability, and pharmacokinetics of single, escalating oral doses of JDTic in healthy male subjects. *Neuropsychopharmacology*. 2015;40(9):1–7. https://doi.org/10.1038/npp.2015.27.

155. Jin-Cheng L, Wen Y, Zhao Y, et al. Anti-arrhythmic effects of kappa-opioid receptor and its changes in ischemia and reperfusion. *Arch Med Res*. 2008;39(5):483–488. https://doi.org/10.1016/j.arcmed.2008.02.011.

156. Pyle WG, Lester JW, Hofmann PA. Effects of kappa-opioid receptor activation on myocardium. *Am J Physiol Heart Circ Physiol*. 2001;281(2):H669–H678. http://www.ncbi.nlm.nih.gov/pubmed/11454571.

157. Melief EJ, Miyatake M, Carroll FI, et al. Duration of action of a broad range of selective -opioid receptor antagonists is positively correlated with c-Jun N-Terminal Kinase-1 activation. *Mol Pharmacol*. 2011;80(5):920–929. https://doi.org/10.1124/mol.111.074195.

158. Lowe SL, Wong CJ, Witcher J, et al. Safety, tolerability, and pharmacokinetic evaluation of single- and multiple-ascending doses of a novel kappa opioid receptor antagonist LY2456302 and drug interaction with ethanol in healthy subjects. *J Clin Pharmacol*. 2014; 54(9):968–978. https://doi.org/10.1002/jcph.286.

159. Reed B, Butelman ER, Fry RS, Kimani R, Kreek MJ. Repeated administration of opra kappa (LY2456302), a novel, short-acting, selective KOP-r antagonist, in persons with and without cocaine dependence. *Neuropsychopharmacology*. 2017:1–12. https://doi.org/10.1038/npp.2017.205.

CHAPTER 2

The Role of Nutrition in Addiction Recovery: What We Know and What We Don't

DAVID A. WISS, MS RDN

INTRODUCTION

The addiction epidemic in the United States has now reached crisis proportions. It is no longer a topic confined to healthcare professionals and is now receiving considerable attention by the press, media, and politicians. Recent data shows widespread use in adolescents and teens.[1] With substance use disorder (SUD) rates rising, there is an urgent need for new and innovative treatment modalities. The concept of using nutrition to treat addiction was proposed as early as 1955[2] but has not yet been accepted in conventional SUD treatment. In 1990, the American Dietetic Association (now called the Academy of Nutrition and Dietetics) published a position paper declaring that nutrition intervention is an essential component of treatment and recovery from SUD.[3,4] Unfortunately, the position statement was never implemented and there has been little progress incorporating nutrition professionals into treatment settings. At the present time, specialized training programs for nutritionists seeking work in addiction treatment settings[5] do not exist. In the past decade, many private sector addiction treatment facilities have begun to incorporate "holistic" approaches to recovery, which include an emphasis on healthful eating, but there are no established standards of practice. Recently, nutrition therapy guidelines have been developed for specific intoxicating substances[6] and this chapter will add to that body of knowledge by emphasizing the latest advances in our understanding of gastrointestinal (GI) health. This paper summarizes the impact of substances on nutritional status and proposes strategies that can be employed to replenish and improve eating behavior in treatment settings. Because drugs and food are both associated with cognitive control and executive functioning in risk/reward decision-making,[7] intervention strategies are grounded in accepted concepts of neuroscience and psychology.

Dietary Patterns and Malnutrition. It is well established that individuals with severe SUD may have inadequate dietary intake leading to malnutrition.[8–11] In a large sample of Canadian intravenous (IV) drug users, 65% met criteria for hunger, which was strongly correlated with depression, and 74% had inadequate housing.[12] Preference for sweets and other easily digestible foods (i.e., refined cereal) and a low intake of fruits and vegetables is a consistent finding in street dwelling drug addicts.[8,9] In one study of 140 heroin and cocaine addicts admitted to a hospital, 18% were considered severely malnourished (serum albumin under 3.5 g/dL and/or serum transferrin under 200 mg/dL), which was worse in females compared to males.[13] These authors also found that the heaviest drug users were also the most malnourished. Research on HIV-infected heroin-addicted females has shown malnutrition in all subjects while using but are able to improve their nutritional status after 6 months of detoxification.[14]

Micronutrient Imbalances. Micronutrient deficiencies have been observed in several studies of patients with SUD.[15–19] Specifically, deficiencies in antioxidant vitamins E, C, and A have been reported. Studies have revealed iron deficiency and anemia.[16,17,19] Elevated levels of serum copper and zinc are commonly seen in subjects with SUD[16] indicative of infection and inflammation,[9,19] slowly returning to normal after abstinence and nutrition intervention.[19] It is possible that imbalances in serum trace minerals alter trace elemental concentrations in the brain which can lead to oxidative damage.[19] Plasma nitric oxide metabolites are higher among persons with substance use disorder compared to controls,[18] suggesting injury by free radicals and an

The Assessment and Treatment of Addiction. https://doi.org/10.1016/B978-0-323-54856-4.00002-X

oxidant–antioxidant disturbance[18,20] that has been implicated in the pathomechanism of relapse.[21]

Weight Concerns. Many persons with SUD report gaining weight during early recovery,[22–25] although there is no established association between lifetime illicit drug abuse and BMI.[26,27] Heavy injection drug users have a lower percent body fat than nondrug users.[28] Hyperphagia has been linked to drug discontinuation as well as smoking cessation.[29] In one study of adolescents in treatment, weight gain occurred independent of smoking and psychotropic medication use.[22] Men in addiction treatment have described dysfunctional eating behaviors such as bingeing and using food to regulate mood in early recovery (1–6 months) as well as distress about efforts to lose weight in later recovery (7–36 months).[23] Women who gain weight in early recovery have expressed interest in incorporating nutrition and exercise into their recovery program.[24,30] In one study (n = 297), 43% of women expressed concern that weight gain could trigger drug relapse[31] and other treatment research (n = 124) has shown that weight-related concerns exist in 70% of women.[32] According to many authors, consideration should be given to prioritizing efforts to improve environmental supports for healthful eating within residential recovery programs.[10,30,33]

ALCOHOL

Chronic Disease. Weight gain and obesity have been associated with an increased risk for lifetime alcohol use disorder (AUD) in men but not women.[27] On the other hand, epidemiological studies support a link between familial alcoholism risk and obesity for women but less so for men.[34] Recent data from a French study suggests that drinking frequency is positively associated with increased BMI and waist circumference independent of drinking patterns.[35] In detoxified patients with AUD, there is evidence of abnormal blood pressure response to variations in salt intake that is similar to sodium-sensitive arterial hypertension, suggesting a possible susceptibility of alcohol abusers to cardiovascular disease (CVD).[36] Other authors have suggested hyperhomocysteinemia may play a role in the development of CVD among patients with alcoholic liver disease (ALD).[37] Investigators in Japan have suggested that ethanol-related colorectal cancer might be linked to the presence of anaerobic bacterial strains that accumulate acetaldehyde under aerobic conditions in the colon and rectum.[38] The data strongly suggests that AUD leads to gut dysbiosis (a condition in which the symbiotic relationship between gut microbiota and host is lost) and peripheral inflammation.

Alcoholic Liver Disease. Recent advances in the assessment of the gut microbiome have changed our understanding of ALD. Evidence suggests that gut health may be linked to ALD by way of a gut-liver axis.[39] Chronic alcohol consumption leads to higher synthesis of bile acids,[40] which may explain the pathogenesis of colonic inflammation in ALD.[41] A recent review summarized the importance of dietary lipids in the progression of ALD.[42] Specifically, proinflammatory omega-6 fatty acids have demonstrated deleterious effects on liver injury in animal models.[43] Additionally, the progression of ALD appears to be linked to the progression of lung disease by way of increased oxidative stress and activation of the inflammatory cascade.[44]

Microbiome. It has been well established that excessive alcohol negatively impacts the microbiome leading to dysbiosis in humans[45–47] and animals.[48–50] Normal gut microbiota appears to be involved in inhibiting the growth of pathogenic bacteria in order to prevent conditions such as small intestinal bacterial overgrowth.[51] Intestinal microbiota function is altered in AUD leading to increased markers of oxidative stress and decreases in the short-chain fatty acids (SCFAs), propionate and isobutyrate, which are important in maintaining intestinal epithelial cell health and barrier integrity.[47]

Immune dysfunction in AUD may be related to a disruption in the integrity of the tight junction (intestinal barrier), allowing bacterial translocation into the portal vein or through gastrointestinal lymphatics.[37,52–56] Lipopolysaccharide (LPS) is a major component of the outer wall of many Gram-negative bacteria which may allow translocation from the lumen of the intestine into the portal circulation and then travel to the liver. Gram-negative bacterial overgrowth results in augmented endotoxin levels that cause hepatic damage.[57] Research has shown that gut "leakiness" and associated inflammation (measured by LPS, TNFα, IL-6, IL-10, and hsCRP) in noncirrhotic alcohol-dependent subjects correlate to measures of depression and alcohol craving.[58] After 3 weeks of abstinence, alcohol-dependent subjects with gut leakiness had higher degrees of depression, anxiety, and craving than those with less gut permeability.[46] These authors suggest that these psychological symptoms may contribute to a negative reinforcement process involved with persistence of AUD. Since not all subjects developed gut leakiness, chronic alcohol consumption by itself is not sufficient to cause gut dysfunction;[46] therefore, other variables (e.g., diet, smoking, genetics, immune status) are likely involved. Other subjects with AUD displayed evidence of alcohol gut dysbiosis that persisted after an extended period of sobriety and in the absence of ALD.[45] A recent review summarized the role of the gut-brain axis in alcohol use disorders.[59] The authors suggest that alcohol-induced gut dysbiosis contributes to neuroinflammation in the amygdala, which contributes directly to withdrawal behavior and symptoms (anxiety and depression). More evidence of the gut-brain axis will be summarized in subsequent sections.

Nutritional Deficiencies. By evaluating gastrointestinal function (assessed by D-xylose breath tests) investigators found that chronic alcohol overconsumption seems to cause malabsorption in the small intestine, comparable to patients with untreated celiac disease.[60] It is likely that compromised gut function leads to reduced absorption of nutrients. Any damage to the liver can compromise the metabolism of micronutrients.[61] Additionally, alcohol instead of food leads to poor nutritional intake,[62] making it difficult to determine if nutrient deficiencies stem from primary malnutrition or secondary malnutrition, which occurs from alterations in the absorption, metabolism, utilization, and excretion of nutrients.

It is well established that thiamine deficiency is linked to alcoholism and can lead to Wernicke—Korsakoff syndrome.[63] Mechanisms of thiamine deficiency include inadequate intake, decreased absorption from the gastrointestinal tract, hypomagnesaemia,[64] and increased utilization in the cells. Intravenous thiamine is routinely administered in hospital settings for AUD. Vitamin B6 may also be deficient due to increased utilization and reduced formation.[61] Serum folic acid concentrations are often low in AUD and some authors have concluded that hyperhomocysteinemia is a probable cause.[65] A recent study showed no differences in folate and vitamin B12 levels between individuals with alcohol dependence and social drinkers.[66] Vitamin B12 deficiencies may be normal or elevated in the serum of AUD patients yet depressed in the liver due to decreased uptake by hepatocytes.[67] Deficiencies of B6, folate, and B12 appear to be linked to ethanol-induced aberrant methionine metabolism[68] yet supplementation with S-adenosylmethionine (SAM) for ALD has led to inconclusive results.[67]

Both human and animal models have demonstrated adverse effects of alcohol on vitamin A metabolism.[69] Low vitamin D levels[70] have been associated with increased fractures in AUD.[71] Links between iron and AUD appear inconclusive. In one investigation, the majority of patients with AUD did not display abnormal iron metabolism; some displayed deficiency while some exhibited iron overload.[66] Micronutrient deficiencies appear inconsistent in human studies since they are retrospective and do not control for dietary intake. Because the prevalence of malnutrition in AUD is high,[72] all patients should be screened for vitamin and mineral deficiencies through conventional laboratory testing and examination of clinical signs and symptoms. Generally, a complete multivitamin/mineral supplement is indicated to augment the diet upon cessation of alcohol, and IV thiamine may be warranted if Wernicke—Korsakoff syndrome is present.

Hormones. Research has shown that circulating leptin levels are increased in a dose-dependent manner in AUD, regardless of nutritional status or the presence of liver disease.[73] These investigators found that leptin levels returned to normal after cessation of ethanol, while other investigators showed that leptin levels increase during the 10-day alcohol withdrawal period.[74] Other research shows rises in leptin that eventually decrease between day 5 and 16, likely attributable to dietary changes (lipid intake).[75] Gut-derived ghrelin appears to play a key role in alcohol-seeking behavior.[76] Alcohol-dependent patients have increased ghrelin levels during early abstinence, increasing during the first week of alcohol withdrawal,[77] whereas other research suggests that ghrelin drops and then rises between day 5 and 16.[75] Similar to leptin, insulin appears to rise between day 2 and 5 and then decrease between day 5 and 16,[75] but failure to adequately control for dietary intake make conclusions difficult to reach. In long-term abstinent alcoholics, investigators observed a significantly blunted response in blood glucose following a glucose infusion.[78] Subjects exhibited trends toward both blunted responses in glucagon and insulin. Authors speculate that nervous system damage attributable to the effects of alcohol exposure is responsible for the insufficient hormonal response, particularly neurons in the hypothalamus. Taken together, the apparent link between alcohol abuse and abnormal hormonal responses highlights the negative impact of alcohol on the endocrine system, providing support for the need for dietary intervention in supporting long-term abstinence and recovery. Further links between hormones and addictive processes are discussed below.

Eating Behavior. Various studies have confirmed that AUD patients display abnormal preference for sweetened foods[79] and beverages.[25,80] Possible mechanisms for increased sweet preference include links between carbohydrates and serotonergic neurotransmission,[79] the dopaminergic impact of sweetened foods,[81] impaired hormonal responses to glucose,[78] links between appetitive hormones and craving,[82] and genetics.[83–85] Tendencies to engage addiction-like eating patterns will be discussed in more detail in subsequent sections, as they cannot be ignored when attempting to improve nutritional habits in this population.

Nutritional Treatment. A recent meta-analysis concluded that nutritional interventions may have beneficial effects on clinical outcomes for patients with alcoholic hepatitis or cirrhosis, including survival and decreased risk of hepatic encephalopathy and infections.[86] Medical interventions for alcoholic hepatitis have been described elsewhere[55] and emerging evidence suggests potential benefit from microbiota-based treatments for ALD including fecal transplants and probiotics/prebiotics,[56] as well as possibly additional polyphenolic compounds such as epigallocatechin gallate (EGCG).[87] In a randomized controlled trial, hospitalized patients with alcoholic hepatitis received 7 days of oral supplementation with cultured *Lactobacillus subtilus/Streptococcus faecium* (1500 mg/day) and had significant restoration of bowel flora and reduction of LPS.[88] Given what is known about the link between dietary fatty acids and inflammation, emphasis on omega-3 essential fatty acids should be considered an important part of nutrition therapy. In animal models, dietary flaxseed oil ameliorates ALD via anti-inflammation and modulating gut microbiota.[89] In other rodent research, polyphenols from olive oil were protective against alcohol-induced oxidative stress.[90] Nutraceutical regimens to ameliorate the toxic effects of alcohol merit further attention.[91] Nutrition intervention strategies specifically for AUD are summarized in Table 2.1. Overall recommendations common for all substance use disorders are summarized in Table 2.2.

STIMULANTS

Cocaine. Similar to AUD, patients with a history of cocaine use disorder (CUD) have a higher preference for sucrose-sweetened beverages[92] and a higher overall intake of carbohydrates.[93] Cases of Wernicke's encephalopathy have been reported in crack-cocaine users who did not regularly consume alcohol, indicative of thiamine malnutrition.[94] Cocaine-dependent men are more likely to skip breakfast than healthy men and to consume higher amounts of fatty foods, reflected by increased levels of monounsaturated and saturated fatty acids in plasma.[93]

In one sample of nonopioid and nonalcohol-dependent persons with cocaine dependence, low

TABLE 2.1
Recommendations for Recovery From Alcohol Use Disorders
• 1.2—1.5 g/kg/day protein
• Full-spectrum multivitamin/mineral broken into at least two separate daily doses
• Additional B-complex vitamin (intravenous thiamine if Wernicke—Korsakoff syndrome is present)
• Additional vitamin D3 if deficient (also direct sunlight for 20 min twice/week)
• Omega-3 DHA-rich 3 g/day, reduced exposure to omega-6 fatty acids
• Probiotic supplement (refrigerated)
Where More Information is Needed:
• If liquid multivitamin/mineral supplements work better for absorption of micronutrients
• If supplemental zinc will be effective in improving gut permeability and optimal dosage
• If supplemental S-adenosylmethionine is effective for alcoholic liver disease and optimal dosage
• If supplements to support liver function are beneficial
• Which particular strains of probiotic bacteria are optimal for alcohol users
• How nutrition interventions should differ based on presence/progression of liver disease
• Link between alcoholism and the insulin-leptin-ghrelin response

polyunsaturated fatty acid (PUFA) levels measured 2 weeks after hospital admission served as a predictor of relapse after 3 months.[95] Investigators suspect that since PUFAs can influence serotonergic and dopaminergic neurotransmission,[96] altered reward mechanisms might influence drug-taking behavior. In a small sample, polysubstance abusers who received 3g omega-3 PUFAs daily for 3 months had significant decreases in measures of anxiety, persisting for at least 3 months post-treatment.[97] While more data on the link between PUFAs and cocaine is needed, this may prove to be a beneficial nutritional strategy.

Cocaine-dependent men exhibit a trend toward lower circulating leptin levels.[93] There is evidence that overeating patterns can precede the recovery process but the effect may be disguised by lack of weight gain.[98] Authors suggest that chronic cocaine use directly interferes with metabolic processes resulting in an imbalance between fat intake and storage.[93] Altered hormones combined with addiction-like eating is likely to explain excessive weight gain upon cessation of the drug. In a large US adult population study, cocaine use has been associated with elevated blood pressure.[99]

TABLE 2.2
Overall Recommendation for Recovery From all Substance Use Disorders

- 2–3 L of water per day, replacing sweetened beverages
- Emphasis on plant proteins from beans, nuts, seeds
- Emphasis on whole grains (oats, farro, quinoa, barley, etc.) over refined grains

- "Anti-inflammatory diet" rich in antioxidant vitamins A, C, E, selenium, iron, omega-3
- Sources of vitamin A: carrots, pumpkin, sweet potatoes, spinach
- Sources of vitamin C: bell peppers, kiwi, broccoli, strawberries
- Sources of vitamin E: almonds, sunflower seeds, avocado, peanut butter
- Sources of selenium: brazil nuts, yellowfin tuna, turkey, halibut
- Sources of iron: red meat, lentils, pumpkin seeds, kidney beans
- Sources of omega-3: fatty fish, chia seeds, flax seeds, walnuts

- Gradual increase in fiber intake to meet daily recommendations: 25 g/day women, 38 g/day men
- Get fiber from whole food over dietary supplements
- Sources of fiber: beans, whole grains, berries, cruciferous vegetables
- For additional fiber, use chia seeds soaked in water

- Eat breakfast within 30 min of waking up
- Eat smaller meals every 2.5–4.5 h (5–6 times/day)
- Fruit or vegetable with every meal/snack
- Raw vegetable daily
- Fermented foods (not fermented beverages!)

- Max 400 mg caffeine/day (3–4 cups of coffee)
- Use green tea over coffee when possible
- Minimize artificial sweeteners

In a small sample of HIV-infected drug users, cocaine users had a higher relative abundance of *Bacteriodetes* in their intestines, suggesting that the drug may contribute to changes in the microbiome.[100] In animal models, alterations in the gut microbiota via antibiotic treatment enhanced behavioral response to cocaine, as modulated by reward circuitry in the brain.[101] Other animal research has led investigators to propose that targeting the microbiota-gut-brain axis has promise in the treatment of co-occurring HIV and cocaine abuse.[102] Taken together, cocaine use is associated with altered physiology in the gut, brain, and endocrine system.

While it is unclear if some of the observable alterations precede drug use, nutrition therapy designed to restore gut flora, stabilize hormones, and reduce addictive neuro-circuitry appears promising in the treatment of CUD. In one small study, supplemental N-Acetylcysteine (NAC) decreased cue-induced cravings in cocaine-dependent individuals.[103] NAC stimulates cysteine-glutamate exchange and can restore glutathione (antioxidant) which appears to be linked to addiction signaling proteins and may have benefits for other substances as well.[104] While rodent research has generated compelling findings, human studies are inconclusive.[105] Additional research linking cocaine to NAC, overall nutritional status, and microbiome is needed.

Methamphetamine. Methamphetamine (MA) use is generally associated with decreased BMI.[106] In rodents, acute administration of MA has led to significant reductions in the appetite hormone NP-Y[107,108] consistent with humans who report lost hunger during MA use. There are published case reports of MA use for weight control in women with eating disorders[109] and larger studies show associations with bulimia nervosa (BN), but not anorexia nervosa.[110] There also exists evidence of hyperphagia and rebound weight gain in amphetamine-treated rodent models during the first month of abstinence.[111] In one study from Australia, amphetamine users were nearly twice as likely to become obese than opioid users.[112] Clinical anecdote suggests that rebound weight gain in humans during first months of abstinence can be as high as 10–30 lbs. per month for previously underweight patients, but eating behaviors and food preference during early recovery from MA has not been adequately described.

An intriguing link between MA and oral health exists. Anything that effects dental health has the potential to impact all areas of nutrition via influence on food choices. Several studies have linked IV MA use with dental problems[113–116] including no visits to the dentist within past year.[113] Other articles have suggested that dentists can play a crucial role in the early detection of MA use.[115,116] It is unknown if the increase in dental disease is due to hygiene habits or from secondary effects of the drug, as dental problems have been linked with other illicit substances including cocaine.[117] It is likely that high intake of sugar sweetened beverages and other sugar-laden foods contributes to this association, as well as increased acidity in the oral cavity.[114] Animal data suggests that MA can cause altered carbohydrate metabolism and cause dysregulation of calcium and iron homeostasis.[118] It is possible that altered calcium metabolism may be linked to MA-induced dental disease but more studies are needed to explore potential underlying mechanisms.

Research on MA-dependent humans in China showed that levels of total cholesterol, triglycerides, and glucose are significantly decreased on the second day of hospital admission, indicative of malnutrition.[106] Consistent with findings of increased oxidative stress in polysubstance users, measures of MA-induced neurotoxicity are reduced by antioxidants selenium[119] and CoQ10.[120] Supplemental antioxidants appear promising, particularly if there are challenges implementing nutrition therapy focused on whole plant foods with high fiber and high antioxidant potential. Similar to alcohol and other intoxicating drugs, MA in high doses disrupts epithelial barrier function by modulating tight junction integrity and epithelial cell viability.[121] To date, links between MA use and gut health have only been explored in animal models, but suggest that administration of the drug leads to dysbiosis.[122] Specifically, propionate-producing genus *Phascolarcobacterium* was repressed by MA and the family Ruminococcaceae (linked to anxiety) was elevated. Investigations exploring links between MA and the microbiome are needed. Nutrition intervention strategies specifically for stimulants cocaine and MA are summarized in Table 2.3. General recommendations for SUD are summarized in Table 2.2.

OPIOIDS

Overview. The cost of opioid use disorder (OUD) represents a substantial and growing economic burden for society in the United States.[123] Increasing IV drug use is one factor that has led to increased rates of overdose and death.[124] Much of the nutrition-related data comes from patients on methadone maintenance.[125] Similar to cocaine, opioids are associated with hormonal abnormalities including decreased serum leptin[126] and rapid weight gain during treatment.[127] Studies have linked prolonged heroin use with oxidant–antioxidant disturbances[20] and lower-than-normal bone mass.[128] Attempts to alleviate the withdrawal and mood symptoms during recovery with supplements containing precursors for neurotransmitters (tyrosine, lecithin, L-glutamine, and 5-HTP) have shown promise,[129] but recent advances in microbiome research indicate that more attention be directed toward prioritizing recovery of GI function.

Gastrointestinal Health. Opioids delay gastric emptying[130] and constipation-related symptoms including straining, hard stools, painful, infrequent,

---

TABLE 2.3
Recommendation for Recovery From Cocaine and Methamphetamine

- Protein-rich diet: 1.2–2.0 g/kg/day (whey or plant-based protein powder can help)
- Minimize refined carbohydrates (use complex carbohydrate)
- Gradual weight gain if underweight (instead of rapid, ideally under 10 lbs./month)
- Full-spectrum multivitamin/mineral broken into at least two separate daily doses
- Additional vitamin D3 if deficient (also direct sunlight for 20 min twice/week)
- Omega-3 DHA-rich 3 g/day, reduced exposure to omega-6 fatty acids
- Probiotic supplement (refrigerated)

Where More Information is Needed:

- If supplemental metals (i.e., iron, copper) in multivitamin/mineral promote oxidative stress
- Which particular strains of probiotic bacteria are optimal for cocaine and meth users
- How compromised oral health can impact nutritional status
- If supplemental N-acetylcysteine (or glutathione) is effective to reduce cravings and optimal dosage

---

and incomplete bowel movements are well known.[131] Opioid-induced bowel dysfunction reflects the impact of opioids on the entire GI tract, which includes symptoms such as: dry mouth, heartburn, nausea, vomiting, chronic abdominal pain, and bloating.[131] In a large retrospective study from a hospital setting, moderate to high use of opioid analgesics are associated with an increased risk of *Clostridium difficile* infection in a dose-dependent manner.[132] It is possible that such association results from interruptions in the rhythmic contraction of the intestine, causing a motionless environment favorable to bacterial growth. Investigators hypothesize that delayed GI transit time may subsequently increase intraluminal concentrations of toxins.[132]

In animal models, morphine disrupts intestinal epithelium increasing the virulence of *Pseudomonas aeruginosa*, capable of causing lethal gut-derived sepsis.[133] In other rodent research, morphine induced bacterial translocation by compromising intestinal barrier function, leading to inflammation in the small intestine.[134] While the mechanism of action behind gastrointestinal imbalance for opioids and alcohol is not identical, the result is the same: inflammatory cascades and compromised immune status. Gut dysbiosis can lead to the overgrowth of specific bacterial strains. Currently, it is unknown if particular strains can influence addictive processes, but it appears possible. In one animal study, *Enterococcus faecalis* was associated with morphine-induced alteration of gut microbiome, with an increase of 100-fold compared to placebo.[135] More research is needed to determine possible links between gut health and opioid-induced pathology.

Nutritional Deficiencies. OUD has been associated with decreased levels of blood glucose,[136] thiamine,[137] vitamin B6,[137,138] folate,[137] vitamin C,[138] potassium,[139] calcium,[139] magnesium,[140] zinc,[141] selenium,[142] and cholesterol.[139] Other data on ex-heroin addicts has shown higher cholesterol levels,[136] suggesting possible differences between using versus abstinence. One group of researchers suggested that cholesterol may be associated with the cognitive aspect of drug craving.[143] Vitamin and mineral values are also inconsistent in published studies, suggesting that confounding variables such as dietary choices make it difficult to associate the drug with any specific deficiencies. In one study, methadone patients received 50,000 IU vitamin D every 2 weeks for 12 weeks and showed significant improvements in psychological symptoms.[144] Notwithstanding, nutrient deficiencies should be confirmed by laboratory testing when available before overzealous administration of supplements. Some researchers believe that medication-assisted treatment is not favorable unless it is coupled with proper diet due to the negative role of vitamin and mineral deficiencies in the withdrawal process.[145] More data is needed on the role of micronutrients in the recovery process from OUD.

Eating Behavior. OUD has been associated with high consumption of sweets and low intake of dietary fiber.[146-148] Given what is known about the impact of opioids on gastrointestinal motility, it is not surprising that this population would select foods requiring minimal digestive efforts. Qualitative research in Australia has revealed that active heroin users have little interest in food and prefer foods that are quick, convenient, and cheap.[149] Other qualitative data indicates that chronic IV drug users are actively involved in managing and improving their health even while continuing to engage in drug use.[150] Once getting sober, some ex-heroin users take pleasure in food preparation and eating, while others express very little interest.

In a small sample, patients on long-term methadone maintenance had higher BMIs than controls, suggesting possible links between endogenous opioid systems and palatable food consumption, leading to overeating.[151] Other research has suggested that mechanisms (e.g., altered hormones) other than addiction-like eating may be responsible for the weight gain associated with methadone.[152] In Turkey, more than a quarter (28%) of patients with heroin use disorder from a detoxification hospital met established criteria for food addiction and 21% met criteria for binge eating disorder (BED) with significant overlap between the two.[153] Co-occurrence of SUD and eating disorder will be discussed in more detail below. More data is needed regarding nutrition intervention strategies during recovery from OUD. Current recommendations for nutritional interventions in OUD can be found in Table 2.4.

CO-OCCURRING SUBSTANCE USE DISORDER AND EATING DISORDER

Background. Co-occurring SUD and eating disorders (ED) have been investigated and described[154-157]

TABLE 2.4
Recommendations for Recovery From Opioids

- Protein-rich diet: 1.2–2.0 g/kg/day (whey or plant-based protein powder can help)
- Use fruit (fresh/frozen/dried) for "sweet tooth"
- Gradual weight gain if underweight (instead of rapid, ideally under 10 lbs./month)
- Full-spectrum multivitamin/mineral broken into at least two daily separate doses
- Additional vitamin D3 if deficient (also direct sunlight for 20 min twice/week)
- Omega-3 DHA-rich 3 g/day, reduced exposure to omega-6 fatty acids
- Probiotic supplement (refrigerated)

Where More Information is Needed:

- If liquid multivitamin/mineral supplements work better for absorption of micronutrients
- If supplemental vitamin B6 is beneficial for heroin users and optimal dosage
- Which particular strains of probiotic bacteria are optimal for heroin users
- How to best manage opioid-induced bowel dysfunction nutritionally
- If digestive enzymes are effective and optimal dosage
- If supplements containing precursors for neurotransmitters are effective and optimal dosage
- Link between opioids, cholesterol, and hormones
- Effectiveness of "sunlight therapy" in recovery from opioid addiction
- Nutritional implications of Suboxone (buprenorphine/naloxone) and Vivitrol (naltrexone)

with data pointing to bidirectional associations. There is significant overlap between SUD and ED both neuro-chemically[158] and behaviorally.[159] Compensatory behaviors such as fasting and self-induced vomiting to avoid weight gain from consuming alcohol have recently been called "drunkorexia".[160] There is evidence of new onset SUDs (primarily alcohol) following bariatric procedures[161–164] suggesting potential for cross-addiction between food and alcohol/drugs.[165] Other authors have suggested that the overlap in maladaptive behaviors may stem from difficulties with emotion regulation[166,167] including tendencies to act rashly in the face of distress[168] and coping with negative affect.[169]

In one small sample of women in long-term addiction treatment, the overlap between SUDs and EDs was 39%.[170] In a study from an ED clinic (n = 50), 100% of patients had a history of psychoactive substance misuse.[171] Overall, the estimated comorbidity of SUD and ED ranges from 3% to 50%.[84,172,173] Despite some data suggesting clinically significant EDs are somewhat rare in SUD populations, problematic eating behaviors such as nibbling, night eating, and dietary restraint are relatively common.[174] Night eating syndrome has been observed in SUD patients[175] with even higher rates in those with nicotine dependence.[176] Misuse of prescription stimulants (Ritalin, Adderral, Concerta), which are known appetite suppressants, has been associated with more severe ED symptomatology.[177] Additional data is needed on the interaction between prescribed medications common in SUD treatment and the development of disordered eating. Anecdotally, there are reports of medications (i.e., Seroquel) leading to nighttime bingeing and distress about weight gain. There are also reports of weight gain from medications that are not linked to dietary change, but rather to adverse effects on metabolism, and potentially alterations in gut microbiota.

Recently, there has been growing interest in an overall integrated treatment approach to SUD and ED, rather than separate sequential treatments.[173,178,179] In SUD populations, loss-of-control binge episodes observed with binge eating disorder (BED) and BN are more common than AN restrictive-type,[156,174,180] with even higher prevalence when there is a post-traumatic stress disorder diagnosis.[181,182] Compulsive exercise has been associated with ED pathology[183] but to date compulsive exercise during SUD recovery is inadequately understood (reviewed below). In the male population, obsessive preoccupation with muscularity coupled with intense exercise and SUD has been described,[184] but the majority of data on co-occurring

SUD and ED exists in women. In adolescents, the use of tobacco, alcohol, and cocaine has been associated with disordered eating behavior.[185] In one study, over half of adolescents who reported substance use engaged in unhealthy weight loss practices such as fasting, diet pills, or laxative use/purging.[186] Taken together, the overlap between disordered eating and substance misuse necessitates that nutritionists and other treatment professionals in SUD settings be adequately trained in ED treatment principles.

Bulimia Nervosa. Shared traits between BN and SUD appear to stem from genetic influences more than environmental factors.[187,188] In a small sample of women, alcohol consumption appears to reduce eating-related urges[189] which is consistent with other findings that women with BN turn to substances to dampen bulimic urges.[157] Conversely, it is also likely that alcohol consumption can act as a trigger for bingeing and purging. Given the neurobiological overlap between BN and drug addiction, some authors have suggested pharmaceutical treatments for BN targeting dopamine, glutamate, or opioid neurotransmitter systems that are effective in treating SUDs.[158] To date, there is no consensus on the frequency and amounts of highly palatable foods to include in the diets of patients with comorbid BN and SUD, but a theoretical model known as the Disordered Eating Food Addiction Nutrition Guide (DEFANG) may be helpful for case conceptualization.[190] Currently, the most common model for nutritional management of BN suggests regular inclusion of highly palatable foods (processed foods with added sugar, salt, fat) because overly restrictive approaches typically are not sustainable and can reinforce an unhealthy relationship to food.

Binge Eating Disorder. Before BED was an official diagnosis, authors described overlaps between SUD and obesity highlighting a need for shared treatment approaches including pharmacology, psychotherapy, mindfulness training, and 12-step.[191] Overlap between BED and SUD has received considerable attention in recent years[192–194] with most conclusions providing support for the food addiction hypothesis. In rodent models, a history of bingeing on high-fat foods led to the development of cocaine seeking and taking behaviors.[195] In young adult women, illicit substance users had a higher likelihood of developing comorbid or substitute binge eating, but the reverse was not true.[191] Despite commonalities between BED and food addiction, there are often distinct characteristics of BED such as shape/weight concerns[196] and dietary restraint that emerge as causal mechanisms in the development of binge eating behavior which suggest that BED, food addiction, and obesity are not always synonymous.[197] A case study and more information about BED/SUD can be found in the DEFANG article.[190]

FOOD ADDICTION

Background. Food addiction (FA) research has been discussed for several decades and much of the research originated in Mark Gold's lab at the University of Florida.[198] In a landmark paper from 2005, Volkow and Wise described overlapping neuroimaging characteristics between obese subjects and SUD subjects, with similar reductions in dopamine (DA) D2 receptors.[199] Other imaging studies using PET scans have shown deficits in DA D2/D3 receptor signaling are related to obesity and addiction susceptibility[200] by making food/drugs less rewarding and more habitual.[201] Although functional imaging techniques are still in their infancy, they hold significant promise for informing intervention strategies for abnormal intake behavior.[202] Animal data suggests that the neurobiological process of relapse into old, unhealthy eating habits has similarities to relapse into drug-seeking during abstinence.[203] Despite the aggregate of convincing data, the FA hypothesis is not without detractors. Important differences between obesity and SUD include the temporal course of relapse across these disorders and respective treatment outcomes.[204] Others prefer to label it as an eating addiction (behavioral addiction) rather than a substance-related addiction.[205]

With the validation of the Yale Food Addiction Scale (YFAS) in 2008[206] and the updated YFAS 2.0 in 2016,[207] there have been hundreds of studies describing FA using this construct in obese patients,[208] adolescents,[209] children,[210] those with eating disorders,[211] and more recently those with SUD.[153,212] It has been established that food restriction enhances the rewarding effect of stimulant drugs in animals[213,214] as well as in humans.[215] Human studies repeatedly show that cessation of drug use leads to rebound hyperphagia and subsequent weight gain.[22–24,29,31] While the "addiction transfer" hypothesis has been described,[216] more research is needed to describe FA in SUD populations, particularly during early abstinence compared to sustained recovery.

In 1996, Blum and colleagues introduced the concept of reward deficiency syndrome (RDS) describing a genetic dysfunction of the DA D2 receptor leading to substance seeking behavior.[217] This framework proposes genetic testing as a means to identify individuals at risk for food and drug addiction[218] and DNA Customized Nutrition (also known as Nutrigenomics) using nutraceuticals (e.g., amino acids) to improve brain dysfunction associated with addiction.[219] The use (including type and dose) of amino acids and other dietary supplements in this research continues to evolve[220–222] and remains controversial. While attempts to induce "dopamine homeostasis" by balancing DA function in the brain's reward circuitry (via genetic expression) through nutraceuticals shows promise for recovery,[223] the use of nutrition therapy (real food) remains difficult to study (small effects require large samples to detect significant change) and underfunded and is therefore virtually unexplored.

An important development in the addiction literature related to both food and reinforcing drugs is the discernment between "wanting" (incentive salience) and "liking" (hedonic impact).[224] Often the addicted individual can strongly "want" for something, which is not cognitively wanted. The "liking" can remain stable, or even decrease, while the "wanting" increases. Wanting is synonymous with craving, which is now part of DSM-5 criteria for SUD, and an important construct considering the contemporary food environment.[225] In one study, highly processed foods were generally related to elevated craving/wanting but not significantly associated with elevated liking.[226] The authors suggest that the term "food addiction" be refined to "highly processed food addiction."

Overactivation of the reward pathways and the subsequent development of compulsive-like behavior[227] causes dysfunction of the prefrontal cortex,[228] which is responsible for executive functioning such as weighing pros and cons. It is not surprising that so many people in early SUD recovery exhibit disordered eating patterns, particularly when rehab settings provide unlimited access to highly palatable foods. The importance of environmental cues on food motivation[229] should necessitate consideration of the food environment at the treatment facility. According to one study, foods with the most addictive potential include: chocolate, ice cream, French fries, pizza, cookie, chips, and cake.[230] These are foods commonly served in SUD treatment settings, which may lead to undesirable patterns of impulsive consumption.[231]

Variations in the DAD2 gene have been associated with impulsive decision-making and delay discounting, which is a preference for small immediate rewards over larger but delayed ones.[232] Delay discounting may be a behavioral marker for pathological disorders across both food and drug use[233] and is an excellent topic for group discussion in treatment settings. Nutrition education that is informed by FA research can target topics like craving, impulsivity, delay discounting, and novelty seeking when providing SUD patients with eating advice. Discussion of the cross-addiction concept by treatment providers can be helpful to normalize concerns about eating behavior during early SUD recovery, particularly as prevention against the development of extreme dieting and EDs. A weekly psychoeducation group led by a registered dietitian nutritionist (RDN) is recommended.

Hormones. A review article suggested that obesity-associated inflammation modulated by leptin in the brain may promote addictive behaviors leading to a self-perpetuating cycle of addiction to food, as well as drugs/alcohol and process addictions such as gambling.[235] Leptin may be implicated in cognition and mood, linking impaired leptin activity to obesity-related depression.[236] In animal models, food deprivation can provoke relapse to heroin seeking via a leptin-dependent mechanism.[237] While still not fully understood, it is known that leptin has action extending to the brain reward circuits contributing to preference for highly palatable foods. It has been suggested that the leptin–dopamine interaction is bidirectional.[238] It is possible that a state of leptin resistance[239] or hypothalamic leptin insufficiency[236] could explain why elevated serum leptin levels activate hedonic mechanisms and fail to promote homeostatic regulation in certain individuals.

Ghrelin has opposing effects with leptin, stimulating appetite by activating orexigenic neurons in the hypothalamus, playing a role in meal initiation.[240] Ghrelin has received attention related to reward mechanisms from alcohol,[76,241] intoxicating drugs,[242–244] and highly palatable food.[242,245] Conclusions suggest that ghrelin increases the incentive value of motivated behaviors (craving) via communication with various DA systems. Similar to leptin and ghrelin, insulin regulates DA neurotransmission calibrating reward processes that motivate consumption behavior.[246] Given that insulin is sensitive to food intake, and that the insulin receptor signaling pathway interferes with leptin signaling,[247] it is likely that high glycemic eating patterns can create a negative reinforcement pathology further perpetuating the cycle of compulsive or binge eating. Prevention of hyperinsulinemia can prevent insulin resistance[248] and therefore should be considered an important target for nutrition interventions, particularly when FA or SUD is present.

Utilizing several small feedings with balanced macronutrient distribution throughout the day (5–6 small meals/day) can be an effective approach toward preventing spikes and subsequent drops in insulin. Given that insulin can block leptin, this strategy may be effective in gradually normalizing leptin levels, although there is no data in the SUD population to support this claim. Similarly, stable insulin levels achieved through regular and consistent feeding patterns may prevent ghrelin from increasing to abnormal levels. Many patients in early recovery report skipping breakfast and postponing eating until they are sufficiently hungry, which makes sense considering the hormone-modulated reward response to food. Gradual increases in fiber intake throughout the recovery process can improve gut function, minimize undesirable insulin spikes, promote satiety, and essentially activate homeostatic mechanisms. Meanwhile, dysregulation of food intake attributed to the complex interplay between neurochemistry and endocrine function remains poorly understood and is yet to be adequately described in SUD populations.

CAFFEINE AND NICOTINE

Excessive intake of nicotine and caffeine have been described in AUD[249] and SUD[250] populations. The stimulant effects of caffeine and nicotine appear to be mediated by DA, explaining their mood-altering appeal in individuals with a history of SUD.[251] Both substances can interact with medications commonly prescribed for mental illness.[252] In one study of AUD inpatients, individuals with a history of alcohol dependence in a first-degree relative had a stronger desire to drink coffee and had a higher coffee consumption than patients without family history,[249] consistent with genetic links.[83] This study also found that a higher consumption of cigarettes was associated with an increased risk of relapse. In one SUD treatment center in Hawaii, caffeine use was associated with depression.[250] While it is conceivable that some depressed individuals may self-medicate with caffeine, no causal relationship has been established. In college students, energy drink consumption was associated with cocaine use, prescription stimulant abuse, and alcohol abuse.[253] The addition of caffeine use disorder to the DSM-5 is likely to promote much needed research on this subject.

In one study, smokers presented with lower levels of docosahexaenoic acid (DHA) compared to controls.[254] Reduced DHA concentrations identified in smokers may affect the dopaminergic system related to compulsion and the perpetuation of dependence, which is consistent with findings of reduced PUFA levels in cocaine addicts[95] and alcoholics.[96] A clinical trial of 3g omega-3 supplement (containing 389.52 mg DHA) brought about a reduction in nicotine dependence.[254] More research on the role of omega-3 in the treatment of addiction is warranted. There is also a shortage of data linking nicotine and gut microbiota. Recent evidence suggests that tobacco consumption impacts the oral microflora[255] and the upper GI tract microbiome[256] but the significance of these findings as well as interactions with dietary factors as well as other substances require further study.

Epidemiological data suggests that overweight and obese men are at decreased risk for both lifetime and past-year nicotine dependence,[27] suggesting an interaction between smoking and food intake. Evidence suggests that nicotine taps into the brain's core sensing and integration mechanisms, controlling both energy intake and energy expenditure.[257] In a population of male smokers, serum leptin concentrations were inversely correlated with nicotine dependence, despite no significant differences in caloric intake.[258] Other research has found that higher serum leptin concentrations among smokers trying to quit were associated with increased craving [259] consistent with craving data for alcohol.[74,260] Recent data found that a subset of adult e-cigarette users (13.5%) reported vaping for weight loss/control.[261] These users were more likely to be overweight, restrict calories, and have poor impulse control. Given what is known about the co-occurrence of ED and SUD, motivations for use of nicotine should be explored in addiction treatment settings. Reduction or cessation should be encouraged.

INTERVENTIONS

Positive associations between nutrition education services and SUD treatment outcomes have been reported within the Veterans Affairs healthcare system.[262] Residents of a SUD program in a United States prison receiving a series of nutrition workshops led to a significant improvement in nutrition practices (increased fiber intake).[263] An Italian study demonstrated that group nutrition education at a residential treatment facility for alcohol led to improved nutrition behaviors (eating more than 3 meals/day) and an 80% self-reported abstinence rate after 6 months.[264] A 6-week environmental and educational intervention (including cooking activities) to improve dietary intake at 6 residential drug treatment facilities for men in Upstate New York led to improved body composition, eating behavior, and overall satisfaction with the education.[265] These investigators documented statistically significant reductions in waist circumference[266] which is important given that men express weight concerns and distress

about efforts to lose weight during later recovery.[23] A 12-week curriculum including group education and take-home assignments targeting thin-ideal internalization, body dissatisfaction, and eating disorder symptoms in women led to improvements in weight-related concerns.[32] A hands-on nutrition and culinary interventions we conducted in a Los Angeles SUD treatment center demonstrates that significant improvements in overall self-efficacy related to food preparation skills and overall enjoyment of cooking can be achieved, despite logistical and monetary constraints.[267]

Exercise. Several small studies have demonstrated positive effects of exercise in the treatment of AUD[268,269] and SUD.[270,271] In a pilot study, a 12-week individually tailored moderate-intensity aerobic exercise intervention resulted in significant increases in percent days abstinent as well as decreases in drinks per drinking day at follow-up.[268] In addition to the well-known overall positive health effects, several authors have described benefits across psychological, behavioral/social, and neurobiological domains.[272,273] Other perceived benefits include more positive outlook and increased self-esteem,[269] as well as more energy and improved body image.[270] It should be considered that compulsive exercise[274] and/or addiction[275] may become a problem given its potential for use as a compensatory mechanism and associated progression into ED behaviors,[274,275] but this has not yet been adequately studied. Despite minimal evidence of exercise as an adjunctive behavioral treatment for SUDs, there is strong theoretical and practical support, particularly given the known link between exercise and nutrition behaviors. Clinical trials examining links between exercise and relapse are needed, as are studies examining the benefits of different types of exercise (e.g., cardio, weights, yoga, etc.) and interaction with other health behaviors (i.e., diet). Studies combining both exercise and nutrition interventions may prove useful.

DISCUSSION

While it is known that medications can influence nutritional status through interacting with absorption, metabolism, utilization, and excretion of nutrients, as well as impacting appetite,[276] less is known about how medications impact the microbiome, and relatively little is known about how illicit drugs impact nutritional status and gut health. The failure to adequately address and improve nutrition behavior among persons with SUD is a major shortcoming of the prevailing treatment model. Kaiser and colleagues believe that "better collaboration among treatment professionals is needed in order to serve the multifaceted needs of chemical dependent patients, and reduce prescriptive care contra-indicated in the condition of substance abuse."[277]

Ravenous food consumption may be due to "rebound appetite" in the wake of the hypothalamic suppression from drug use. Making healthful food choices after abstinence has been achieved may be very challenging. Sobriety is associated with new emotions, anxiety, and uncertainty. It is easy to seek a predictable and comforting response from food. This may lead to overeating, relapse, compromised quality of life, and the development of chronic disease. Weight gain during SUD recovery should be monitored and controlled (gradual rather than drastic) in order to counter the associated adaptations in nutrition-related hormones[33] and to mediate body image concerns. Most authors agree that craving for highly palatable food could be considered a form of dopamine-opioid-related addiction,[278] but there is no consensus on the extent to which we should intervene on eating habits during SUD recovery. Conventional wisdom from Alcoholics Anonymous literature (1939) suggests that sweets and chocolate should be used liberally in early abstinence,[279] and while there appears to be resistance against a paradigm shift, emerging evidence suggests individuals in recovery are increasingly interested in healthier eating.[30,267] Meanwhile, extreme dieting should be discouraged.

An understanding of how various substances impact GI health, hormones, and reward pathways is critical for a comprehensive picture of the role of nutrition in SUD recovery. Research on the potential modulation of leptin signaling cascades via nutrition therapy during SUD withdrawal and recovery is warranted. Hormonal improvements toward homeostasis may be achievable through gradual yet progressive changes in eating behavior that promote stable blood sugar, although there is limited data to support this approach, particularly given the inevitable presence of confounding variables over time.

Restoration of nutritional status in SUD recovery should look beyond correction of vitamin/mineral status and body weight and should account also for recovery of gut function and dysfunctional neurohormonal circuitry. Future research targeting the "gut-brain" axis in addiction by considering the vagus nerve, production of neurotransmitters serotonin and DA in the gut, and the hypothalamic-pituitary-adrenal (HPA) axis may lead to novel "psychobiotic" treatments designed to target the "ecology within."[280] A recent review article provides an overview of the link between gut and brain by summarizing findings related to the "crosstalk" between microbes and the central nervous system function, with specific focus on anxiety and depression.[281] A recent meta-analysis found that probiotics were associated with a significant reduction in depression.[282] We are in the beginning stages of understanding how bacteria and microbes in the human gut play a fundamental role in immune function, adaptive stress responding, and brain function. There are studies pointing to a meaningful influence of gut microbes on eating behavior,[283,284] as well as papers suggesting possible biological links to EDs.[281]

Unfortunately, to date relatively few studies examine the direct impact of diet on human gut health, likely due to known difficulties controlling variables in prospective nutrition research (reviewed elsewhere Ref. 285). Most authors suggest antibiotics (in some cases), probiotics, fermented foods, and encourage further exploration on the role of fecal transplants. The market is currently flooded with dietary supplements from functional medicine communities, most lacking empirical evidence. High-quality studies on alternative approaches to healing gut function are needed. Perhaps more importantly, we need to know more about how common ingredients in contemporary Western foods,[286] such as processed meats, added fats, refined grains, added sugars, artificial sweeteners, artificial colors/flavors, and emulsifiers/stabilizers, cause dysbiosis. We also need human studies to confirm that chronic low-fiber diets degrade the colonic mucus barrier enhancing pathogen susceptibility[287] and impair production of SCFAs by gut microbes.[288]

Before a successful nutrition intervention can occur, it is of paramount importance to heal gut function to promote optimal nutrient absorption throughout the GI tract. Reducing highly processed foods is a good start. With alcohol, increased swelling of the gut can cause decreased absorption of nutrients and increase exposure of toxins to the liver promoting systemic inflammation. With cocaine and MA, we have evidence of dysbiosis, altered oral health, and oxidative stress. With opioids, we see impaired GI function leading to inflammatory cascades and a compromised immune system. All intoxicating substances are associated with suboptimal eating patterns and nutrient deficiencies.

Currently, there is no requirement for nutrition education and counseling in SUD treatment. There have been proposed pilot projects intended to assess nutritional deficiencies associated with OUD and provide the necessary nutrients to return the person to a more stable state, and improve social functioning.[289] Well-designed studies are needed to substantiate the role of nutrition into the current paradigm for SUD treatment. Meanwhile, anecdotal reports suggest that most treatment centers allow unlimited or excessive amounts of highly palatable foods and seldom include nutrition education. Our research showed that in Los Angeles, less than one-third of treatment centers offered any nutrition services, and of those that do, less than a quarter utilize an RDN.[236a]

While food restriction can lead to relapse,[237] overindulgence can perpetuate the cycle of addictive behavior and contribute significantly to healthcare burden. The best strategy appears to lie somewhere in between these extremes, which will require clinical expertise in treatment settings. To accomplish this, exposure to highly palatable foods with addictive potential should be monitored and high-fiber foods should be encouraged. The focus should be on what to eat, instead of what not to eat. Nutritional interventions should never feel punitive, but rather a helpful component of the physiological healing process. The need for commitment to intervention protocols as well as ongoing supervision and consultation is warranted for successful program implementation in residential treatment facilities.

RDNs should be integrated members of the treatment team. Specific topics for group education in SUD treatment settings have been suggested elsewhere.[234] A summary of information currently needed can be found in Table 2.5.

Nutrition interventions during recovery may promote abstinence and prevent or minimize the onset of chronic illness, improving resource allocation. A review article from the UK on the role of healthy eating advice as part of drug treatment in prisons sums it: "substance-misuse is a major factor in recidivism and if this could be reduced through improvement of nutritional status, it could be a cost effective means of helping to tackle this problem."[290] Ersche and colleagues state: "the most substantial health burden arising from drug addiction lies not in the direct effect of intoxication but in the secondary effects on physical health."[93]

CONCLUSION

In summary, nutrition interventions have not yet been standardized or widely implemented as a treatment modality for SUDs. Given the evidence reviewed herein,

---

TABLE 2.5
Overall Where More Information is Needed

- Optimal rate to increase fiber intake for to improve fiber tolerance
- If antioxidant supplements such as turmeric/curcumin, coenzyme Q10, alpha lipoic acid, resveratrol, and flavonoid polyphenols are beneficial and optimal dosage
- If supplements for "leaky gut" used by functional medicine practitioners are effective and optimal dosage
- If supplements for "immune support" are effective and optimal dosage
- Which probiotic strains are best for AUD/SUD and optimal dosage
- If stool samples will soon be able to inform nutrition intervention strategies
- The role of magnesium in recovery from AUD/SUD
- How genetic testing can inform nutrition intervention strategies
- If high-dose amino acid therapies are effective and optimal dosage
- How to best treat co-occurring AUD/SUD and ED
- How to determine necessity for referring to ED treatment
- How to best treat co-occurring AUD/SUD and FA
- Best ways to address body image concerns in AUD/SUD treatment
- Best strategies to reduce nighttime eating in treatment settings
- How "mindful eating" can benefit individuals with AUD/SUD
- If long-term nutrition therapy with consistent eating patterns can impact hormones sufficient to normalize reward processing in the brain
- Long-term nutritional implications of medications, and how to best counsel patients on it
- Best topics for group education in treatment settings
- Best practices for implementation of cooking classes and other "life skills" workshops
- Best practices for implementation of nutrition guidelines in treatment settings
- How smoking/vaping impacts taste preferences and relationship to food
- Best strategies to encourage reduction/cessation of caffeine/nicotine
- Best strategies for incorporating exercise into treatment settings
- Best ways to collect data and publish findings

AUD, alcohol use disorder; *ED*, eating disorder; *FA*, food addiction; *SUD*, substance use disorder.

individual nutrition counseling, group education, and food service improvements are likely to improve treatment outcomes. Nutrition therapy should address the most serious medical and nutrition conditions first and then target the psychological and behavioral aspects of eating. Cooking classes and life skills development are important to the application of new nutrition knowledge. Emphasis should be placed on gastrointestinal health and reintroduction of foods high in fiber and antioxidants such as fruits, vegetables, whole grains, beans, nuts, and seeds. Adequate intake of protein and omega-3 essential fatty acids should be consumed daily. Regular meal patterns can help to stabilize blood sugar. Water should replace sweetened beverages. Caffeine and nicotine intake should be monitored. Dietary supplements can be very helpful in the recovery process, but should not supplant whole foods. Once nutrition behavior has improved, use of dietary supplements should be reevaluated. Laboratory tests and stool samples assessing gut function should provide valuable insights in upcoming years. In addition to expertise with the interaction between specific substances and nutritional status, RDNs working in treatment settings should specialize in gastrointestinal health, eating disorders, and should be keeping up to date with food addiction research. There is a timely need for specialized nutrition expertise in SUD treatment settings, including outpatient clinics and "sober living" environments. Public health campaigns and specialized training programs targeting primary care physicians, mental health professionals, and other SUD treatment professionals are warranted.

REFERENCES

1. Center for Behavioral Health Statistics and Quality. *Key Substance Use and Mental Health Indicators in the United States: Results from the 2015 National Survey on Drug Use and Health (HHS Publication No. SMA 16–4984, NSDUH Series H-51)*. 2016.
2. Verzar F. Nutrition as a factor against addiction. *Am J Clin Nutr*. 1955;3(5):363–374.
3. American Dietetic Association. Position of the American Dietetic Association: nutrition intervention in treatment and recovery from chemical dependency. *J Am Diet Assoc*. 1990;90(9):1274–1277.
4. Mohs ME, Watson RR, Leonard-Green T. Nutritional effects of marijuana, heroin, cocaine, and nicotine. *J Am Diet Assoc*. 1990;90(9):1261–1267.
5. Pelican S, et al. Nutrition services for alcohol/substance abuse clients. Indian Health Service's tribal survey provides insight. *J Am Diet Assoc*. 1994;94(8):835–836.
6. Wiss DA, Waterhous TS. *Nutrition therapy for eating disorders, substance use disorders, and addictions*. 2014:509–532.
7. Hammond CJ, Mayes LC, Potenza MN. Neurobiology of adolescent substance use and addictive behaviors: treatment implications. *Adolesc Med*. 2014;025:15–32.
8. Baptiste F. Drugs and diet among women street sex workers and injection drugs user in Quebec city. *Canadian J Urban Res*. 2009;18(2):78–95.
9. Saeland M, et al. High sugar consumption and poor nutrient intake among drug addicts in Oslo, Norway. *Br J Nutr*. 2011;105(4):618–624.
10. Noble C, McCombie L. Nutritional considerations in intravenous drug misusers: a review of the literature and current issues for dietitians. *J Hum Nutr Diet*. 1997;10:181–191.
11. Tang AM, et al. Malnutrition in a population of HIV-positive and HIV-negative drug users living in Chennai, South India. *Drug Alcohol Depend*. 2011;118(1):73–77.
12. Anema A, et al. Hunger and associated harms among injection drug users in an urban Canadian setting. *Subst Abuse Treat Prev Policy*. 2010;5(20).
13. Santolaria-Fernandez FJ, et al. Nutritional assessment of drug addicts. *Drug Alcohol Depend*. 1995;38(1):11–18.
14. Varela P, et al. Human immunodeficiency virus infection and nutritional status in female drug addicts undergoing detoxification: anthropometric and immunologic assessments. *Am J Clin Nutr*. 1997;191997(66):504S–508S.
15. Islam SKN, Hossain KJ, Ahsan M. Serum vitamin E, C and A status of the drug addicts undergoing detoxification: influence of drug habit, sexual practice and lifestyle factors. *Eur J Clin Nutr*. 2001;55:1022–1027.
16. Hossain KJ, et al. Serum antioxidant micromineral (Cu, Zn, Fe) status of drug dependent subjects: influence of illicit drugs and lifestyle. *Subst Abuse Treat Prev Policy*. 2007;2:12.
17. Ross LJ, et al. Prevalence of malnutrition and nutritional risk factors in patients undergoing alcohol and drug treatment. *Nutrition*. 2012;28(7–8):738–743.
18. Verweij KJ, et al. Genetic and environmental influences on cannabis use initiation and problematic use: a meta-analysis of twin studies. *Addiction*. 2010;105(3):417–430.
19. Mannan SJ, et al. Investigation of serum trace element, malondialdehyde and immune status in drug abuser patients undergoing detoxification. *Biol Trace Elem Res*. 2011;140(3):272–283.
20. Zhou JF, et al. Heroin abuse and nitric oxide, oxidation, peroxidation, lipoperoxidation. *Biomed Environ Sci*. 2000;13(2):131–139.
21. Budzynski J, et al. Oxidoreductive homeostasis in alcohol-dependent male patients and the risk of alcohol drinking relapse in a 6-month follow-up. *Alcohol*. 2016;50:57–64.
22. Hodgkins C, Frost-Pineda K, Gold MS. Weight gain during substance abuse treatment: the dual problem of addiction and overeating in an adolescent population. *J Addict Dis*. 2007;26(suppl 1):41–50.
23. Cowan JA, Devine CM. Food, eating, and weight concerns of men in recovery from substance addiction. *Appetite*. 2008;50(1):33–42.

24. Emerson M, et al. Unhealthy weight gain during treatment for alcohol and drug use in four residential programs for Latina and African American women. *Subst Use Misuse.* 2009;44(11):1553–1565.

25. Krahn D, et al. Sweet intake, sweet-liking, urges to eat, and weight change: relationship to alcohol dependence and abstinence. *Addict Behav.* 2006;31(4):622–631.

26. Petry NM, et al. Overweight and obesity are associated with psychiatric disorders: results from the national epidemiologic survey on alcohol and related conditions. *Psychosom Med.* 2008;70(3):288–297.

27. Barry D, Petry NM. Associations between body mass index and substance use disorders differ by gender: results from the national epidemiologic survey on alcohol and related conditions. *Addict Behav.* 2009;34(1):51–60.

28. Tang AM, et al. Heavy injection drug use is associated with lower percent body fat in a multi-ethnic cohort of HIV-positive and HIV-negative drug users from three U.S. cities. *Am J Drug Alcohol Abuse.* 2010;36(1):78–86.

29. Edge PJ, Gold MS. Drug withdrawal and hyperphagia: lessons from tobacco and other drugs. *Curr Pharm Des.* 2011;17(12):1173–1179.

30. Wall-Bassett ED, Robinson MA, Knight S. "Moving toward healthy": insights into food choices of mothers in residential recovery. *Glob Qual Nurs Res.* 2016;3: 2333393616680902.

31. Warren CS, et al. Weight-related concerns related to drug use for women in substance abuse treatment: prevalence and relationships with eating pathology. *J Subst Abuse Treat.* 2013;44(5):494–501.

32. Lindsay AR, et al. A gender-specific approach to improving substance abuse treatment for women: the healthy steps to freedom program. *J Subst Abuse Treat.* 2012;43(1):61–69.

33. Jeynes KD, Gibson EL. The importance of nutrition in aiding recovery from substance use disorders: a review. *Drug Alcohol Depend.* 2017;179:229–239.

34. Grucza RA, et al. The emerging link between alcoholism risk and obesity in the United States. *Arch Gen Psychiatry.* 2010;67(12):1301–1308.

35. Dumesnil C, et al. Alcohol consumption patterns and body weight. *Ann Nutr Metab.* 2013;62(2):91–97.

36. Di Gennaro C, et al. Sodium sensitivity of blood pressure in long-term detoxified alcoholics. *Hypertension.* 2000; 35(4):869–874.

37. Park B, Lee HR, Lee YJ. Alcoholic liver disease: focus on prodromal gut health. *J Dig Dis.* 2016;17(8):493–500.

38. Tsuruya A, et al. Major anaerobic bacteria responsible for the production of carcinogenic acetaldehyde from ethanol in the colon and rectum. *Alcohol Alcohol.* 2016; 51(4):395–401.

39. Khalsa J, et al. Omics for understanding the gut-liver-microbiome axis and precision medicine. *Clin Pharmacol Drug Dev.* 2017;6(2):176–185.

40. Betrapally NS, Gillevet PM, Bajaj JS. Changes in the intestinal microbiome and alcoholic and nonalcoholic liver diseases: causes or effects? *Gastroenterology.* 2016; 150(8):1745–1755.

41. Kakiyama G, et al. Colonic inflammation and secondary bile acids in alcoholic cirrhosis. *Am J Physiol Gastrointest Liver Physiol.* 2014;306(11):G929–G937.

42. Kirpich IA, et al. Alcoholic liver disease: update on the role of dietary fat. *Biomolecules.* 2016;6(1):1.

43. Kirpich IA, et al. Saturated and unsaturated dietary fats differentially modulate ethanol-induced changes in gut microbiome and metabolome in a mouse model of alcoholic liver disease. *Am J Pathol.* 2016;186(4): 765–776.

44. Massey VL, et al. Potential role of the gut/liver/lung axis in alcohol-induced tissue pathology. *Biomolecules.* 2015; 5(4):2477–2503.

45. Mutlu EA, et al. Colonic microbiome is altered in alcoholism. *Am J Physiol Gastrointest Liver Physiol.* 2012; 302(9):G966–G978.

46. Leclercq S, et al. Intestinal permeability, gut-bacterial dysbiosis, and behavioral markers of alcohol-dependence severity. *Proc Natl Acad Sci USA.* 2014;111(42): E4485–E4493.

47. Couch RD, et al. Alcohol induced alterations to the human fecal VOC metabolome. *PLoS One.* 2015;10(3): e0119362.

48. Xie G, et al. Chronic ethanol consumption alters mammalian gastrointestinal content metabolites. *J Proteome Res.* 2013;12(7):3297–3306.

49. Labrecque MT, et al. Impact of ethanol and saccharin on fecal microbiome in pregnant and non-pregnant mice. *J Pregnancy Child Health.* 2015;2(5).

50. Lowe PP, et al. Alcohol-related changes in the intestinal microbiome influence neutrophil infiltration, inflammation and steatosis in early alcoholic hepatitis in mice. *PLoS One.* 2017;12(3):e0174544.

51. Vassallo G, et al. Review article: alcohol and gut microbiota – the possible role of gut microbiota modulation in the treatment of alcoholic liver disease. *Aliment Pharmacol Ther.* 2015;41(10):917–927.

52. Dhanda AD, Collins PL. Immune dysfunction in acute alcoholic hepatitis. *World J Gastroenterol.* 2015;21(42): 11904–11913.

53. Chen P, Schnabl B. Host-microbiome interactions in alcoholic liver disease. *Gut Liver.* 2014;8(3):237–241.

54. Hartmann P, Seebauer CT, Schnabl B. Alcoholic liver disease: the gut microbiome and liver cross talk. *Alcohol Clin Exp Res.* 2015;39(5):763–775.

55. Shasthry SM, Sarin SK. New treatment options for alcoholic hepatitis. *World J Gastroenterol.* 2016;22(15): 3892–3906.

56. Sung H, et al. Microbiota-based treatments in alcoholic liver disease. *World J Gastroenterol.* 2016;22(29): 6673–6682.

57. Malaguarnera G, et al. Gut microbiota in alcoholic liver disease: pathogenetic role and therapeutic perspectives. *World J Gastroenterol.* 2014;20(44):16639–16648.

58. Leclercq S, et al. Role of intestinal permeability and inflammation in the biological and behavioral control of alcohol-dependent subjects. *Brain Behav Immun.* 2012;26(6):911–918.

59. Gorky J, Schwaber J. The role of the gut-brain axis in alcohol use disorders. *Prog Neuropsychopharmacol Biol Psychiatry*. 2016;65:234—241.

60. Bjorkhaug ST, et al. Chronic alcohol overconsumption may alter gut microbial metabolism: a retrospective study of 719 13C-D-xylose breath test results. *Microb Ecol Health Dis*. 2017;28(1):1301725.

61. Lieber CS. Alcohol: its metabolism and interaction with nutrients. *Annu Rev Nutr*. 2000;20:395—430.

62. Santolaria F, et al. Nutritional assessment in alcoholic patients. Its relationship with alcoholic intake, feeding habits, organic complications and social problems. *Drug Alcohol Dependence*. 2000;59:295—304.

63. Martin PR, Singleton CK, Hiller-Sturmhofel S. The role of thiamine deficiency in alcoholic brain disease. *Alcohol Res Health*. 2003;27(2):134—142.

64. Dingwall KM, et al. Hypomagnesaemia and its potential impact on thiamine utilisation in patients with alcohol misuse at the Alice Springs Hospital. *Drug Alcohol Rev*. 2015;34(3):323—328.

65. Kopczynska E, et al. [The concentrations of homocysteine, folic acid and vitamin B12 in alcohol dependent male patients]. *Psychiatr Pol*. 2004;38(5):947—956.

66. Lieb M, et al. Effects of alcohol consumption on iron metabolism. *Am J Drug Alcohol Abuse*. 2011;37(1): 68—73.

67. Halsted CH, Medici V. Vitamin-dependent methionine metabolism and alcoholic liver disease. *Adv Nutr*. 2011; 2(5):421—427.

68. Halsted CH. B-Vitamin dependent methionine metabolism and alcoholic liver disease. *Clin Chem Lab Med*. 2013;51(3):457—465.

69. Clugston RD, Blaner WS. The adverse effects of alcohol on vitamin A metabolism. *Nutrients*. 2012;4(5): 356—371.

70. Quintero-Platt G, et al. Vitamin D, vascular calcification and mortality among alcoholics. *Alcohol Alcohol*. 2015; 50(1):18—23.

71. Gonzalez-Reimers E, et al. Vitamin D and nutritional status are related to bone fractures in alcoholics. *Alcohol Alcohol*. 2011;46(2):148—155.

72. Teixeira J, Mota T, Fernandes JC. Nutritional evaluation of alcoholic inpatients admitted for alcohol detoxification. *Alcohol Alcohol*. 2011;46(5):558—560.

73. Nicolas JM, et al. Increased circulating leptin levels in chronic alcoholism. *Alcohol Clin Exp Res*. 2001;25(1): 83—88.

74. Kraus T, et al. Leptin is associated with craving in females with alcoholism. *Addict Biol*. 2004;9(3—4):213—219.

75. de Timary P, et al. The loss of metabolic control on alcohol drinking in heavy drinking alcohol-dependent subjects. *PLoS One*. 2012;7(7):e38682.

76. Leggio L, et al. Ghrelin system in alcohol-dependent subjects: role of plasma ghrelin levels in alcohol drinking and craving. *Addict Biol*. 2012;17(2):452—464.

77. Kraus T, et al. Ghrelin levels are increased in alcoholism. *Alcohol Clin Exp Res*. 2005;29(12):2154—2157.

78. Umhau JC, et al. Long-term abstinent alcoholics have a blunted blood glucose response to 2-deoxy-D-glucose. *Alcohol Alcohol*. 2002;37(6):586—590.

79. D., M, et al. Carbohydrate craving by alcohol-dependent men during sobriety: relationship to nutrition and serotonergic function. *Alcohol Clin Exp Res*. 2000;24(5): 635—643.

80. Kampov-Polevoy A, Garbutt JC, Janowsky D. Evidence of preference for a high-concentration sucrose solution in alcoholic men. *Am J Psychiatry*. 1997;154(2):269—270.

81. Fortuna JL. Sweet preference, sugar addiction and the familial history of alcohol dependence: shared neural pathways and genes. *J Psychoact Drugs*. 2011;42(2): 147—151.

82. Kenna GA, et al. The relationship of appetitive, reproductive and posterior pituitary hormones to alcoholism and craving in humans. *Neuropsychol Rev*. 2012;22(3): 211—228.

83. Munn-Chernoff MA, et al. A twin study of alcohol dependence, binge eating, and compensatory behaviors. *J Stud Alcohol Drugs*. 2013;74(5):664—673.

84. Munn-Chernoff MA, Baker JH. A primer on the genetics of comorbid eating disorders and substance use disorders. *Eur Eat Disord Rev*. 2016;24(2):91—100.

85. Mennella JA, et al. Sweet preferences and analgesia during childhood: effects of family history of alcoholism and depression. *Addiction*. 2010;105(4):666—675.

86. Fialla AD, et al. Nutritional therapy in cirrhosis or alcoholic hepatitis: a systematic review and meta-analysis. *Liver Int*. 2015;35(9):2072—2078.

87. Rishi P, et al. Better management of alcohol liver disease using a "microstructured synbox" system comprising L. plantarum and EGCG. *PLoS One*. 2017;12(1):e0168459.

88. Han SH, et al. Effects of probiotics (cultured *Lactobacillus subtilis/Streptococcus faecium*) in the treatment of alcoholic hepatitis: randomized-controlled multicenter study. *Eur J Gastroenterol Hepatol*. 2015;27(11):1300—1306.

89. Zhang X, et al. Flaxseed oil ameliorates alcoholic liver disease via anti-inflammation and modulating gut microbiota in mice. *Lipids Health Dis*. 2017;16(1):44.

90. Carito V, et al. Olive polyphenol effects in a mouse model of chronic ethanol addiction. *Nutrition*. 2017;33: 65—69.

91. McCarty MF. Nutraceutical strategies for ameliorating the toxic effects of alcohol. *Med Hypotheses*. 2013;80(4): 456—462.

92. Janowsky DS, Pucilowski O, Buyinza M. Preference for higher sucrose concentrations in cocaine abusing-dependent patients. *J Psychiatr Res*. 2003;37(1):35—41.

93. Ersche KD, et al. The skinny on cocaine: insights into eating behavior and body weight in cocaine-dependent men. *Appetite*. 2013;71:75—80.

94. Sukop PH, et al. Wernicke's encephalopathy in crack-cocaine addiction. *Med Hypotheses*. 2016;89:68—71.

95. Buydens-Branchey L, et al. Polyunsaturated fatty acid status and relapse vulnerability in cocaine addicts. *Psychiatry Res*. 2003;120(1):29—35.

96. Hibbeln JR, et al. Essential fatty acids predict metabolites of serotonin and dopamine in cerebrospinal fluid among healthy control subjects, and early- and late-onset alcoholics. *Biol Psychiatry*. 1998;44(4):235−242.

97. Buydens-Branchey L, Branchey M. n-3 polyunsaturated fatty acids decrease anxiety feelings in a population of substance abusers. *J Clin Psychopharmacol*. 2006;26(6):661−665.

98. Billing L, Ersche KD. Cocaine's appetite for fat and the consequences on body weight. *Am J Drug Alcohol Abuse*. 2015;41(2):115−118.

99. Akkina SK, et al. Illicit drug use, hypertension, and chronic kidney disease in the US adult population. *Transl Res*. 2012;160(6):391−398.

100. Volpe GE, et al. Associations of cocaine use and HIV infection with the intestinal microbiota, microbial translocation, and inflammation. *J Stud Alcohol Drugs*. 2014;75(2):347−357.

101. Kiraly DD, et al. Alterations of the host microbiome affect behavioral responses to cocaine. *Sci Rep*. 2016;6:35455.

102. Harrod SB, et al. The microbiota-gut-brain axis as a potential therapeutic approach for HIV-1+ cocaine abuse. *Drug & Alcohol Dependence*. 2015;156:e90−e91.

103. LaRowe SD, et al. Is cocaine desire reduced by N-Acetylcysteine? *Am J Psychiatry*. 2007;164(1115−1117).

104. Uys JD, Mulholland PJ, Townsend DM. Glutathione and redox signaling in substance abuse. *Biomed Pharmacother*. 2014;68(6):799−807.

105. McClure EA, et al. Potential role of N-acetylcysteine in the management of substance use disorders. *CNS Drugs*. 2014;28(2):95−106.

106. Lv D, et al. The body mass index, blood pressure, and fasting blood glucose in patients with methamphetamine dependence. *Med Baltim*. 2016;95(12):e3152.

107. Kobeissy FH, et al. Changes in leptin, ghrelin, growth hormone and neuropeptide-Y after an acute model of MDMA and methamphetamine exposure in rats. *Addict Biol*. 2008;13(1):15−25.

108. Goncalves J, et al. Effects of drugs of abuse on the central neuropeptide Y system. *Addict Biol*. 2016;21(4):755−765.

109. Neale A, Abraham S, Russell J. "Ice" use and eating disorders: a report of three cases. *Int J Eat Disord*. 2009;42(2):188−191.

110. Glasner-Edwards S, et al. Bulimia nervosa among methamphetamine dependent adults: association with outcomes three years after treatment. *Eat Disord*. 2011;19(3):259−269.

111. Orsini CA, et al. Food consumption and weight gain after cessation of chronic amphetamine administration. *Appetite*. 2014;78:76−80.

112. McIlwraith F, et al. Is low BMI associated with specific drug use among injecting drug users? *Subst Use Misuse*. 2014;49(4):374−382.

113. Laslett AM, Dietze P, Dwyer R. The oral health of street-recruited injecting drug users: prevalence and correlates of problems. *Addiction*. 2008;103(11):1821−1825.

114. Hamamoto DT, Rhodus NL. Methamphetamine abuse and dentistry. *Oral Dis*. 2009;15(1):27−37.

115. Shetty V, et al. The relationship between methamphetamine use and increased dental disease. *JADA*. 2010;141(3):307−318.

116. Riemer L, Holmes R. Under the influence: informing oral health care providers about substance abuse. *J Evid Based Dent Pract*. 2014;14:127−135.

117. Cury PR, et al. Dental health status in crack/cocaine-addicted men: a cross-sectional study. *Environ Sci Pollut Res*. 2017;24(8):7585−7590.

118. Sun L, et al. Systems-scale analysis reveals pathways involved in cellular response to methamphetamine. *PLoS One*. 2011;6(4):e18215.

119. Imam SZ, Ali SF. Selenium, an antioxidant, attenuates methamphetamine-induced dopaminergic toxicity and peroxynitrite generation. *Brain Res*. 2000;855(1):186−191.

120. Klongpanichapak S, et al. Attenuation of cocaine and methamphetamine neurotoxicity by coenzyme Q10. *Neurochem Res*. 2006;31(3):303−311.

121. Bennet BL, Ma J, Roy S. Effect of methamphetamine on the gut epithelial barrier function. In: *Showcase of Undergraduate Research and Creative Endeavors*. Winthrop University; 2016.

122. Ning T, et al. Gut microbiota analysis in rats with methamphetamine-induced conditioned place preference. *bioRxiv*. 2017. https://www.ncbi.nlm.nih.gov/pmc/articles/PMC5575146/.

123. Birnbaum H, et al. Societal costs of opioid abuse, dependence, and misuse in the United States: PMH38. *Value Health*. 2010;13(3):A111.

124. U.S. Department of Health and Human Services Centers for Disease Control and Prevention. Increases in heroin overdose deaths − 28 states, 2010 to 2012. *Morb Mortal Wkly Rep*. 2014;63(29):849−854.

125. Fenn JM, Laurent JS, Sigmon SC. Increases in body mass index following initiation of methadone treatment. *J Subst Abuse Treat*. 2015;51:59−63.

126. Housova J, et al. Adipocyte-derived hormones in heroin addicts: the influence of methadone maintenance treatment. *Physiol Res*. 2005;54(1):73−78.

127. Peles E, et al. Risk factors for weight gain during methadone maintenance treatment. *Subst Abus*. 2016;37(4):613−618.

128. Dursteler-MacFarland KM, et al. Patients on injectable diacetylmorphine maintenance have low bone mass. *Drug Alcohol Rev*. 2011;30(6):577−582.

129. Chen D, et al. Neurotransmitter-precursor-supplement intervention for detoxified heroin addicts. *J Huazhong Univ Sci Technol Med Sci*. 2012;32(3):422−427.

130. Nimmo WS, et al. Inhibition of gastric emptying and drug absorption by narcotic analgesics. *Br J Clin Pharmacol*. 1975;2(6):509−513.

131. Leppert W. Emerging therapies for patients with symptoms of opioid-induced bowel dysfunction. *Drug Des Devel Ther*. 2015;9:2215−2231.

132. Mora AL, et al. Moderate to high use of opioid analgesics are associated with an increased risk of *Clostridium difficile* infection. *Am J Med Sci.* 2012;343(4):277–280.

133. Babrowski T, et al. *Pseudomonas aeruginosa* virulence expression is directly activated by morphine and is capable of causing lethal gut-derived sepsis in mice during chronic morphine administration. *Ann Surg.* 2012; 255(2):386–393.

134. Meng J, et al. Morphine induces bacterial translocation in mice by compromising intestinal barrier function in a TLR-dependent manner. *PLoS One.* 2013;8(1):e54040.

135. Wang F. *Temporal Modulation of Gut Microbiome and Metabolome by Morphine.* 2015.

136. Divsalar K, et al. Serum biochemical parameters following heroin withdrawal: an exploratory study. *Am J Addict.* 2014;23(1):48–52.

137. el-Nakah A, et al. A vitamin profile of heroin addiction. *Am J Public Health.* 1979;69(10):1058–1060.

138. Heathcote J, Taylor KB. Immunity and nutrition in heroin addicts. *Drug Alcohol Depend.* 1981;8(3):245–255.

139. Kouros D, et al. Opium and heroin alter biochemical parameters of human's serum. *Am J Drug Alcohol Abuse.* 2010;36(3):135–139.

140. Daini S, et al. Serum magnesium profile in heroin addicts: according to psychiatric comorbidity. *Magnesium Res.* 2006;19(3):162–166.

141. Ciubotariu D, Ghiciuc CM, Lupusoru CE. Zinc involvement in opioid addiction and analgesia—should zinc supplementation be recommended for opioid-treated persons? *Subst Abuse Treat Prev Policy.* 2015;10:29.

142. Diaz-Flores Estevez JF, et al. Application of linear discriminant analysis to the biochemical and haematological differentiation of opiate addicts from healthy subjects: a case-control study. *Eur J Clin Nutr.* 2004;58(3):449–455.

143. Lin S-H, et al. Association between cholesterol plasma levels and craving among heroin users. *J Addict Med.* 2012;6(4):287–291.

144. Ghaderi A, et al. Clinical trial of the effects of vitamin D supplementation on psychological symptoms and metabolic profiles in maintenance methadone treatment patients. *Prog Neuropsychopharmacol Biol Psychiatry.* 2017; 79(Pt B):84–89.

145. Nabipour S, Ayu Said M, Hussain Habil M. Burden and nutritional deficiencies in opiate addiction- systematic review article. *Iran J Public Health.* 2014;43(8): 1022–1032.

146. Morabia A, et al. Diet and opiate addiction: a quantitative assessment of the diet of non-institutionalized opiate addicts. *Br J Addict.* 1989;84:173–180.

147. Zador D, Lyons Wall PM, Webster I. High sugar intake in a group of women on methadone maintenance in South Western Sydney, Australia. *Addiction.* 1996;91(7): 1053–1061.

148. Alves D, et al. Housing and employment situation, body mass index and dietary habits of heroin addicts in methadone maintenance treatment. *Heroin Addict Relat Clin Probl.* 2011;13(1):11–14.

149. Neale J, et al. Eating patterns among heroin users: a qualitative study with implications for nutritional interventions. *Addiction.* 2012;107(3):635–641.

150. Drumm RD, et al. "I'm a health nut!" Street drug users' accounts of self-care strategies. *J Drug Issues.* 2005; 35(3):607–630.

151. Nolan LJ, Scagnelli LM. Preference for sweet foods and higher body mass index in patients being treated in long-term methadone maintenance. *Subst Use Misuse.* 2007;42(10):1555–1566.

152. McDonald E. *Hedonic Mechanisms for Weight Changes in Medication Assisted Treatment for Opioid Addiction.* 2017.

153. Canan F, et al. Eating disorders and food addiction in men with heroin use disorder: a controlled study. *Eat Weight Disord.* 2017. https://www.ncbi.nlm.nih.gov/pubmed/28434177.

154. Grilo CM, et al. Eating disorders in female inpatients with versus without substance use disorders. *Addict Behav.* 1995;20(2):255–260.

155. Gadalla T, Piran N. Eating disorders and substance abuse in Canadian men and women: a national study. *Eat Disord.* 2007;15(3):189–203.

156. Root TL, et al. Patterns of co-morbidity of eating disorders and substance use in Swedish females. *Psychol Med.* 2010;40(1):105–115.

157. Baker JH, et al. Eating disorder symptomatology and substance use disorders: prevalence and shared risk in a population based twin sample. *Int J Eat Disord.* 2010; 43(7):648–658.

158. Hadad NA, Knackstedt LA. Addicted to palatable foods: comparing the neurobiology of Bulimia Nervosa to that of drug addiction. *Psychopharmacol Berl.* 2014;231(9): 1897–1912.

159. Courbasson CM, Rizea C, Weiskopf N. Emotional eating among individuals with concurrent eating and substance use disorders. *Int J Ment Health Addict.* 2008;6(3): 378–388.

160. Hunt TK, Forbush KT. Is "drunkorexia" an eating disorder, substance use disorder, or both? *Eat Behav.* 2016; 22:40–45.

161. Fowler L, Ivezaj V, Saules KK. Problematic intake of high-sugar/low-fat and high glycemic index foods by bariatric patients is associated with development of post-surgical new onset substance use disorders. *Eat Behav.* 2014; 15(3):505–508.

162. King WC, et al. Prevalence of alcohol use disorders before and after bariatric surgery. *JAMA.* 2012;307(23): 2516–2525.

163. Reslan S, et al. Substance misuse following Roux-en-Y gastric bypass surgery. *Subst Use Misuse.* 2014;49(4): 405–417.

164. Wiedemann AA, Saules KK, Ivezaj V. Emergence of new onset substance use disorders among post-weight loss surgery patients. *Clin Obes.* 2013;3(6):194–201.

165. Ivezaj V, et al. Obesity and addiction: can a complication of surgery help us understand the connection? *Obes Rev.* 2017;18(7):765–775.

166. Buckholdt KE, et al. Emotion regulation difficulties and maladaptive behaviors: examination of deliberate self-harm, disordered eating, and substance misuse in two samples. *Cognitive Ther Res.* 2015;39:140−152.

167. Stewart SH, et al. Why do women with alcohol problems binge eat? Exploring connections between binge eating and heavy drinking in women receiving treatment for alcohol problems. *J Health Psychol.* 2006;11(3): 409−425.

168. Fischer S, Anderson KG, Smith GT. Coping with distress by eating or drinking: role of trait urgency and expectancies. *Psychol Addict Behav.* 2004;18(3):269−274.

169. Luce KH, Engler PA, Crowther JH. Eating disorders and alcohol use: group differences in consumption rates and drinking motives. *Eat Behav.* 2007;8:177−184.

170. Czarlinski JA, Aase DM, Jason LA. Eating disorders, normative eating self-efficacy and body image self-efficacy: women in recovery homes. *Eur Eat Disord Rev.* 2012;20(3):190−195.

171. Beitscher-Campbell H, et al. Pilot clinical observations between food and drug seeking derived from fifty cases attending an eating disorder clinic. *J Behav Addict.* 2016; 5(3):533−541.

172. Bulik CM, Slof M, Sullivan P. Comorbidity of eating disorders and substance-related disorders. *Med Psychiatry.* 2004;27:317−348.

173. Bonfa F, et al. Treatment dropout in drug-addicted women: are eating disorders implicated? *Eat Weight Disord.* 2008;13(2):81−86.

174. Calero-Elvira A, et al. Meta-analysis on drugs in people with eating disorders. *Eur Eat Disord Rev.* 2009;17(4): 243−259.

175. Lundgren JD, et al. Prevalence of the night eating syndrome in a psychiatric population. *Am J Psychiatry.* 2006;163(1):156−158.

176. Saracli O, et al. The prevalence and clinical features of the night eating syndrome in psychiatric out-patient population. *Compr Psychiatry.* 2015;57:79−84.

177. Kilwein TM, et al. Nonmedical prescription stimulant use for suppressing appetite and controlling body weight is uniquely associated with more severe eating disorder symptomatology. *Int J Eat Disord.* 2016;49(8):813−816.

178. Dennis AB, Pryor T, Brewerton TD. *Integrated treatment principles and strategies for patients with eating disorders, substance use disorder, and addictions.* 2014:461−489.

179. Ho V, Arbour S, Hambley JM. Eating disorders and addiction: comparing eating disorder treatment outcomes among clients with and without comorbid substance use disorder. *J Addict Nurs.* 2011;22(3):130−137.

180. Root TL, et al. Substance use disorders in women with anorexia nervosa. *Int J Eat Disord.* 2010;43(1):14−21.

181. Cohen LR, et al. Survey of eating disorder symptoms among women in treatment for substance abuse. *Am J Addict.* 2010;19(3):245−251.

182. Brewerton TD. Posttraumatic stress disorder and disordered eating: food addiction as self-medication. *J Womens Health (Larchmt).* 2011;20(8):1133−1134.

183. Muller A, et al. Risk for exercise dependence, eating disorders pathology, alcohol use disorder and addictive behaviors among clients of fitness centers. *J Behav Addict.* 2015;4(4):273−280.

184. Specter SE, Wiss DA. Muscle dysmorphia: where body image obsession, compulsive exercise, disordered eating, and substance abuse intersect in susceptible males. In: *Eating Disorders, Addictions and Substance Use Disorders.* 2014:439−457.

185. Eichen DM, et al. Weight perception, substance use, and disordered eating behaviors: comparing normal weight and overweight high-school students. *J Youth Adolesc.* 2012;41(1):1−13.

186. Vidot DC, et al. Relationship between current substance use and unhealthy weight loss practices among adolescents. *Matern Child Health J.* 2016;20(4):870−877.

187. Baker JH, Mazzeo SE, Kendler KS. Association between broadly defined bulimia nervosa and drug use disorders: common genetic and environmental influences. *Int J Eat Disord.* 2007;40:673−678.

188. Slane JD, Burt SA, Klump KL. Bulimic behaviors and alcohol use: shared genetic influences. *Behav Genet.* 2012;42(4):603−613.

189. Bruce KR, et al. Effects of acute alcohol intoxication on eating-related urges among women with bulimia nervosa. *Int J Eat Disord.* 2011;44:333−339.

190. Wiss DA, Brewerton TD. Incorporating food addiction into disordered eating: the disordered eating food addiction nutrition guide (DEFANG). *Eat Weight Disord.* 2017; 22(1):49−59.

191. Vanbuskirk KA, Potenza MN. The treatment of obesity and its Co-occurrence with substance use disorders. *J Addict Med.* 2010;4(1):1−10.

192. Schreiber LRN, Odlaug BL, Grant JE. The overlap between binge eating disorder and substance use disorders: diagnosis and neurobiology. *J Behav Addict.* 2013;2(4): 191−198.

193. Becker DF, Grilo CM. Comorbidity of mood and substance use disorders in patients with binge-eating disorder: associations with personality disorder and eating disorder pathology. *J Psychosom Res.* 2015;79(2): 159−164.

194. Davis C, et al. Binge eating disorder (BED) in relation to addictive behaviors and personality risk factors. *Front Psychol.* 2017;8:579.

195. Puhl MD, et al. A history of bingeing on fat enhances cocaine seeking and taking. *Behav Neurosci.* 2011; 125(6):930−942.

196. Eichen DM, et al. Addiction vulnerability and binge eating in women: exploring reward sensitivity, affect regulation, impulsivity & weight/shape concerns. *Pers Individ Dif.* 2016;100:16−22.

197. Schulte EM, Grilo CM, Gearhardt AN. Shared and unique mechanisms underlying binge eating disorder and addictive disorders. *Clin Psychol Rev.* 2016;44:125−139.

198. Gold MS. From bedside to bench and back again: a 30-year saga. *Physiol Behav.* 2011;104(1):157−161.

199. Volkow ND, Wise RA. How can drug addiction help us understand obesity? *Nat Neurosci.* 2005;8(5):555–560.

200. Michaelides M, et al. PET imaging predicts future body weight and cocaine preference. *Neuroimage.* 2012;59(2):1508–1513.

201. Guo J, et al. Striatal dopamine D2-like receptor correlation patterns with human obesity and opportunistic eating behavior. *Mol Psychiatry.* 2014;19(10):1078–1084.

202. Michaelides M, et al. Translational neuroimaging in drug addiction and obesity. *ILAR J.* 2012;53(1):59–68.

203. Nair SG, et al. The neuropharmacology of relapse to food seeking: methodology, main findings, and comparison with relapse to drug seeking. *Prog Neurobiol.* 2009;89(1):18–45.

204. Wilson GT. Eating disorders, obesity and addiction. *Eur Eat Disord Rev.* 2010;18(5):341–351.

205. Hebebrand J, et al. "Eating addiction", rather than "food addiction", better captures addictive-like eating behavior. *Neurosci Biobehav Rev.* 2014;47:295–306.

206. Gearhardt AN, Corbin WR, Brownell KD. Preliminary validation of the Yale food addiction scale. *Appetite.* 2009;52(2):430–436.

207. Gearhardt AN, Corbin WR, Brownell KD. Development of the Yale food addiction scale version 2.0. *Psychol Addict Behav.* 2016;30(1):113–121.

208. Chao AM, et al. Prevalence and psychosocial correlates of food addiction in persons with obesity seeking weight reduction. *Compr Psychiatry.* 2017;73:97–104.

209. Muele A, Hermann T, Kubler A. Food addiction in overweight and obese adolescents seeking weight-loss treatment. *Eur Eat Disord Rev.* 2015;23:193–198.

210. Burrows T, et al. Food addiction in children: associations with obesity, parental food addiction and feeding practices. *Eat Behav.* 2017;26:114–120.

211. Meule A, von Rezori V, Blechert J. Food addiction and bulimia nervosa. *Eur Eat Disord Rev.* 2014;22(5):331–337.

212. Mies GW, et al. The prevalence of food addiction in a large sample of adolescents and its association with addictive substances. *Appetite.* 2017;118:97–105.

213. Cabeza de Vaca S, Carr KD. Food restriction enhances the central rewarding effect of abused drugs. *J Neurosci.* 1998;18(18):7502–7510.

214. D'Cunha TM, et al. The effects of chronic food restriction on cue-induced heroin seeking in abstinent male rats. *Psychopharmacol Berl.* 2013;225(1):241–250.

215. Avena NM, Murray S, Gold MS. Comparing the effects of food restriction and overeating on brain reward systems. *Exp Gerontol.* 2013;48(10):1062–1067.

216. Brunault P, et al. Why do liver transplant patients so often become obese? The addiction transfer hypothesis. *Med Hypotheses.* 2015;85(1):68–75.

217. Blum K, et al. The D2 dopamine receptor gene as a determinant of reward deficiency syndrome. *J R Soc Med.* 1996;89:396–400.

218. Blum K, et al. Dopamine genetics and function in food and substance abuse. *J Genet Syndr Gene Ther.* 2013;4(121).

219. Blum K, et al. The benefits of customized DNA directed nutrition to balance the brain reward circuitry and reduce addictive behaviors. *Precis Med (Bangalore).* 2016;1(1):18–33.

220. Blum K, et al. Neurogenetic impairments of brain reward circuitry links to reward deficiency syndrome (RDS): potential nutrigenomic induced dopaminergic activation. *J Genet Syndr Gene Ther.* 2012;3(4).

221. Blum K, et al. Neurogenomics and Nutrigenomics of neuro-nutrient therapy for reward deficiency syndrome (RDS): clinical ramifications as a function of molecular neurobiological mechanisms. *J Addict Res Ther.* 2012;3(5):139.

222. Chen TJH, et al. Gene narcotic attenuation program attenuates substance use disorder, a clinical subtype of reward deficiency syndrome. *Adv Ther.* 2007;24(2):402–414.

223. Blum K, et al. Pro-dopamine regulator - (KB220) to balance brain reward circuitry in reward deficiency syndrome. *J Reward Defic Syndrome Addict Sci.* 2017;3(1):3–13.

224. Berridge KC, Robinson TE, Aldridge JW. Dissecting components of reward: 'liking', 'wanting', and learning. *Curr Opin Pharmacol.* 2009;9(1):65–73.

225. Potenza MN, Grilo CM. How relevant is food craving to obesity and its treatment? *Front Psychiatry.* 2014;5:164.

226. Polk SE, et al. Wanting and liking: separable components in problematic eating behavior? *Appetite.* 2016;115:45–53.

227. Garcia-Garcia I, et al. Reward processing in obesity, substance addiction and non-substance addiction. *Obes Rev.* 2014;15(11):853–869.

228. Goldstein RZ, Volkow ND. Dysfunction of the prefrontal cortex in addiction: neuroimaging findings and clinical implications. *Nat Rev Neurosci.* 2011;12(11):652–669.

229. Stojek MK, Fischer S, MacKillop J. Stress, cues, and eating behavior. Using drug addiction paradigms to understand motivation for food. *Appetite.* 2015;92:252–260.

230. Schulte EM, Avena NM, Gearhardt AN. Which foods may be addictive? The roles of processing, fat content, and glycemic load. *PLoS One.* 2015;10(2):e0117959.

231. Dawe S, Loxton NJ. The role of impulsivity in the development of substance use and eating disorders. *Neurosci Behav Rev.* 2004;28:343–351.

232. Kawamura Y, et al. Variation in the *DRD2* gene affects impulsivity in intertemporal choice. *Open J Psychiatry.* 2013;03(01):26–31.

233. Mole TB, et al. Impulsivity in disorders of food and drug misuse. *Psychol Med.* 2014;45(4):771–782.

234. Wiss DA, Schellenberger M, Prelip ML. Registered dietitian nutritionists in substance use disorder treatment centers. *J Acad Nutr Diet.* 2017. https://www.ncbi.nlm.nih.gov/pubmed/29102421.

235. Heber D, Carpenter CL. Addictive genes and the relationship to obesity and inflammation. *Mol Neurobiol.* 2011; 44(2):160–165.

236. Amitani M, et al. The role of leptin in the control of insulin-glucose axis. *Front Neurosci.* 2013;7:51.

236a. Wiss DA, Schellenberger M, Prelip ML. Rapid assessment of nutrition services in Los Angeles substance use disorder treatment centers. *J Community Health.* 2018. https://doi.org/10.1007/s10900-018-0557-2.

237. Shalev U, Yap J, Shaham Y. Leptin attenuates acute food deprivation-induced relapse to heroin seeking. *J Neurosci.* 2001;21(4):RC129.

238. Leininger GM. Lateral thinking about leptin: a review of leptin action via the lateral hypothalamus. *Physiol Behav.* 2011;104(4):572–581.

239. Pandit R, et al. Dietary factors affect food reward and motivation to eat. *Obes Facts.* 2012;5(2):221–242.

240. Shan X, Yeo GS. Central leptin and ghrelin signalling: comparing and contrasting their mechanisms of action in the brain. *Rev Endocr Metab Disord.* 2011;12(3): 197–209.

241. Jerlhag E, et al. Requirement of central ghrelin signaling for alcohol reward. *Proc Natl Acad Sci USA.* 2009; 106(27):11318–11323.

242. Dickson SL, et al. The role of the central ghrelin system in reward from food and chemical drugs. *Mol Cell Endocrinol.* 2011;340(1):80–87.

243. Vengeliene V. The role of ghrelin in drug and natural reward. *Addict Biol.* 2013;18(5):897–900.

244. Maric T, et al. A limited role for ghrelin in heroin self-administration and food deprivation-induced reinstatement of heroin seeking in rats. *Addict Biol.* 2012;17(3): 613–622.

245. Skibicka KP, Dickson SL. Ghrelin and food reward: the story of potential underlying substrates. *Peptides.* 2011; 32(11):2265–2273.

246. Daws LC, et al. Insulin signaling and addiction. *Neuropharmacology.* 2011;61(7):1123–1128.

247. Kellerer M, et al. Insulin inhibits leptin receptor signalling in HEK293 cells at the level of janus kinase-2: a potential mechanism for hyperinsulinaemia-associated leptin resistance. *Diabetolgia.* 2001;44(1125–1132).

248. Ye J. Mechanisms of insulin resistance in obesity. *Front Med.* 2013;7(1):14–24.

249. Junghanns K, et al. The consumption of cigarettes, coffee and sweets in detoxified alcoholics and its association with relapse and a family history of alcoholism. *Eur Psychiatry.* 2005;20(5–6):451–455.

250. Yudko E, McNiece SI. Relationship between coffee use and depression and anxiety in a population of adult polysubstance abusers. *J Addict Med.* 2014;8(6):438–442.

251. Garrett BE, Griffiths RR. Intravenous nicotine and caffeine: subjective and physiological effects in cocaine abusers. *J Pharmacol Exp Ther.* 2001;296:486–494.

252. Hilton T. Pharmacological issues in the management of people with mental illness and problems with alcohol and illicit drug misuse. *Crim Behav Ment Health.* 2007; 17(4):215–224.

253. Arria AM, et al. Trajectories of energy drink consumption and subsequent drug use during young adulthood. *Drug & Alcohol Dependence.* 2017. https://www.ncbi.nlm.nih.gov/pubmed/28797805.

254. Zaparoli JX, et al. Omega-3 levels and nicotine dependence: a cross-sectional study and clinical trial. *Eur Addict Res.* 2016;22(3):153–162.

255. Sheth CC, et al. Alcohol and tobacco consumption affect the oral carriage of Candida albicans and mutans streptococci. *Lett Appl Microbiol.* 2016;63(4):254–259.

256. Vogtmann E, et al. Association between tobacco use and the upper gastrointestinal microbiome among Chinese men. *Cancer Causes Control.* 2015;26(4):581–588.

257. Novak CM, Gavini CK. Smokeless weight loss. *Diabetes.* 2012;61(4):776–777.

258. Suhaimi MZ, et al. Leptin and calorie intake among different nicotine dependent groups. *Ann Saudi Med.* 2016;36(6):404–408.

259. Gomes Ada S, et al. Influence of the leptin and cortisol levels on craving and smoking cessation. *Psychiatry Res.* 2015;229(1–2):126–132.

260. Lenz B, et al. Association of V89L SRD5A2 polymorphism with craving and serum leptin levels in male alcohol addicts. *Psychopharmacol Berl.* 2012;224(3): 421–429.

261. Morean ME, Wedel AV. Vaping to lose weight: predictors of adult e-cigarette use for weight loss or control. *Addict Behav.* 2017;66:55–59.

262. Grant LP, Haughton B, Sachan DS. Nutrition education is positively associated with substance abuse treatment program outcomes. *J Am Diet Assoc.* 2004;104(4):604–610.

263. Curd P, Ohlmann K, Bush H. Effectiveness of a voluntary nutrition education workshop in a state prison. *J Correct Health Care.* 2013;19(2):144–150.

264. Barbadoro P, et al. The effects of educational intervention on nutritional behaviour in alcohol-dependent patients. *Alcohol Alcohol.* 2011;46(1):77–79.

265. Cowan JA, Devine CM. Process evaluation of an environmental and educational nutrition intervention in residential drug-treatment facilities. *Public Health Nutr.* 2012;15(7):1159–1167.

266. Cowan JA, Devine CM. Diet and body composition outcomes of an environmental and educational intervention among men in treatment for substance addiction. *J Nutr Education Behav.* 2013;45(2):154–158.

267. Moore K, et al. Hands-on nutrition and culinary intervention within a substance use disorder residential treatment facility. *J Acad Nutr Diet.* 2016;116(9):A20.

268. Brown RA, et al. Aerobic exercise for alcohol recovery: rationale, program description, and preliminary findings. *Behav Modif.* 2009;33(2):220–249.

269. Read JP, et al. Exercise attitudes and behaviors among persons in treatment for alcohol use disorders. *J Subst Abuse Treat.* 2001;21:199–206.

270. Roessler KK. Exercise treatment for drug abuse—a Danish pilot study. *Scand J Public Health*. 2010;38(6):664—669.

271. Brown RA, et al. A pilot study of aerobic exercise as an adjunctive treatment for drug dependence. *Ment Health Phys Act*. 2010;3(1):27—34.

272. Linke SE, Ussher M. Exercise-based treatments for substance use disorders: evidence, theory, and practicality. *Am J Drug Alcohol Abuse*. 2015;41(1):7—15.

273. Read JP, Brown RA. The role of physical exercise in alcoholism treatment and recovery. professional psychology: *Res Pract*. 2003;34(1):49—56.

274. Allegre B, et al. Definitions and measures of exercise dependence. *Addict Res Theor*. 2009;14(6):631—646.

275. Terry A, Szabo A, Griffiths M. The exercise addiction inventory: a new brief screening tool. *Addict Res Theor*. 2004;12(5):489—499.

276. White R. Drugs and nutrition: how side effects can influence nutritional intake. *Proc Nutr Soc*. 2010;69(4): 558—564.

277. Kaiser SK, Prendergast K, Ruter TJ. Nutritional links to substance abuse recovery. *J Addict Nurs*. 2008;19(3): 125—129.

278. Campbell H, et al. Common phenotype in patients with both food and substance dependence: case reports. *J Genet Syndr Gene Ther*. 2013;4(122):1—7.

279. *Alcoholics Anonymous World Services, Alcoholics Anonymous*. New York City: Alcoholics Anonymous World Services, Inc; 2001.

280. Skosnik PD, Cortes-Briones JA. Targeting the ecology within: the role of the gut-brain axis and human microbiota in drug addiction. *Med Hypotheses*. 2016;93:77—80.

281. Rieder R, et al. Microbes and mental health: a review. *Brain Behav Immun*. 2017. https://www.ncbi.nlm.nih.gov/pubmed/28131791.

282. Huang R, Wang K, Hu J. Effect of probiotics on depression: a systematic review and meta-analysis of randomized controlled trials. *Nutrients*. 2016;8(8).

283. Alcock J, Maley CC, Aktipis CA. Is eating behavior manipulated by the gastrointestinal microbiota? Evolutionary pressures and potential mechanisms. *Bioessays*. 2014; 36(10):940—949.

284. Wasielewski H, Alcock J, Aktipis A. Resource conflict and cooperation between human host and gut microbiota: implications for nutrition and health. *Ann NY Acad Sci*. 2016;1372(1):20—28.

285. Singh RK, et al. Influence of diet on the gut microbiome and implications for human health. *J Transl Med*. 2017; 15(1):73.

286. Rodriguez-Castano GP, et al. Advances in gut microbiome research, opening new strategies to cope with a western lifestyle. *Front Genet*. 2016;7:224.

287. Desai MS, et al. A dietary fiber-deprived gut microbiota degrades the colonic mucus barrier and enhances pathogen susceptibility. *Cell*. 2016;167(5):1339—1353.

288. Vonk RJ, Reckman G. Progress in the biology and analysis of short chain fatty acids. *J Physiol*. 2017;595(2): 419—420.

289. Cunningham PM. The use of sobriety nutritional therapy in the treatment of opioid addiction. *J Addict Res Ther*. 2016;7(3).

290. Sandwell H, Wheatley M. Healthy eating advice as part of drug treatment in prisons. *Prison Serv J*. 2009;182:15—26.

CHAPTER 3

E-Cigarettes

DARBY LOWE, BSC • ALEXANDRIA S. COLES, BA • TONY P. GEORGE, MD, FRCPC • KAROLINA KOZAK, MSC

INTRODUCTION

Background of Electronic Nicotine Delivery Systems

Invented in 2003 by Chinese pharmacist Hon Lik, electronic nicotine delivery systems (ENDS), also referred to as electronic cigarettes (e-cigarettes or ECIGS), constituted a 10 billion US dollar global market in 2015.[1] Most e-cigarette sales occur online, consisting of extensive advertisement and multiple platforms for social communities surrounding e-cigarettes, which further facilitates the putative expansion of e-cigarette use by both adult and adolescent cliental.[2–4] The market for e-cigarettes has rapidly grown with rates of expansion such as 132.5% over a 1 year span ending in 2013.[5]

Typically, e-cigarettes are comprised of a cartridge for the e-cigarette liquid (e-liquid), a heating element, and a battery. The e-liquid is a solution of humectants (either propylene glycol and/or glycerol), distilled water, nicotine, flavoring, and other optional additives.[6,7]

The mechanism by which the e-cigarette can allow for e-liquid inhalation involves the process of rapid heating and then cooling of the solution, producing an aerosol mist.[8] A battery-powered electric current runs through a coiled resistance system within an atomizer where the e-liquid is stored, which saturates and, consequentially, heats the e-liquid.[8,9] The liquid then vaporizes into an aerosol mist, a mixture of liquid droplets and gas, which is then inhaled or "vaped" by the user through a mouthpiece.[6,8,10] The activation of this process can be initiated by either an air sensor upon inhaling, mimicking a cigarette, or manually initiated by pressing a button.[3,11]

There is immense variation in terms of e-cigarette manufacturing and their use—there are roughly 460 brands and 8000 distinct e-liquid flavors, such as the popular menthol flavor as well as those resembling flavors of fruits, sweets and beverages.[5,7,8,11,12] E-liquid solutions not only differ in flavoring, but also can vary in terms of nicotine concentrations, pH levels and additional additives.[1,6] Nicotine concentration ranges from 0 to 24 mg/mL and to a maximum of 36 mg/mL; however, the typical concentration of nicotine-containing e-cigarettes has been averaged around 18 mg/mL[2,6,8,13]; this is notably much higher, in comparison with a domestic cigarette of which contains ~6–13 mg of nicotine (an average of 12 mg), depending on the brand and manufacturer.[14] Despite this, however, the actual nicotine concentration delivered to one's bloodstream after inhalation is overall lower in comparison with levels following tobacco cigarette use.[4]

Other points of variation exist due to the different e-cigarette models, the style of inhalation used as well as device manipulation by the user.[4] E-cigarettes are being used for purposes that extend beyond nicotine consumption, including flavor manipulation, smoke tricks, and the inhalation of other substances.[15] For example, substances, such as cannabis, vitamins, herbs and vodka, have been reportedly inhaled using e-cigarettes.[2,16,17] A trend in e-cigarette use is for cannabis consumption, a popular substance choice to vape, due to the decreased amounts of smoke and odor.[16] One risk that exists with consumption of cannabis via e-cigarettes is that tetrahydrocannabinol (THC) levels can exceed combustion-produced methods by 4- to 30-fold.[16] Furthermore, e-cigarettes are also being used for "dripping," which involves dripping a few drops of a choice substance directly onto the coil atomizer of the e-cigarette and inhaling what is immediately and directly vaporized from the high temperature, leading to better product delivery or experienced "throat hit."[10,15]

Overall, e-cigarettes generate a smokeless aerosol absent of carbon monoxide.[3] The aerosol's further constituents, however, depend directly on the e-liquid ingredients, the electrical processes (e.g., resistance and voltage), the temperature of heating, and the type of coil or wire used as a conductor.[8]

The Assessment and Treatment of Addiction. https://doi.org/10.1016/B978-0-323-54856-4.00003-1

E-cigarettes have potential risk factors associated with their use. Nonetheless, there have also been suggested benefits, especially among individuals with tobacco use disorder and the possibility of the device being used for smoking cessation and reduction.[18–20] Such benefits include that nicotine in an aerosol may be self-administered with fewer tobacco toxicants compared to tobacco smoke resulting in reduced health risk.[21] The most prominent barrier for e-cigarette regulation and consensus is the current limited experimental evidence as well as the predicted advanced and rapid evolution of the devices and their use, further contributing to variation.[8] There are also three different e-cigarette generations that consist of various device characteristics and manipulation abilities, which facilitates even more variation in the e-cigarette discussion.[18,22] Not only do these factors contribute to the difficulty in regulation, but they also contribute to the difficulty in generalizing the risks and benefits, the specific ingredients, and details of drug delivery.[7]

Reasons for Use of E-Cigarettes

In general, e-cigarettes are perceived to be a healthier, less harmful/toxic, and less addictive alternative to tobacco cigarettes.[2,3,23–31] Moreover, e-cigarettes are generally perceived to be a useful aid in smoking cessation or reduction.[2–4,25,27,32] One of the most common reasons for e-cigarette use is to address tobacco cravings and withdrawal in attempts of smoking reduction or cessation,[4,13,23,31,33–37] as use of e-cigarettes has been perceived as or even more efficacious in comparison with nicotine replacement therapies (NRTs).[12] Interestingly, adolescents do not use e-cigarettes primarily for smoking cessation, unlike the general adult population.[6] Flavoring is a major appeal for youth, as well as for adults, supporting the migration away from tobacco flavoring preferences.[1]

Other reasons for use of e-cigarettes include evading smoke-free policies and second-hand disturbances that are normally associated with the smoke from tobacco cigarettes.[4,13,23,33–35,37] Further reasons include curiosity, accessibility, social influence, manageable cost, and the preferred taste or smell.[2,4,34,37] Some individuals also report using e-cigarettes because of resemblances to the sensations surrounding oral inhalation and experience of nicotine delivery in comparison with smoking tobacco cigarettes.[8] Another major appeal for all e-cigarette users is the adjustability and reuse of the device. For example, replaceable coils and voltage variance can affect current flow and heating of the coil, promoting different throat hits or aerosol amounts, respectively.[1,6,18]

Among individuals who discontinue using e-cigarettes, initial use is more likely to be for experimentation rather than for a specific goal, such as smoking cessation. Other reasons for no longer using e-cigarettes involve the negative health perceptions, manual characteristics of the device, as well as the taste, vapor, look or feel, and cost of the device.[34,37]

E-Cigarette Prevalence Trends in the Global Population

There has been an increase in the prevalence of e-cigarette use throughout several countries including Canada, Australia, the United States (US), and the United Kingdom (UK)[23,24,27,31,32,34,35,38–52] (Table 3.1). From 2010 to 2013, there was a rise in 1.8%–13% of adults in the United States who reported having ever tried an e-cigarette[50] with similar results found within the United Kingdom and Australia.[35,40] However, only a small proportion of single-use or first-time users of e-cigarettes, however, progress to consistent use.[11,53] Nonetheless, there has been substantial increases in the rates of prevalence for e-cigarette use among adults in the US regardless of concurrent smoking levels, age, race, sex, or education.[50] This trend has been observed in other countries besides the United States, such as in Great Britain; however, less prominent growth trajectories have been observed within countries with more regulation, such as in Canada and Australia.[40,50]

There is significant concurrent substance use among e-cigarette users with substances including marijuana, alcohol and, specifically, tobacco products.[4,54–56] A high proportion of e-cigarette users, including high frequency users, consist of current and former tobacco smokers, while the minority of users are nonsmokers[4,24,28,30,32,35,37,42,57–61] (Table 3.1). In 2013, for example, over one-third of smokers in the US reported using e-cigarettes.[38] Current smokers are the most prevalent population to qualify as having ever used or as currently using e-cigarettes, compared to both nonsmokers and former smokers.[32,36,50] Specifically, current smokers, as well as former smokers who have quit within the past year, were most likely to be current e-cigarette users, in comparison with those who quit more than 1 year prior or who have never smoked.[36,51] Additionally, daily use is also more frequently reported by those who have recently quit in comparison with concurrent smokers.[62]

In terms of demography, e-cigarette use is prevalent within older adolescents and young adults, as well as male and Caucasian individuals.[2,3,28,32,35–37,45,48,57–59,63] Both awareness and use of e-cigarettes is prevalent

TABLE 3.1
Demographics of E-Cigarette Users and Prevalence Rates

Year	Canada %	Australia %[a]	US %	UK %
2010–13	2 (2013) [1]	0.6–6.6 (2010–13) [2]	0.3–6.8 (2010–13) [3]	7.2 (2012) [4] 9.6–39.9[a](2010–13) [2]
2014–16	3 (2015) [1]	–	3.7 (2014) [5]	11.6 (2014) [4] 5.6 (2016) [6]
AGE				
Adolescents	2.6 (16–19) [7]	–	2 [8]	5.8 [6]
Young Adults	7.0 (20–24) [7]	0.31 (18–24) [2]	5.1 [5]	5.8 (16–24) [6]
Adults	6.3 (25–30) [7]	0.51 (25–39) 0.53 (40–55) [2]	4.7% (25–44), 3.5%(45–64) [5]	6.9 (25–34) 7.1 (35–49) 6.5 (50–59) [6]
Elders	–	1 (55+) [2]	1.2 (65+) [5]	2.9 [6]
SMOKERS VERSUS NONSMOKERS				
Smokers	15 [7]	8.9 [2]	30.3 [3]	20.7 [2]
Nonsmokers	0.8 [7]	–	1.4 [3]	–

1, Canada, H. *Canadian Tobacco Alcohol and Drugs (CTADS): 2015 Summary*. 2015. Available from: https://www.canada.ca/en/health-canada/services/canadian-tobacco-alcohol-drugs-survey/2015-summary.html; 2, Yong H-H, et al. Trends in e-cigarette awareness, trial, and use under the different regulatory environments of Australia and the United Kingdom. *Nicotine Tob Res*, 2014;17(10):1203–1211; 3, McMillen RC, et al. Trends in electronic cigarette use among US adults: use is increasing in both smokers and nonsmokers. *Nicotine Tob Res*. 2014;17(10):1195–1202; 4, Filippidis FT, et al. Two-year trends and predictors of e-cigarette use in 27 European Union member states. *Tob Control*. 2017; 26(1):98–104; 5, Schoenborn CA, Gindi RM. Electronic cigarette use among adults: United States, 2014. 2015: US Department of Health and Human Services, Centers for Disease Control and Prevention, National Center for Health Statistics; 6, England PH. Adult smoking habits in the UK: 2016. Cigarette smoking among adults including the proportion of people who smoke, their demographic breakdowns, changes over time, and e-cigarettes. 2016. Available from: https://www.ons.gov.uk/peoplepopulationandcommunity/healthandsocialcare/healthandlifeexpectancies/bulletins/adultsmokinghabitsingreatbritain/2016; 7, Czoli CD, Hammond D, White CM. Electronic cigarettes in Canada: prevalence of use and perceptions among youth and young adults. *Can J Public Health*. 2014;105(2):e97–e102; 8, Dutra LM, Glantz SA. Electronic cigarettes and conventional cigarette use among US adolescents: a cross-sectional study. *JAMA Pediatr*. 2014;168(7):610–617.
[a] Statistics are among a smoking cohort (ex-smokers or current smokers in the population).

within populations of individuals with intermediate to high levels of education, who are employed or who have substantial socioeconomic status.[2,3,11,23,35,39,57,58,62,63] There have been, however, notable increases among those with lower levels of education.[50]

In the subpopulation of nonsmoking e-cigarette users, young adults predominate, with an average age range of 18–24.[18,51] Adolescents, especially among high school students, also highly populate this category.[1,28,59,64,65] Additionally, in both 2014 and 2015, e-cigarettes were the most used tobacco product by adolescents.[8,41] Adolescents may populate the frequent user group due to naturally higher impulsivity as well as peer pressure and technological interests that reside within the current adolescent generation.[65,66] E-cigarettes are also very accessible for purchase with minimal regulation, and online advertisements that are specifically aimed to capture youth interest have

increased by 356% from 2011 to 2013.[8,64–66] Additionally, positive perceptions on e-cigarettes with a lack of knowledge regarding nicotine addiction and the associated risks pose a threat to this population.[28,65–67] A major concern involves the potential of e-cigarette use in early adolescence being associated with a higher likelihood of transitioning to combustible tobacco cigarette use.[67–69] E-cigarettes are also commonly being manipulated by this population to vaporize cannabis.[16,17] Despite highly occupying the nonsmoker e-cigarette user group, there are still reportedly high levels of concurrent or former cigarette smoking in adolescents who use e-cigarettes.[52,70]

Individuals with mental disorders, as well as substance use disorders, depict another subpopulation of which have high prevalence rates of e-cigarette use, specifically with twice the prevalence of ever using e-cigarettes in comparison with those without mental health conditions.[8,71–74] Individuals with mental health concerns are more likely to both try and use e-cigarettes compared to the general population; however, there are similarities including the reasoning for use, such as smoking cessation or reduction aid, and the higher trends in prevalence rates among concurrent smokers.[71] E-cigarette consumption has also been shown to increase over time by users with mental illness despite the specific diagnosis, especially among individuals within the age range of 18–25,[75] which may relate to the higher successful smoking cessation and reduction attempts found among this subpopulation.[71,76]

Generations of E-Cigarettes

Despite consistent demographic trends among e-cigarette users, device brands and styles are diverse

and continue to grow.[7] Companies include Joye, Vapor4Life, Janty, Totally Wicked, and PureSmoker, as well as a large variety of e-liquids.[2] Further, a variety of e-cigarette models on the market include the 510, eGo, KR808, 901, and Tornado along with the ability to personalize and manipulate the devices to one's preference.[2,7] As such, e-cigarettes have been divided into "generations" to classify the different types, generally enhancing in size, complexity and modifiability as one moves from one generation to the next[1,18,77–81] (Table 3.2).

First-generation devices are activated through inhalation pressure, mechanistically resembling tobacco cigarettes in addition to their physical resemblance and are powered by disposable or replaceable lithium batteries

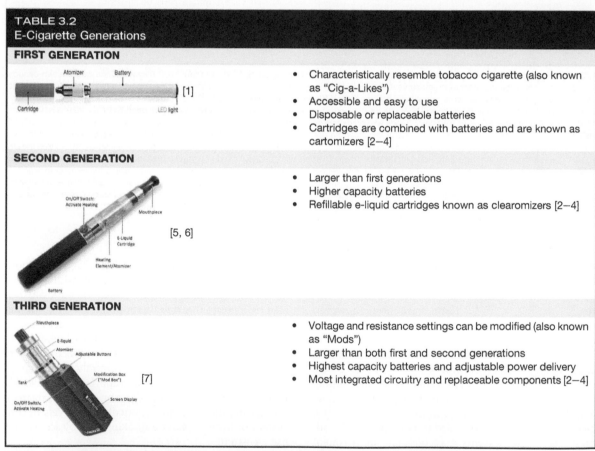

TABLE 3.2
E-Cigarette Generations

FIRST GENERATION

- Characteristically resemble tobacco cigarette (also known as "Cig-a-Likes")
- Accessible and easy to use
- Disposable or replaceable batteries
- Cartridges are combined with batteries and are known as cartomizers [2–4]

SECOND GENERATION

- Larger than first generations
- Higher capacity batteries
- Refillable e-liquid cartridges known as clearomizers [2–4]

THIRD GENERATION

- Voltage and resistance settings can be modified (also known as "Mods")
- Larger than both first and second generations
- Highest capacity batteries and adjustable power delivery
- Most integrated circuitry and replaceable components [2–4]

1, first_generation_ecig; 2, B, M. *The 4 Generations of Electronic Cigarettes*. 2015. Available from: http://ecigclopedia.com/the-4-generations-of-electronic-cigarettes/; 3, Dawkins L, et al. First-versus second-generation electronic cigarettes: predictors of choice and effects on urge to smoke and withdrawal symptoms. *Addiction*. 2015;110(4):669–677; 4, Farsalinos KE, Polosa R. Safety evaluation and risk assessment of electronic cigarettes as tobacco cigarette substitutes: a systematic review. *Ther Adv Drug Saf*. 2014;5(2):67–86; Administration, U.S.F. *Electronic Cigarette Fires and Explosions*. Available from: http://moon-vapes.com/what-is-vaping/first_generation_ecig/; 6, *How Long Do E-cigarettes Last?* Available from: https://www.quora.com/How-long-do-e-cigarettes-last; 7, *Boom In E-Cigarettes Sparks Calls For Regulation*.

via cartomizers, which are prefilled cartridges that surround an atomizer.[11,18,22] **Second-generation** devices, no longer specifically resembling tobacco cigarettes, contain higher-capacity lithium batteries and atomizers as well as refillable e-liquid cartridges, collectively known as clearomizers.[18,22] **Third-generation** devices are described by their modifiable voltage delivery and resistance settings by means of enhanced circuitry in the device as well as replaceable and personalized components.[18,22] The "advanced generation devices" (AGD), which include third-generation e-cigarettes, have higher-powered batteries and the user must press a button before inhalation, which further allows for manipulation via heating and timing of e-liquid vaporization.[11]

The smoking sensation that a user experiences, in part, largely depends on the model that is used. Some e-cigarettes are produced to mirror both behavioral and stimulatory sensations that reflect tobacco cigarette use.[3] For example, first-generation devices mimic tobacco cigarettes in their shape, size, method of inhalation as well as in occasionally having ends that glow either red or blue, stimulating the burning end of a tobacco cigarette.[3] Depending on the generation, however, alterations can be made to the type of e-liquid, the style of inhalation vapers use, and how the device vaporizes the liquid, which can all manipulate the overall smoking sensation and level of nicotine delivery.[1,8]

Furthermore, e-cigarettes are progressively becoming more personalized, as certain parts of the AGDs have been manufactured for the user to match one's preference.[6,7] E-cigarette users have the ability to rebuild atomizers and set desirable resistance and voltage in the electrical circuitry system.[18] Individuals can also manipulate the replaceable coils, which can affect the resistance or flow of the current and heat within the coil, as well as the voltage variance, in order to change the overall amount of aerosol produced, for example.[6,8] Engineering differences correlate with differences in the heating and conversion of nicotine-containing e-liquid, which also can alter the nicotine concentrations and chemical profile of the aerosol that is delivered to one's bloodstream.[12] More powerful, longer-lasting batteries as well as the act of preactivating a manual switch for inhalation are both associated with a more intense vapor or amount inhaled per "puff."[3,9] Because of this, the AGDs can support higher plasma concentrations of nicotine or a more satisfactory "hit"; however, there is a much slower absorption rate in comparison with what is facilitated by tobacco cigarettes.[4]

Due to better delivery, the AGDs have also been correlated with better craving reduction and overall satisfaction compared to first-generation devices as well as with use by regular users.[3,11] Through this user-device correlation and practice, more experienced vapers tend to be able to achieve the highest reported concentrations of nicotine delivery of which can compare or exceed combustible cigarette levels.[4,82] In a study using 18 mg/mL nicotine containing e-cigarettes, 35 min of vaping with AGDs was calculated to achieve the same nicotine plasma concentrations after smoking a tobacco cigarette for 5 min.[9] First-generation devices were associated with a longer time-frame for vaping of 65 minutes in order to reach the same nicotine plasma concentrations similar to those from 5 min of smoking.[9] Despite this, the most popular model is the first-generation, "cigalike" model, which is also the generation that is correlated to preference by individuals who are rare or first-time e-cigarette users.[3,11] Most individuals who continue to use e-cigarettes, however, progress to using AGDs or continue using an AGD if that was the initial generation used.[11]

Risks Associated With Use of E-Cigarettes

There are a number of risks that can be associated with e-cigarette possession and use; however, serious adverse events are not common.[20,53,83,84] The most common side effects subjectively reported from e-cigarette use include throat and mouth irritations as well as nausea, vomiting, dizziness, headaches and dry coughing[2,4,6,18,45,84,85] (Table 3.3). There is considerably less adverse physiological affect reported from e-cigarette use compared to tobacco cigarettes in terms of cardiovascular and respiratory functioning.[18] Some respiratory concerns may be presented, due to glycol and glycerin exposure, which include total periphery resistance, potential oxidative stress in lung epithelial cells, and inflammatory responses.[6,86] Furthermore, flavorings are usually aldehydes that at certain concentrations can also be irritants associating with respiratory disease[8] and influencing airway inflammation, infection susceptibility and overall cytotoxicity.[1,86]

Many of the negative consequences that ensue due to e-cigarette use manifests from improper use and experimentation.[4] For example, adverse consequences that can arise from "dripping" include exposures to high temperature and potential toxic chemicals, such as aldehydes, which can be increased to levels comparable, if not higher, to those from combustible cigarettes.[10,15] Further concerns exist in regard to an enhanced nicotine delivery with advanced e-cigarette generations and users, which, in turn, poses increased risk for nicotine dependence and addiction due to a more comparable delivery to that from smoking.[15]

TABLE 3.3
Summary of Side Effects Reported by E-Cigarette Users

Side Effects	Etter, J.F. & C. Bullen (2011) [N = 3587]	Farsalinos et al. (2013) [N = 111]	Dawkins et al. (2013) [N = 1347]	Bullen et al. (2010) [N = 40]	Caponnetto et al. (2013) [N = 14]	Caponnetto et al. (2013) Eclat [N = 300]	Polosa et al. (2011) [N = 34]	Polosa et al. (2014) [N = 27]
Throat/mouth irritations	22%	27%	0.5%	38%	14.4%	17%/22%	32.4%/20.6%	14.8%/7.4%
Nausea/vomiting	–	–	0.3%	29%	0%	–	14.7%	3.7%
Dizziness (includes vertigo, light headedness)	–	–	0.2%	21%	0%	–	14.7%	3.7%
Headaches	–	<5%	0.2%	18%	7.2%	17%	11.8%	3.7%
Dry coughing	–	13.5%	–	–	28.6%	26%	32.4%	11.1%
Stomach pain	–	7.2%	0.5%	–	–	–	–	–
Bloating/flatulence	–	–	0.7%	5%	–	–	–	–
Heartburn	–	–	0.4%	5%	–	–	–	–
Shortness of breath	–	–	–	–	–	20%	–	–

Other potential adverse consequences include nicotine exposure from accidental ingestion or topical overexposure, as well as electrical accidents and fires relating to overheating and batter explosions from defective or overcharged batteries,[6,8,18,53,87] which can physically lead to risk of burns, lacerations and smoke inhalation.[4] In the US, there has also been an exponential rise in exposures reported to Poison Centers starting in 2010. This has been specifically in children under 5 years of age and adults ranging from 20 to 39 years of age, consisting of reports of nausea and vomiting,[43,88] as well as headaches, eye pain, and conjunctivitis.[43] Certain trace levels of toxic compounds have been found in e-liquids as well as the aerosol counterpart. Most health concerns originate from aerosol components including glycols, carbonyl compounds (formaldehyde and acetaldehyde), volatile organic compounds, polycyclic aromatic hydrocarbon, tobacco-specific nitrosamines, metals, and silicate particles.[1,3,4,18,89,90] Toxicant production is overall much lower in e-cigarettes compared to cigarette smoke with 4000 chemicals in tobacco smoke, which are emitted via the combustion process, that are absent in e-cigarette vapor.[1,18] Metal, however, is found at more comparable levels in aerosol compared to smoke, which includes lead, formaldehyde, chromium, and nickel.[1,89] Other similar toxins that have been reported in e-liquids include tobacco-specific nitrosamines and tobacco impurities; however, these reports are at insignificant levels compared to those in cigarettes.[6,8,18,53,91] In terms of the different flavors associated with e-liquids, some are considered more cytotoxic than others, such as cinnamon, for example, but this is an under-researched area with further studies needing to be conducted.[4,91] In general, there are lower levels of tobacco-specific nitrosamines, volatile organic compounds, carbonyls and heavy metals as well as overall cytotoxicity in the aerosol produced by e-cigarettes in comparison with tobacco cigarettes.[91–93] The range of less toxic elements from e-cigarettes is between 9 and 450 times lower compared to cigarette smoke.[92] Overall, peer-reviewed analyses of e-cigarette toxicity is not well established in the literature and marketed brands lack robust evaluations of toxicology, as standard testing paradigms are not concretely available.[91]

Another major risk produced by the majority of e-cigarettes surrounds nicotine concentrations in e-liquids.[4] Nicotine overdose is uncommon due to low concentrations of nicotine in e-cigarettes, but is associated with other potential negative consequences.[18] Nicotine poses risks during pregnancy and childhood development and can be a threat due to its dependence liability, link with cardiovascular disease, and evidenced role in tumor promotion, despite not being classified as a carcinogen.[1] E-cigarette products have a much lower dependence liability in comparison with tobacco cigarettes.[94] In comparison with nicotine gum, e-cigarettes may have similar, if not lower, dependence liability, which is fairly insignificant.[94] Additionally, subjective reports by users who consume e-cigarettes for long periods of time depict reasons for use that are unrelated to dependence.[94] However, because nicotine delivery depends on the user, device, and amount "vaped," dependence liability and product experience varies depending on both the product and user.[4,6,53,95–97] The risk for dependence is overall lower for e-cigarette use compared to cigarette use, as cigarette smoking provides the most rapid form nicotine delivery; however, the device also allows for the most direct and efficient mode of administration via pulmonary absorption similar to cigarettes and AGDs are continually supporting more efficient nicotine delivery.[4,6,98] A seemingly large determinant of nicotine levels delivered to e-cigarette users involves experience in using e-cigarettes, as more experienced users have been documented in attaining higher nicotine levels compared to inexperienced users based on different intensities of use.[92,98] Concern has been raised for the nonconcurrent smoking population in terms of primary nicotine addiction that could potentially develop with e-cigarette use.[8,50,99] With concurrent smokers, there is also the risk of maintaining dependence to nicotine; however, there is a much lower overall concern for this population within the discussion of addiction.[18,50]

Long-term use of e-cigarettes, although inconclusively investigated, can be associated with variable risk of disease, such as cardiovascular disease, obstructive pulmonary disease, and lung cancer, all of which exist at much lower risk than for cigarette users, but are still notable.[1] Because consequences of long-term use are largely unknown, there is a lack of proper knowledge translation to users, which is a risk in itself for those planning to become an e-cigarette user.[3,53] Secondhand adverse health effects have also been suggested due to certain trace levels of metals, nicotine, and some volatile organic compounds; although these are generally insignificant compared to secondhand tobacco smoke, they require more research.[1,90,100,101]

Overall, it is difficult to make assured assessments on the risks with e-cigarette use, especially concerning toxicology of e-cigarettes, as the minimal reports that have been done are on specific brands, generations, and e-liquids, which cannot be generalized to overarching e-cigarettes.[91] Nonetheless, if e-cigarette products are regulated and used properly, the aerosol is much less toxic than cigarette smoke; however, this does not make the product or use of the device completely harmless or absent of any risk.[1,91,93,96,100,101] Thus, being aware of the mentioned risks is critical to ensure any associated safety and health issues are minimized.

Potential Benefits Associated With Use of E-Cigarettes

Harm reduction and smoking cessation evidence-based treatment for tobacco use disorder

E-cigarettes have been considered as potential smoking and reduction cessation interventions; however, e-cigarettes are not approved as smoking cessation devices by major health organizations, such as Health Canada or the Food and Drug Administration.[33] Tobacco harm reduction, with the goal to reduce the major negative consequences associated with smoking, has been a suggested mechanism through which e-cigarettes may aid individuals in smoking reduction and, potentially, smoking cessation.[18,19] There is an attraction to these devices for this application due to their greatly reduced toxicity levels and adverse health consequences in comparison with tobacco cigarettes as well as the psycho-behavioral and chemical (i.e., nicotine delivery) stimulation that resembles those of tobacco cigarettes.[1,9,18,22,85,96,102,103]

A main reason for use by the general adult population surrounds smoking cessation and the belief that e-cigarettes are helpful in the cessation process. Subjective survey analyses and population trend collections, although solely anecdotal, have described supportive evidence in the use of e-cigarettes aiding with smoking cessation, craving, and frequency[2,3,12,13,22,23,25,34,44,45,60] (Table 3.4). It is suggested that if regulated, manufactured and used properly, e-cigarettes could have the same efficacy as Nicotine Replacement Therapies (NRTs), as they have been shown to have similar, if not better, nicotine delivery rates.[9,104] Population surveys have depicted support for this use of e-cigarettes, describing correlations of both reductions and cessation in smokers concurrently using e-cigarettes.[105–108] Other survey-based studies with follow-up have found similar correlations of increased attempts to stop smoking as well as reductions in smoking behavior; however, there were not significant correlations found with complete cessation.[23,62] One longitudinal study, using exhaled carbon monoxide (CO) to monitor smoking levels, showed reductions of 50%, overall abstinence in 40% and a general reduction in exhaled CO levels across e-cigarette

participants after 24 months, who interestingly had no original intention of quitting.[109] Additional longitudinal studies with objective smoking measurements have shown similar results of high reduction rates and moderate cessation levels in smokers.[83]

There is a modest collection of randomized, controlled trials with mixed findings that either support or oppose the use of e-cigarettes for smoking cessation. In one study, participants with no intentions of quitting were given e-cigarettes and showed reduction in cravings, similar to those exhibited after smoking a cigarette, few withdrawal symptoms, as well as substantial reduction (60%) and cessation (34%) supported by carbon monoxide measurements.[110] A randomized, double-blind controlled experiment, involving 300 cigarette smokers with no intentions of quitting, explored the efficacy and safety concerns of e-cigarettes of differing nicotine concentrations over the span of 52 weeks.[111] By the end of the study, 73.1% of the participants were no longer dependent on tobacco cigarettes and there was an abstinence rate of 8.7% at the 52-week follow-up in addition to minimal reports of withdrawal, craving, and reported adverse events.[111] Other studies have described the advantage of non-nicotinic e-cigarettes in smoking reduction as well as the additional reports of superior mood, physical symptoms, working memory, attention/visual-spatial processing, and common lack of withdrawal and craving in smokers using nicotinic e-cigarettes.[112–114]

A select few studies have investigated e-cigarettes by comparing the devices to NRTs. One such study involved 600 smokers with motivation to quit and randomized into a 16 mg nicotine e-cigarette group, a daily nicotine patch (21 mg) group, and a placebo e-cigarette group.[115] Most participants relapsed; however, the active e-cigarette group relapsed later than the patch and placebo group, had a slightly greater decrease in the amount of cigarettes smoked per day and a greater abstinence rate, and were more likely to adhere to the study's protocol.[115] Another study analyzed heavy smokers assigned to groups involving the use of 16 mg nicotine e-cigarettes, 0 mg nicotine e-cigarettes, a Nicorette nicotine inhaler (10 mg of nicotine per cartridge), or only cigarettes.[114] The 16 mg e-cigarette group had sustained decreases in desire to smoke, decreases in irritability, restlessness, and concentration difficulties, as well as similar withdrawal symptom affect, pharmacokinetics and desire to smoke levels as the inhaler group; however, nicotine e-cigarettes were preferred more by participants in comparison with the classic NRT.[114]

TABLE 3.4
Randomized, Controlled Trials of E-Cigarette Results

First-Generation E-Cigarette

Study	Sample (N)	Sample Demographics	Smoking Reduction	Smoking Cessation	Withdrawal	Craving	Adverse Effects	Notes
Tseng et al. (2016)	N = 99	Young adult smokers; not intending to quit	✓	✓	NR	NR	–	Nicotine versus non-nicotine e-cig
Bullen et al. (2013)	N = 657	Smokers willing to quit	✓	✓	✗	NR	–	Nicotine e-cig, placebo e-cig, nicotine patch (6 mo)
Dawkins et al. (2012)	N = 86	Smokers	NR	NR	✗	✗	NR	Nicotine e-cig, non-nicotine e-cig, just hold e-cig (1 hour ab)
Bullen et al. (2010)	N = 40	Smokers	NR	NR	✗	✗	✗	Nicotine e-cig, non-nicotine e-cig, Nicorette nicotine inhaler (overnight ab)
Caponnetto et al. (2013)	N = 14	Smokers with schizophrenia; not intending to quit	✓	✓	NR	NR	✗	Discusses results in a specific population (smokers with schizophrenia)

Second-Generation E-Cigarettes

Study	Sample (N)	Sample Demographics	Smoking Reduction	Smoking Cessation	Withdrawal	Craving	Adverse Effects	Notes
Adriaens et al. 2014	N = 48	Smokers not intending to quit (e-cig naïve)	✓	✓	✗	✗	–	Short-term abstinence on craving/withdrawal
Pacifici et al. 2015	N = 34	Smokers not intending to quit	✓	✓	NR	NR	–	Assurance of successful nicotine intake via educational introduction to cigarette use
O'Brien et al. 2015	N = 657	Smokers willing to quit (those with and without mental illness)	✓	✓	NR	NR	✓	No differences across population with and without mental illness; minimal adverse effects

NR, Not reported; –, none; ✓, yes; ✗, none.

Apart from some support in the form of surveys, longitudinal population analyses, and experimental trials, there is also evidence that does not support the use of e-cigarettes as smoking cessation devices. One study analyzed a population undergoing standard smoking cessation treatment, and at the 3-month follow-up date, concurrent e-cigarette users had lower quit rates, had lower rates of >50% reductions in smoking, and were 30% less likely to report abstinence compared to the group not using e-cigarettes for cessation.[33] Another study looking at the California Smokers Cohort over a 3-year span found that smokers were more likely to use e-cigarettes; however, a history of e-cigarette use did not correlate with successful cessation and those users were not as likely to reduce cigarette consumption.[116] Further evidence against the role of e-cigarettes in smoking cessation in the form of a 2014 online survey described how e-cigarette use at baseline was not correlated to individuals having more intention of quitting, to predicting quit rates 1 year later, nor to changes in cigarette consumption over the year.[117] Furthermore, one systematic review surrounding e-cigarettes and smoking cessation, consisting of 18 real-world studies and 2 clinical trials, found a 28% lower chance of smoking cessation in e-cigarette users compared to nonusers, suggesting a negative correlation between smoking cessation and e-cigarette use.[118] There are also studies that describe mixed results for support of the efficacy of e-cigarette's role in cessation. For example, a UK study comparing the efficacy of e-cigarettes to NRT and to no treatment over a time span ranging between 2009 and 2014 found that e-cigarette users were more likely to smoke more cigarettes per day and have more dependence in the form of urges in comparison with those who used no aids.[119] Nonetheless, the e-cigarette group had higher abstinence rates in comparison with the two other groups.[119]

An issue that has risen regarding e-cigarettes and smoking cessation evidence is the variability in the methods by which participants use the device, as this changes with experience and type of device used.[7,34,113] An 8-month pilot study attempted to control for the style of e-cigarette usage, such as inhalation duration, frequency and strength, by training participants to properly monitor nicotine intake by means of a standard method of inhalation.[97] At the 4- and 8-month follow-ups, there was a significant decrease in the biomarker for tobacco cigarette consumption, decreased exhaled carbon monoxide, but similar nicotine levels, depicting evidence for accurate nicotine replacement.[97]

Harm reduction and smoking cessation using e-cigarette in mental health populations

Recently, the use of e-cigarettes has been a focus in populations with mental disorders who not only exhibit a higher smoking prevalence compared to the general population but who also have less successful smoking reduction or cessation rates, lower response to standard treatment options, as well as greater sensitivity to potential psychiatric side effects that certain pharmacological, first-line medications possess.[75,102,120,121] For example, individuals with schizophrenia have robustly lower smoking cessation rates, and NRTs are not highly effective in this population.[18] With this said, e-cigarettes could be an additional nonmedicinal cessation tool for this population, along with other populations or individuals, who do not respond as well to classic therapies.[18] In one study, smokers with chronic schizophrenia were enrolled in an uncontrolled study that distributed e-cigarettes to use ad libitum and assessed the participants five additional times across a 12-month period.[121] At week 52, a 50% reduction in smoking cigarettes was exhibited in half of the participants and another 14% of users completely quit smoking, which occurred in an absence of side effects from smoking reduction and cessation.[121] Another study enrolled motivated to quit smokers, both with and without mental illness, who were allocated to either 0 or 16 mg nicotine e-cigarette groups (requested to use ad libitum) or a 21 mg nicotine patch group (users were asked to use once daily).[102] Cessation and relapse rates were comparable between the three experimental groups in the population with mental illness. The 16 mg nicotine e-cigarette groups across the study were correlated with better reduction, compliance, and acceptance in comparison with the nicotine patch group and 0 mg nicotine groups, suggesting its plausible harm reduction implementation.[102] An additional case study investigated two heavy smokers suffering from depression (51-year-old man; 50-year-old woman) who had unsuccessfully attempted smoking cessation through means of both counseling and first-line treatment methods. Both individuals received e-cigarettes to aid them in another cessation attempt.[76] The two individuals were able to quit and remain abstinent for 6 months after starting e-cigarette use.[76] Other studies have shown similar results of e-cigarettes aiding individuals with severe mental illness as well as concurrent addiction toward substantial smoking reductions.[122,123]

Overall, despite the evidence for the efficacy of e-cigarette use for smoking reduction and cessation, there is also a collection of counter evidence and the overall conclusion possesses little certainty.[20,108,116] The World

Health Organization has claimed that there have been no firm inferences made in regard to e-cigarettes and their efficacy in smoking cessation.[1,3] It is suggested that certain steps must be made in order to properly assess the harm reduction and cessation status of e-cigarettes, such as device safety standards as well as nicotine content, carrier compound, and additive disclosure.[104] Additionally, it is quite difficult to make confident conclusions regarding the device and its application due to the immense variation between studies and the type of device and e-liquids used as well as across e-cigarette models and users in the general population.[96]

CONCLUSIONS AND FUTURE DIRECTIONS

E-cigarettes are not only becoming more prevalent in use and awareness among the general population, but are also undergoing rapid technological advancement and consequently are subject to manipulation with other substances used (i.e., cannabis) and vaping style. Variability is a very common topic in the discussion surrounding e-cigarettes. The frequency and duration of e-cigarette use can lead to variable user experience and nicotine delivery, which has implications in understanding the device's efficacy for smoking cessation and generalizing any conclusions about e-cigarettes.[5,33,108] There are also many different e-liquid combinations and nicotine concentrations that have been commonly reported as mislabeled, which poses further difficulties in regulation of this device's application in clinical settings.[1,12] Furthermore, the long-term effects of e-cigarettes are widely unknown,[124] which is an important consideration such that patients are urged to plan use as only a temporary intervention.[12] Additionally, there have also been reported differences between genders in e-cigarette use and experiences with smoking cessation that are notable, but lack assured conclusions.[108,112] Overall, e-cigarettes may be a safer alternative for users in comparison with tobacco cigarettes, which makes them attractive for harm reduction and replacement when considering smoking cessation, but more research to establish their safety and efficacy is needed.

REFERENCES

1. Organization WH. *Electronic Nicotine Delivery Systems and Electronic Non-nicotine*. Delivery Systems (ENDS/ENNDS); 2016.
2. Etter JF, Bullen C. Electronic cigarette: users profile, utilization, satisfaction and perceived efficacy. *Addiction*. 2011;106(11):2017–2028.
3. Foulds J, Veldheer S, Berg A. Electronic cigarettes (e-cigs): views of aficionados and clinical/public health perspectives. *Int J Clin Pract*. 2011;65(10):1037–1042.
4. Glasser AM, et al. Overview of electronic nicotine delivery systems: a systematic review. *Am J Prev Med*. 2017;52(2):e33–e66.
5. Giovenco DP, et al. E-cigarette market trends in traditional US retail channels, 2012–2013. *Nicotine Tob Res*. 2014;17(10):1279–1283.
6. Kaisar MA, et al. A decade of e-cigarettes: limited research & unresolved safety concerns. *Toxicology*. 2016;365:67–75.
7. Zhu S-H, et al. Four hundred and sixty brands of e-cigarettes and counting: implications for product regulation. *Tob Control*. 2014;23(suppl 3):iii3–iii9.
8. Dinakar C, O'Connor GT. The health effects of electronic cigarettes. *N Engl J Med*. 2016;375(14):1372–1381.
9. Farsalinos KE, et al. Nicotine absorption from electronic cigarette use: comparison between first and new-generation devices. *Sci Rep*. 2014;4.
10. Talih S, et al. "Direct Dripping": a high-temperature, high-formaldehyde emission electronic cigarette use method. *Nicotine Tob Res*. 2015;18(4):453–459.
11. Yingst JM, et al. Factors associated with electronic cigarette users' device preferences and transition from first generation to advanced generation devices. *Nicotine Tob Res*. 2015;17(10):1242–1246.
12. Grana R, Benowitz N, Glantz SA. E-cigarettes: a scientific review. *Circulation*. 2014;129(19):1972–1986.
13. Etter J-F. Electronic cigarettes: a survey of users. *BMC Public Health*. 2010;10(1):231.
14. Taghavi S, et al. Nicotine content of domestic cigarettes, imported cigarettes and pipe tobacco in Iran. *Addict Health*. 2012;4(1–2):28.
15. Krishnan-Sarin S, et al. E-cigarettes and "dripping" among high-school youth. *Pediatrics*. 2017;139(3):e20163224.
16. Morean ME, et al. High school students' use of electronic cigarettes to vaporize cannabis. *Pediatrics*. 2015;136(4):611–616.
17. Giroud C, et al. E-cigarettes: a review of new trends in cannabis use. *Int J Environ Res Public Health*. 2015;12(8):9988–10008.
18. Farsalinos KE, Polosa R. Safety evaluation and risk assessment of electronic cigarettes as tobacco cigarette substitutes: a systematic review. *Ther Adv Drug Saf*. 2014;5(2):67–86.
19. Cahn Z, Siegel M. Electronic cigarettes as a harm reduction strategy for tobacco control: a step forward or a repeat of past mistakes? *J Public Health Policy*. 2011;32(1):16–31.
20. Franck C, et al. Electronic cigarettes in North America. *Circulation*. 2014;129(19):1945–1952.
21. Pisinger C, Godtfredsen NS. Is there a health benefit of reduced tobacco consumption? A systematic review. *Nicotine Tobacco Res*. 2007;9(6):631–646.
22. Dawkins L, et al. First-versus second-generation electronic cigarettes: predictors of choice and effects on urge to smoke and withdrawal symptoms. *Addiction*. 2015;110(4):669–677.

23. Adkison SE, et al. Electronic nicotine delivery systems: international tobacco control four-country survey. *Am J Prev Med*. 2013;44(3):207–215.

24. Xu Y, et al. E-cigarette awareness, use, and harm perception among adults: a meta-analysis of observational studies. *PLoS One*. 2016;11(11):e0165938.

25. Berg CJ, et al. Attitudes toward e-cigarettes, reasons for initiating e-cigarette use, and changes in smoking behavior after initiation: a pilot longitudinal study of regular cigarette smokers. *Open J Prevent Med*. 2014;4(10):789.

26. Li J, et al. The use and acceptability of electronic cigarettes among New Zealand smokers. *New Zeal Med J (Online)*. 2013;126(1375).

27. Choi K, Forster J. Characteristics associated with awareness, perceptions, and use of electronic nicotine delivery systems among young US Midwestern adults. *Am J Public Health*. 2013;103(3):556–561.

28. Dobbs PD, Hammig B, Henry LJ. E-cigarette use among US adolescents: perceptions of relative addiction and harm. *Health Edu J*. 2017;76(3):293–301.

29. O'Connor RJ, et al. Smoker awareness of and beliefs about supposedly less-harmful tobacco products. *Am J Prevent Med*. 2005;29(2):85–90.

30. Zhu S-H, et al. The use and perception of electronic cigarettes and snus among the US population. *PLoS One*. 2013;8(10):e79332.

31. England PH. *Adult Smoking Habits in the UK: 2016. Cigarette Smoking Among Adults Including the Proportion of People who Smoke, Their Demographic Breakdowns, Changes Over Time, and E-Cigarettes*. 2016. Available from: https://www.ons.gov.uk/peoplepopulationandcommunity/healthandsocialcare/healthandlifeexpectancies/bulletins/adultsmokinghabitsingreatbritain/2016.

32. Czoli CD, Hammond D, White CM. Electronic cigarettes in Canada: prevalence of use and perceptions among youth and young adults. *Can J Public Health*. 2014;105(2):e97–e102.

33. Zawertailo L, et al. Concurrent E-cigarette use during tobacco dependence treatment in primary care settings: association with smoking cessation at three and six months. *Nicotine Tob Res*. 2016;19(2):183–189.

34. Biener L, Hargraves JL. A longitudinal study of electronic cigarette use among a population-based sample of adult smokers: association with smoking cessation and motivation to quit. *Nicotine Tob Res*. 2014;17(2):127–133.

35. Filippidis FT, et al. Two-year trends and predictors of e-cigarette use in 27 European Union member states. *Tob Control*. 2017;26(1):98–104.

36. Vardavas CI, Filippidis FT, Agaku IT. Determinants and prevalence of e-cigarette use throughout the European Union: a secondary analysis of 26 566 youth and adults from 27 Countries. *Tob Control*. 2015;24(5):442–448.

37. Pepper JK, et al. Reasons for starting and stopping electronic cigarette use. *Int J Environ Res Public Health*. 2014;11(10):10345–10361.

38. King BA, et al. Trends in awareness and use of electronic cigarettes among US adults, 2010–2013. *Nicotine Tob Res*. 2014;17(2):219–227.

39. Huerta TR, et al. Trends in e-cigarette awareness and perceived harmfulness in the US. *Am J Prevent Med*. 2017;52(3):339–346.

40. Yong H-H, et al. Trends in e-cigarette awareness, trial, and use under the different regulatory environments of Australia and the United Kingdom. *Nicotine Tob Res*. 2014;17(10):1203–1211.

41. Arrazola RA, et al. Tobacco use among middle and high school students-United States, 2011–2014. *MMWR Morb Mortality Weekly Rep*. 2015;64(14):381–385.

42. Regan AK, et al. Electronic nicotine delivery systems: adult use and awareness of the 'e-cigarette' in the USA. *Tob Control*. 2011. https://doi.org/10.1136/tobaccocontrol-2011–050044.

43. Chatham-Stephens K, et al. Exposure Calls to US Poison Centers involving electronic cigarettes and conventional cigarettes—September 2010–December 2014. *J Med Toxicol*. 2016;12(4):350–357.

44. Pepper JK, Brewer NT. Electronic nicotine delivery system (electronic cigarette) awareness, use, reactions and beliefs: a systematic review. *Tob Control*. 2014;23(5):375–384.

45. Dawkins L, et al. 'Vaping' profiles and preferences: an online survey of electronic cigarette users. *Addiction*. 2013;108(6):1115–1125.

46. Dockrell M, et al. E-cigarettes: prevalence and attitudes in Great Britain. *Nicotine Tob Res*. 2013;15(10):1737–1744.

47. Pearson JL, et al. E-Cigarette awareness, use, and harm perceptions in US adults. *Am J Public Health*. 2012;102(9):1758–1766.

48. White J, et al. Tripling use of electronic cigarettes among New Zealand adolescents between 2012 and 2014. *J Adolesc Health*. 2015;56(5):522–528.

49. Canada H. *Canadian Tobacco Alcohol and Drugs (CTADS): 2015 Summary*. 2015; August 30, 2017. Available from: https://www.canada.ca/en/health-canada/services/canadian-tobacco-alcohol-drugs-survey/2015-summary.html.

50. McMillen RC, et al. Trends in electronic cigarette use among US adults: use is increasing in both smokers and nonsmokers. *Nicotine Tob Res*. 2014;17(10):1195–1202.

51. Schoenborn CA, Gindi RM, Electronic cigarette use among adults: United States, 2014. *US Department of Health and Human Services, Centers for Disease Control and Prevention*. National Center for Health Statistics; 2015.

52. Dutra LM, Glantz SA. Electronic cigarettes and conventional cigarette use among US adolescents: a cross-sectional study. *JAMA Pediatr*. 2014;168(7):610–617.

53. Hajek P, et al. Electronic cigarettes: review of use, content, safety, effects on smokers and potential for harm and benefit. *Addiction*. 2014;109(11):1801–1810.

54. Cohn A, et al. The association between alcohol, marijuana use, and new and emerging tobacco products in a young adult population. *Addict Behav.* 2015;48:79–88.

55. Berg CJ, et al. Perceived harm, addictiveness, and social acceptability of tobacco products and marijuana among young adults: marijuana, hookah, and electronic cigarettes win. *Subst Use Misuse.* 2015;50(1):79–89.

56. Hughes K, et al. Associations between e-cigarette access and smoking and drinking behaviours in teenagers. *BMC Public Health.* 2015;15(1):244.

57. Kilibarda B, Mravcik V, Martens MS. E-cigarette use among Serbian adults: prevalence and user characteristics. *Int J Public Health.* 2016;61(2):167–175.

58. Ooms GI, et al. Sociodemographic differences in the use of electronic nicotine delivery systems in the European Union. *Nicotine Tob Res.* 2015;18(5):724–729.

59. Reid JL, et al. Who is using e-cigarettes in Canada? Nationally representative data on the prevalence of e-cigarette use among Canadians. *Prev Med.* 2015;81: 180–183.

60. West R, Brown J, Beard E. *Trends in Electronic Cigarette use in England.* Vol. 21. 2014. University College London, Smoking Toolkit Study.

61. Sutfin EL, et al. Electronic cigarette use by college students. *Drug Alcohol Depend.* 2013;131(3): 214–221.

62. Brose LS, et al. Is the use of electronic cigarettes while smoking associated with smoking cessation attempts, cessation and reduced cigarette consumption? A survey with a 1-year follow-up. *Addiction.* 2015;110(7): 1160–1168.

63. Hartwell G, et al. E-cigarettes and equity: a systematic review of differences in awareness and use between sociodemographic groups. *Tob Control.* 2016: tobaccocontrol-2016–053222.

64. Bostean G, Trinidad DR, McCarthy WJ. E-cigarette use among never-smoking California students. *Am J Public Health.* 2015;105(12):2423–2425.

65. Ahern NR, Mechling B. E-cigarettes: a rising trend among youth. *J Psychosocial Nursing Mental Health Services.* 2014; 52(6):27–31.

66. Cho JH, Shin E, Moon S-S. Electronic-cigarette smoking experience among adolescents. *J Adolesc Health.* 2011; 49(5):542–546.

67. Miech R, et al. E-cigarette use as a predictor of cigarette smoking: results from a 1-year follow-up of a national sample of 12th grade students. *Tob Control.* 2017: tobaccocontrol-2016–053291.

68. Leventhal AM, et al. Association of electronic cigarette use with initiation of combustible tobacco product smoking in early adolescence. *JAMA.* 2015;314(7):700–707.

69. Primack BA, et al. Progression to traditional cigarette smoking after electronic cigarette use among US adolescents and young adults. *JAMA Pediatr.* 2015;169(11): 1018–1023.

70. Eastwood B, et al. Electronic cigarette use in young people in Great Britain 2013–2014. *Public Health.* 2015; 129(9):1150–1156.

71. Cummins SE, et al. Use of e-cigarettes by individuals with mental health conditions. *Tob Control.* 2014: tobaccocontrol-2013–051511.

72. Hefner K, et al. E-cigarette use in veterans seeking mental health and/or substance use services. *J Dual Diagnosis.* 2016;12(2):109–117.

73. Peters EN, et al. Electronic cigarettes in adults in outpatient substance use treatment: awareness, perceptions, use, and reasons for use. *Am J Addict.* 2015;24(3): 233–239.

74. Leventhal AM, et al. Psychiatric comorbidity in adolescent electronic and conventional cigarette use. *J Psychiat Res.* 2016;73:71–78.

75. Prochaska JJ, Grana RA. E-cigarette use among smokers with serious mental illness. *PLoS One.* 2014;9(11): e113013.

76. Caponnetto P, et al. Smoking cessation with e-cigarettes in smokers with a documented history of depression and recurring relapses. *Int J Clin Med.* 2011;2(03):281.

77. first_generation_ecig.

78. B M. *The 4 Generations of Electronic Cigarettes*; 2015. Available from: http://ecigclopedia.com/the-4-generations-of-electronic-cigarettes/.

79. Administration, U.S.F. Electronic Cigarette Fires and Explosions. Available from: http://moon-vapes.com/what-is-vaping/first_generation_ecig/.

80. How long do e-cigarettes last? Available from: https://www.quora.com/How-long-do-e-cigarettes-last.

81. Boom In E-Cigarettes Sparks Calls For Regulation.

82. Vansickel AR, Eissenberg T. Electronic cigarettes: effective nicotine delivery after acute administration. *Nicotine Tob Res.* 2012;15(1):267–270.

83. Polosa R, et al. Effect of an electronic nicotine delivery device (e-Cigarette) on smoking reduction and cessation: a prospective 6-month pilot study. *BMC Public Health.* 2011;11(1):786.

84. Farsalinos KE, et al. Evaluating nicotine levels selection and patterns of electronic cigarette use in a group of "vapers" who had achieved complete substitution of smoking. *Subst Abuse Res Treat.* 2013;7:139.

85. Dawkins L, Corcoran O. Acute electronic cigarette use: nicotine delivery and subjective effects in regular users. *Psychopharmacology.* 2014;231(2):401–407.

86. Schweitzer KS, et al. Endothelial disruptive proinflammatory effects of nicotine and e-cigarette vapor exposures. *Am J Physiol Lung Cell Mol Physiol.* 2015;309(2): L175–L187.

87. Bartschat S, et al. Not only smoking is deadly: fatal ingestion of e-juice—a case report. *Int J Legal Med.* 2015; 129(3):481–486.

88. Vakkalanka J, Hardison Jr L, Holstege C. Epidemiological trends in electronic cigarette exposures reported to US Poison Centers. *Clin Toxicol.* 2014;52(5):542–548.

89. Williams M, et al. Metal and silicate particles including nanoparticles are present in electronic cigarette cartomizer fluid and aerosol. *PLoS One.* 2013;8(3):e57987.

90. Schripp T, et al. Does e-cigarette consumption cause passive vaping? *Indoor Air.* 2013;23(1):25–31.

91. Orr MS. Electronic cigarettes in the USA: a summary of available toxicology data and suggestions for the future. *Tob Control*. 2014;23(suppl 2):ii18–ii22.

92. Goniewicz ML, et al. Levels of selected carcinogens and toxicants in vapour from electronic cigarettes. *Tob Control*. 2013: tobaccocontrol-2012–050859.

93. Romagna G, et al. Cytotoxicity evaluation of electronic cigarette vapor extract on cultured mammalian fibroblasts (ClearStream-LIFE): comparison with tobacco cigarette smoke extract. *Inhal Toxicol*. 2013;25(6):354–361.

94. Etter JF, Eissenberg T. Dependence levels in users of electronic cigarettes, nicotine gums and tobacco cigarettes. *Drug Alcohol Depend*. 2015;147:68–75.

95. Farsalinos KE, et al. Evaluation of electronic cigarette use (vaping) topography and estimation of liquid consumption: implications for research protocol standards definition and for public health authorities' regulation. *Int J Environ Res Public Health*. 2013;10(6):2500–2514.

96. Polosa R, et al. A fresh look at tobacco harm reduction: the case for the electronic cigarette. *Harm Reduct J*. 2013;10(1):19.

97. Pacifici R, et al. Successful nicotine intake in medical assisted use of e-cigarettes: a pilot study. *Int J Environ Res Public Health*. 2015;12(7):7638–7646.

98. Schroeder MJ, Hoffman AC. Electronic cigarettes and nicotine clinical pharmacology. *Tob Control*. 2014;23(suppl 2):ii30–ii35.

99. Coleman BN, et al. Association between electronic cigarette use and openness to cigarette smoking among US young adults. *Nicotine Tob Res*. 2014;17(2):212–218.

100. Nutt DJ, et al. Estimating the harms of nicotine-containing products using the MCDA approach. *Eur Addict Res*. 2014;20(5):218–225.

101. McAuley TR, et al. Comparison of the effects of e-cigarette vapor and cigarette smoke on indoor air quality. *Inhal Toxicol*. 2012;24(12):850–857.

102. O'Brien B, et al. E-cigarettes versus NRT for smoking reduction or cessation in people with mental illness: secondary analysis of data from the ASCEND trial. *Tob Induced Dis*. 2015;13(1):5.

103. Hartmann-Boyce J, et al. Electronic cigarettes for smoking cessation. *Cochrane Libr*. 2016.

104. Cobb NK, Abrams DB. The FDA, e-cigarettes, and the demise of combusted tobacco. *N Engl J Med*. 2014;371(16):1469–1471.

105. Etter J-F, Bullen C. A longitudinal study of electronic cigarette users. *Addict Behav*. 2014;39(2):491–494.

106. Siegel MB, Tanwar KL, Wood KS. Electronic cigarettes as a smoking-cessation tool: results from an online survey. *Am J Prevent Med*. 2011;40(4):472–475.

107. Beard E, et al. Association between electronic cigarette use and changes in quit attempts, success of quit attempts, use of smoking cessation pharmacotherapy, and use of stop smoking services in England: time series analysis of population trends. *BMJ*. 2016;354:i4645.

108. Jorenby DE, et al. Nicotine levels, withdrawal symptoms, and smoking reduction success in real world use: a comparison of cigarette smokers and dual users of both cigarettes and E-cigarettes. *Drug Alcohol Depend*. 2017;170:93–101.

109. Polosa R, et al. Effectiveness and tolerability of electronic cigarette in real-life: a 24-month prospective observational study. *Intern Emerg Med*. 2014;9(5):537–546.

110. Adriaens K, et al. Effectiveness of the electronic cigarette: an eight-week Flemish study with six-month follow-up on smoking reduction, craving and experienced benefits and complaints. *Int J Environ Res Public Health*. 2014;11(11):11220–11248.

111. Caponnetto P, et al. EffiCiency and Safety of an eLectronic cigAreTte (ECLAT) as tobacco cigarettes substitute: a prospective 12-month randomized control design study. *PLoS One*. 2013;8(6):e66317.

112. Dawkins L, et al. The electronic-cigarette: effects on desire to smoke, withdrawal symptoms and cognition. *Addict Behav*. 2012;37(8):970–973.

113. Tseng T-Y, et al. A randomized trial comparing the effect of nicotine versus placebo electronic cigarettes on smoking reduction among young adult smokers. *Nicotine Tob Res*. 2016;18(10):1937–1943.

114. Bullen C, et al. Effect of an electronic nicotine delivery device (e cigarette) on desire to smoke and withdrawal, user preferences and nicotine delivery: randomised cross-over trial. *Tob Control*. 2010;19(2):98–103.

115. Bullen C, et al. Electronic cigarettes for smoking cessation: a randomised controlled trial. *Lancet*. 2013;382(9905):1629–1637.

116. Al-Delaimy WK, et al. E-cigarette use in the past and quitting behavior in the future: a population-based study. *Am J Public Health*. 2015;105(6):1213–1219.

117. Grana RA, Popova L, Ling PM. A longitudinal analysis of electronic cigarette use and smoking cessation. *JAMA Intern Med*. 2014;174(5):812–813.

118. Kalkhoran S, Glantz SA. E-cigarettes and smoking cessation in real-world and clinical settings: a systematic review and meta-analysis. *Lancet Respir Med*. 2016;4(2):116–128.

119. Brown J, et al. Real-world effectiveness of e-cigarettes when used to aid smoking cessation: a cross-sectional population study. *Addiction*. 2014;109(9):1531–1540.

120. Tidey JW, Miller ME. Smoking cessation and reduction in people with chronic mental illness. *BMJ*. 2015;351(1):h4065.

121. Caponnetto P, et al. Impact of an electronic cigarette on smoking reduction and cessation in schizophrenic smokers: a prospective 12-month pilot study. *Int J Environ Res Public Health*. 2013;10(2):446–461.

122. Pratt SI, et al. Appeal of electronic cigarettes in smokers with serious mental illness. *Addict Behav*. 2016;59:30–34.

123. Stein MD, et al. An open trial of electronic cigarettes for smoking cessation among methadone-maintained smokers. *Nicotine Tob Res*. 2015;18(5):1157–1162.

124. Hefner K, Valentine G, Sofuoglu M. Electronic cigarettes and mental illness: Reviewing the evidence for help and harm among those with psychiatric and substance use disorders. *Am J Addict*. 2017.

CHAPTER 4

The Neuropsychoendocrinology of Substance Use Disorders

ELIE G. AOUN, MD • KRISTEN SCHMIDT, MD, MAPH

CHAPTER INTRO

Our understanding of the neurobiological basis of substance use disorders (SUD) is limited, so are available treatment options. Patterns of substance use intersect with stress, appetite, sleep, anxiety and sex. These physiologic drives are regulated predominantly by endocrine pathways. As such, it makes sense to examine whether hormonal systems play a role in the initiation or maintenance of substance use disorders. Exploring and exploiting these pathways confers the potential to better understand and target the neurophysiology of addictions. Hormones are circulating compounds that may be objectively measured and tracked. As such, with a growing body of knowledge about their role in addictions, hormones may be used as potential biomarkers to gauge SUD predisposition or prognosis. Similarly, these pathways can be investigated for the development of safe and novel therapeutic targets for SUD. This chapter will survey and review preclinical and clinical studies addressing the relationship between substance use disorders and hormones implicated in regulating stress, water volume, appetite, sleep, reproduction, and parturition.

APPETITE REGULATING HORMONES

Appetite regulating hormones including ghrelin, leptin, glucagon-like peptide 1 (GLP-1) and insulin are known to govern the metabolism of ingested nutrients. In addition, research supports their role in modulating cognitive function, stress, and reward processing that affects hedonic drive. The involvement between appetite regulating hormones and substance use has been most extensively documented with alcohol. Indeed, alcohol is both a source of calories and a substance of abuse.

GHRELIN

Ghrelin is a 28-amino acid peptide hormone produced primarily by gastric endocrine cells. It is frequently labeled as the "hunger hormone" because of its primary role in increasing appetite and food intake. Ghrelin produces its effect by binding the growth hormone secretagogue receptor 1a (GHS-R1a), which is expressed in peripheral organs as well as in the brain. As such, ghrelin's actions are mediated by direct peripheral as well as central effects when it crosses the blood—brain barrier. The latter is postulated to modulate dopamine transmission in the reward processing for food and other reinforcers. Ghrelin also interacts with the hypothalamic—pituitary—adrenal (HPA) axis modulating stress responses and anxiety. It is thought that ghrelin's interactions with both the reward and stress pathways explain its role in addictive behaviors.

GHRELIN AND ALCOHOL

Early data from rodent models shows that blood ghrelin concentration is lowered in rats exposed to alcohol, and this reduction is blunted in alcohol preferring rats.[1] Conversely, ghrelin administration to rats is shown to increase alcohol consumption.[2]

Molecular studies found that following exposure to alcohol, alcohol preferring rats show an upregulation of the ghrelin receptors in the parts of the brain regulating the reward pathway, namely, in the prefrontal cortex, the nucleus accumbens, hippocampus, amygdala, and ventral tegmental area.[1] To test this finding, central ghrelin infusions directly in the ventral tegmental area, the laterodorsal tegmental nucleus, or cerebral ventricles led to increased alcohol drinking in rodents.[3,4]

It is thought that ghrelin's central effects on the amygdala modulate GABA and serotonin pathways and this is responsible for its relationship with alcohol drinking behaviors.[5,6] Peripheral ghrelin signaling, on the other hand, does not appear to play a role.

Human studies show similar findings. Indeed, alcohol consumption in adults without Alcohol Use

Disorder (AUD) lowers plasma ghrelin levels.[7,8] Similarly, early abstinence from alcohol in subjects with AUD is associated with increased circulating ghrelin levels.[9,10] Observational studies are inconclusive as it has been suggested that individuals with AUD have higher ghrelin levels,[11] while others demonstrated opposite findings.[12]

Ghrelin was also found to affect craving for alcohol. A positive correlation has been identified in numerous studies between the urges to drink alcohol and ghrelin plasma concentration.[10,12,13] In order to examine whether there is a cause and effect relationship between craving and ghrelin levels, Leggio et al. used a placebo-controlled double-blind design where participants were randomized to receive intravenous injections of ghrelin or placebo followed by measurements of craving for alcohol. They demonstrated that subjects who received ghrelin injections had higher measures of cravings for alcohol but not for neutral cues such as juice. In addition, craving measure scores correlated with plasma ghrelin concentration.[14] Single-nucleotide polymorphism studies examining variability in the gene coding for the ghrelin receptor identified a gene missense polymorphism to be associated significantly with a diagnosis of AUD.[15]

The research summarized above highlights a role for ghrelin and the ghrelin receptor as potential pharmacological targets for the treatment of AUD. Ghrelin antagonists have been developed and studied in rodent models of AUD. Early findings demonstrate a reduction in alcohol consumption and alcohol seeking behaviors associated with the systemic administration of these compounds.[16–18] Similar results were seen in ghrelin receptor knockout mice.[19] Human studies examining the effects of ghrelin receptor antagonists are currently underway.

GHRELIN AND STIMULANTS

Not unlike the alcohol data, early evidence of ghrelin's role in stimulant use is derived from animal and translational studies. In rodent models, exposure to methamphetamine or MDMA was found to correlate with higher plasma ghrelin levels.[20,21] Similarly, ghrelin levels were found to correlate with cocaine seeking behaviors following a period of extinction.[22] Ghrelin injection in the ventral tegmental area in rats is associated with increased preference for cocaine.[23] Similarly, exogenous ghrelin led to cocaine-induced hyperlocomotion when infused intraperitoneally[24] or directly into the nucleus accumbens.[25]

In one human gene polymorphism study, a single-nucleotide polymorphism (SNP) in the gene coding for ghrelin was found to be associated with the severity of stimulant use. Another SNP polymorphism in the gene coding for the ghrelin receptor correlated with the incidence of stimulant use disorder in a sample of amphetamine using adults.[26]

These findings support the consideration of ghrelin receptor antagonists to reduce stimulant use. One such compound was tested prior to an injection of cocaine or methamphetamine in a rodent model. It led to reduction in dopamine release in the nucleus accumbens as well as decreased conditioned place preference for stimulants.[27] In another study, the compound was associated with reduced stimulant-induced hyperlocomotion.[28]

GHRELIN AND NICOTINE

Ghrelin potentiates dopamine release in rats' striatum in response to nicotine.[29] Conversely, nicotine exposure leads to increased ghrelin levels in rats.[30,31] In humans, there is some evidence of increased ghrelin levels immediately after smoking.[32] Ghrelin levels in individuals with tobacco use disorders were found to correlate with the years of smoking and were predictive of relapse to tobacco use.[33,34] In a rodent model of tobacco use disorder, the administration of a ghrelin receptor antagonist diminished nicotine associated behaviors and dopamine release.[35,36]

GHRELIN AND OPIOIDS

The research examining the role of ghrelin in modulating opioid use is very limited. In a rat model of opioid use, the direct injection of ghrelin in the CSF led to increased heroin seeking and consumption.[37] Conversely, the administration of ghrelin receptor antagonists is associated with increased levels of endogenous opioid levels in brain tissue as well as decreased opioid seeking behaviors and accumbal dopamine release.[38] New data suggests these effects might be mediated by ghrelin's role in modulating the interaction between the opioid and endocannabinoid pathways.[39]

GHRELIN AND CANNABIS

Cannabis administration in a rat model led to increased serum ghrelin levels as well as food consumption.[40] Similarly, in a study, men who smoke cannabis to increase appetite in the context of HIV infection were found to have higher ghrelin levels.[41] More research is necessary to better understand the role of ghrelin in cannabis use.

LEPTIN

Leptin is a peptide hormone produced by adipose tissue with appetite regulating function opposite to that of ghrelin. Leptin causes diminished appetite and reward associated with eating. Such opposing effects suggest a "cross-talk" between ghrelin and leptin in regulating appetite, and in turn, a role for leptin in addictive behaviors. Leptin receptors are expressed in the central reward processing pathway, namely, the ventral tegmental area, the substantia nigra, and the arcuate nucleus of the hypothalamus. Leptin was found to regulate the stress responses via the HPA axis, which is suggested as one mechanism explaining its role in addictive behaviors.[42]

LEPTIN AND ALCOHOL

Studies of individuals with AUD show a correlation between serum leptin levels and craving for alcohol.[43,44] Conversely, treating persons with AUD with acamprosate or naltrexone leads to lower leptin levels, suggesting that leptin concentration can potentially play a role in prognostic determinations and treatment response (I, 13). In humans, leptin levels were found to be elevated with chronic alcohol use[45] and correlated significantly with craving for alcohol.[43,46] In a study of subjects with AUD, Haass-Koffler et al. demonstrated that a ghrelin infusion leads to lower leptin levels. The change in leptin levels correlated with craving for alcohol.[47]

LEPTIN AND STIMULANTS

Animal models are instrumental for understanding the role of leptin in stimulant use. In rodent models, exposure to methamphetamine or MDMA was found to correlate with lower plasma leptin levels.[20,21] Similarly, leptin infusion causes the blunting of dopaminergic signaling in the nucleus accumbens and a reduction of the rewarding effects of cocaine in rats.[48–50]

In humans with a stimulant use disorder, Martinotti et al.[51] demonstrated a correlation between leptin levels and cocaine use and craving for cocaine in early abstinence.

LEPTIN AND NICOTINE

In a rat model of nicotine use, rodents exposed to nicotine were observed to eat less and had lower leptin plasma levels[30] that normalized following nicotine abstinence.[52] In a study of humans who have never smoked, nicotine administration was found to correlate with leptin levels in the mesocorticolimbic system and

was associated with decreased appetite.[53] Another study demonstrated increased plasma leptin levels in individuals who had stopped smoking for 2 months.[54] Al'Absi et al.[55] found that in smokers, circulating leptin levels correlated significantly with craving for nicotine and withdrawal symptoms.

LEPTIN AND OPIOIDS

Little is known on the effects of leptin on opioid use. One human study identified reduced circulating leptin levels in subjects with opioid use disorder maintained on methadone.[56]

LEPTIN AND CANNABIS

Cannabis use was found to be associated with elevated leptin levels in adults with HIV.[41] No other studies have examined this relationship.

GLUCAGON-LIKE PEPTIDE-1 (GLP-1)

GLP-1 is a neuropeptide hormone produced in the intestinal L-cells following food intake with central and peripheral effects leading to insulin release and reduced appetite. As such, GLP-1 receptor agonists have been developed and approved by the FDA for the treatment of diabetes. In the CNS, GLP-1 receptors are found in the nucleus accumbens, the globus pallidus, and the ventral tegmental area suggesting that it may play a role in the reward pathway.[57]

GLP-1 AND ALCOHOL

Significant data coming from animal models suggests that GLP-1 plays an important role in the regulation of alcohol drinking. GLP-1 receptor agonists were found to reduce dopamine release and diminish alcohol mediated rewards in mice leading to decreased spontaneous alcohol intake.[58–61] In a model of alcohol preferring mice, alcohol deprivation is used as a paradigm to study the aversive effects of withdrawal as well as craving. GLP-1 agonist treatment in these mice prevented the expected increase in alcohol intake following re-exposure to alcohol.[62] Similarly, rats with increased circulating levels of GLP-1 following a gastric bypass procedure reduced their alcohol intake.[63] Conversely, GLP-1 receptor antagonists led to increased alcohol self-administration.[59]

Human studies examining the role of GLP-1 in alcohol drinking behaviors are limited. Suchankova et al.[64] tested SNP variability in the gene coding for the GLP-1 receptor in a large sample of individuals with AUD. They identified a functional mutation that is significantly associated with AUD. Individuals with the mutation were also more likely to seek intravenous alcohol self-administration and on fMRI to show a strong response mapping to the globus pallidus.

GLP-1 AND STIMULANTS

Not unlike the studies examining the effects of GLP-1 on alcohol intake, rodent models were used to examine the role of GLP-1 receptor agonists in stimulant use. Indeed, the administration of such compounds was found to be associated with diminished amphetamine-induced hyperlocomotion, cocaine-induced conditioned place preference, and dopamine release in the nucleus accumbens.[65–67] Similarly, GLP-1 receptor agonist administration led to decreased cocaine self-administration.[68]

In humans, a study of individuals with a stimulant use disorder demonstrated that circulating GLP-1 levels were reduced following IV administration of cocaine.[69]

GLP-1 AND NICOTINE

Little is known about the role of GLP-1 in nicotine use. One study examined the effect of a GLP-1 receptor agonist in mice. The compound blocked the rewarding effects of nicotine as well as nicotine-induced locomotor sensitization.[70]

VOLUME REGULATING HORMONES

Volume regulating hormones include renin, angiotensin, aldosterone, vasopressin, and some other natriuretic peptides such as atrial natriuretic peptide (ANP) that play a key role in the control and homeostasis of blood pressure in the arteries, tissue perfusion, and extracellular volume. These hormones interact with each other to control the total blood volume and blood pressure. For example, with dehydration, hyponatremia or hypotension, the renin—angiotensin aldosterone system is activated. Renin, which is produced by the kidneys, stimulates the hydrolysis of angiotensin I by the liver. The lungs produce angiotensin converting enzyme (ACE) that is responsible for angiotensin I becoming angiotensin II. The latter stimulates the zona glomerulosa of the adrenal cortex to produce aldosterone, a mineralocorticoid. Mineralocorticoid receptors (MR) that are encoded by the gene NR3C2 are found in the kidneys where they regulate water reabsorption, but also, they have been identified in the central nervous system mainly in limbic brain regions as the amygdala and the prefrontal cortex (PFC). Volume regulating

hormones, aldosterone in particular, have been identified as playing a role in alcohol use disorder, but not with other substance use disorders.

VOLUME REGULATING HORMONES AND ALCOHOL

Available research supports a role for aldosterone in alcohol drinking behaviors and anxiety responses; it is hypothesized that central MR signaling modulates this effect. Indeed, central MR localization maps to brain areas involved in the development and maintenance of maladaptive drinking.[71] In addition, the central nucleus of the amygdala (CeA) that is known to play a major role in stress and anxiety-induced alcohol drinking was demonstrated to express greater levels of the MR than other amygdala nuclei. Structural changes in the CeA result in disinhibition of alcohol-drinking behaviors via functional changes in central nuclei that are downstream from the CeA.

Early human studies demonstrated that in adults with AUD, early withdrawal from alcohol is associated with higher aldosterone as well as renin and angiotensin II levels that later normalize during recovery.[72–74] In the subset of patients who developed severe withdrawal including delirium tremens, investigators identified elevated ANP levels in early abstinence that did not normalize until 2 weeks later.[75] Similarly, in that subgroup, the renin activity was noted to start higher than the general sample of adults with AUD in acute withdrawal, but dips to significantly lower activity by 10 days compared to those who do not develop DT. Such findings support a possible protective role against severe withdrawal for these volume regulating hormones. As such, renin and aldosterone could be viewed as compensating mechanisms for the physiological stress associated with withdrawal by conserving sodium.

Another study examined the relationship between alcohol craving and the actual volume of alcohol that a person consumes, regardless of alcohol content and percentage in a sample of adults with AUD.[76] The investigators found that the severity of craving correlates directly and significantly with the volume of alcohol containing beverages consumed. This highlights a possible effect of volume regulating hormones on craving for alcohol. Leggio et al. followed a sample of adults with AUD for 3 months of abstinence and identified significant direct correlations between measures of craving and renin activity and circulating aldosterone levels.[74]

A recently published study by Aoun et al.[77] examined these relationships across three species. In a macaque model of alcohol use, aldosterone levels increased significantly from predrinking baseline after these monkeys were trained to self-administer alcohol. Before they could experience any symptoms of withdrawal, their brains were analyzed for gene expression of NR3C2, the gene for MR. The investigators identified a significant negative correlation between the amount of alcohol consumed and the gene expression in the CeA. This suggests that the CeA *NR3C2* gene expression is sensitive to alcohol consumption. The negative correlation identified along with the higher circulating levels of aldosterone is consistent with a negative feedback loop whereby alcohol use could be triggering an increased production of aldosterone, which in turn, inhibits the production of MR in the CeA.

In a rodent model of alcohol use, a significant negative correlation was identified between the expression of NR3C2 in the CeA and compulsive alcohol consumption by alcohol dependent rats. In contrast, rats with lower NR3C2 expression were noted to have less anxiety and stress-induced drinking.[77] This suggests that high expression of this NR3C2 gene may be protective against compulsive drinking or stress-induced drinking.

Finally, in the third part of the study, adults with AUD were followed for 3 months after they stopped drinking. Study participants who relapsed were found to have significantly higher aldosterone levels that those who were abstinent and the amount of drinks consumed correlated with circulating aldosterone concentration. A significant direct correlation was also identified between aldosterone levels and measures of alcohol craving and anxiety.[77]

STRESS HORMONES

Any clinician who has worked with individuals with SUD can appreciate the significant relationship between stress and substance use. Indeed, using substances such as stimulants or hallucinogens often leads to states of anxiety and hyperarousal. On the other hand, many reports using drugs or alcohol to "self-medicate." The term is somewhat of a misnomer because substance use does not alleviate the stressors, rather, it can blunt one's cognitive abilities, distracting from the stressor. As such, external stressors are often identified as tightly related to initial experimentation with substance use and relapses. Similarly, internal stressors including the physiological stress imposed by substance withdrawal is often managed by using the same substance to relieve the symptoms. In such situations, using alcohol or drugs to lessen a person's anxiety is an example of negative reinforcement that increases the likelihood of continued use. Such clinical

observations suggest that stress physiology plays a role in substance use disorders.

The body's response to stress is mediated by a complicated system of hormones, second messengers, and neurotransmitters. Among endocrine pathways known to play a major role in the stress response is the HPA axis. Stress triggers hypothalamic neurons in the periventricular nucleus to produce corticotropin-releasing factor (CRF). CRF stimulates the anterior pituitary to secrete proopiomelanocortin that is enzymatically modified into adrenocorticotropin hormone (ACTH). The ACTH is released in the bloodstream and interacts with receptors on the adrenal medulla stimulating the production of glucocorticoids such as cortisol. Kiefer and colleagues suggested a model explaining the interrelationship between the HPA axis and addictions.[78] Stressor stimulation of the HPA axis is a known contributor to states of anxiety and mood alteration. These are known risk factors for substance use causing further neuroendocrine dysregulation. In turn, the chronic use of drugs and alcohol is associated with emerging anxiety and depressive disorders causing altered sensitivity of the hormone/receptor sensitivity in the HPA axis with such changes increasing craving for substance use. Understanding how drug use is influenced by the HPA axis is valuable for identifying potential biomarkers of relapse as well as new treatment targets.

Stress was shown to be associated with increased craving as well as increased likelihood for relapse in abstinent individuals with AUD and those with OUD receiving naltrexone.[79,80] There is data supporting a role for the body stress response in modulating emotional and altered hedonic responses in individuals with SUD.[81] In those subjects with AUD or a stimulant use disorder, stress cues or drug cues result in more pronounced craving, anxiety, and negative emotions than in their counterpart without a SUD diagnosis.[81] This exemplifies the association between stress, drug cues, craving, and changes in the biomarkers of stress response such as the HPA axis. Human studies have demonstrated that corticosterone release mediated by the HPA axis activation plays a role in drug self-administration.[81]

The interaction between stress pathways and addiction appears to be mediated by the kappa-opioid receptor as well as dopamine.[82] Indeed, stress-induced glucocorticoid receptor activation has been shown to lead to increased dopamine production,[83] and dopamine is known to play an essential role in addictions. Given the complexity of the stress pathways and the multidimensional relationships between the different hormones involved, we will discuss the collective role of stress hormones in addictions instead of looking at individual hormones.

STRESS HORMONES AND ALCOHOL

When individuals with AUD are exposed to a validated stress paradigm, they were found to exhibit increased craving to alcohol, as well as a blunted salivary cortisol response.[84] Stress cues were found to render these subjects more likely to relapse to alcohol and more likely to drink larger amounts of alcohol when they relapse. As is the case with stimulants, elevated basal levels of CRF, ACTH, and cortisol were demonstrated in early withdrawal from alcohol[85,86] along with a blunted response to stressful experimental designs.[87–89] This physiologic stress response manifesting as HPA hyperactivity was noted to be sustained for at least 1 month. Abstinent subjects with AUD have increased salivary cortisol levels 4 weeks after their last drink compared to a control group of social drinkers.[90] With alcohol and stress-cue exposure, this same group was noted to experience more significant feelings of distress and craving, but a blunted HPA response to stress. This blunted HPA response to stress-cues, along with negative mood and stress-induced craving have been shown in numerous studies to be associated with drinking outcomes such as relapse.[88,91–94]

STRESS HORMONES AND STIMULANTS

In a rodent model of cocaine and morphine self-administration, suppression of corticosterone by adrenalectomy was associated with a reduced locomotor hyperactivity normally associated with these substances.[95] Corticosterone replacement reversed these effects. Central glucocorticoid receptors (GR) are hypothesized to play a role. Indeed, models of GR gene knockout in mice showed a decreased motivation for cocaine self-administration.[96] When given amphetamines, individuals without SUD were found to have increased plasma cortisol levels.[97] Similarly, Wand et al.[98] showed that amphetamine-induced cortisol level elevation was correlated with the level of amphetamine-induced euphoria in individuals without SUDs receiving amphetamine. Interestingly, chronic cocaine use was demonstrated to cause sustained increases in the HPA axis functions.[99]

Changes in HPA axis functions are also observed in withdrawal states. Indeed, early withdrawal from cocaine was shown to be associated with elevated basal levels of CRF, ACTH, cortisol as well as epinephrine and norepinephrine.[100,101] Similarly, these hormones are

noted to be hyperreactive to experimental stress paradigms.[81] In one study, subjects with a stimulant use disorder using cocaine were followed for 3 months following inpatient treatment.[102] The study investigators showed that the severity of stress-induced craving following stress-cues experimental designs serves as a predictor for time to relapse. ACTH as well as cortisol levels were correlated with the amount of cocaine used following relapse. This suggests that stress-cues along with drug-cues contribute to the emergence of compulsive drug-seeking behaviors, making the individual more vulnerable to relapse. As such, it is reasonable to consider ACTH and cortisol as potential biomarkers for addiction severity, risk of relapse, and response to treatment.

STRESS HORMONES AND NICOTINE

Nicotine delivery to individuals without a tobacco use disorder was found to stimulate the HPA axis resulting in increased levels of cortisol and ACTH.[81,82,103] This in turn triggers inhibition of the production of these hormones by way of a negative feedback loop. Early withdrawal from nicotine is also associated with elevated basal levels of CRF, ACTH, and cortisol[104] along with a suppressed ACTH and cortisol response to stressful experimental designs.[105,106] These markers of abnormal stress response were identified as predictors of nicotine relapse.[105]

STRESS HORMONES AND OPIOIDS

In a rodent model of opioid use, a central injection of a GR antagonist was found to be associated with decreased locomotor activity associated with morphine use.[107] This finding supports a role of the GR in dopaminergic pathways. A study examined the effect of drug cues in individuals with opioid use disorder (OUD) treated with methadone maintenance or buprenorphine.[108] In these subjects, drug cues were found to be associated with increased levels of cortisol, and higher cortisol response predicted relapses to nonprescribed opioid use. On the other hand, the use of opioids leads to lower cortisol levels,[81,109,110] in contrast to the effect of other substances discussed above on cortisol level. When subjects with OUD are exposed to stress in experimental models, they are noted to have a blunted HPA response.[111]

STRESS HORMONES AND CANNABIS

In one study, individuals with co-occurring alcohol, cannabis and stimulant use disorder were compared to a control group with alcohol and stimulant use disorder, without a cannabis use disorder. In the former group, exposure to alcohol or cocaine cues was found to be associated with increased anxiety and craving as well as increased circulating levels of cortisol and ACTH in response to stress cues compared to the control group.[112]

REPRODUCTIVE HORMONES

Sex differences in substance use disorders exist. Clinically, a telescoping phenomenon has been observed whereby females achieve disordered substance use faster than males.[113] Females also suffer physiologic consequences like end-organ damage at a quicker pace.[113] While some sex variance may be mediated by culture, preclinical studies have consistently demonstrated differences between male and female substance use in multiple domains.

Animal studies reflect the disparity in disordered substance use observed clinically in males versus females. For instance, female animals show increased substance acquisition, dysregulation, and drug reinstatement compared to males.[113] This is particularly true of stimulants, where female rats self-administer more cocaine than males until diurnal control becomes dysregulated.[114,115] Similarly, females escalate their alcohol intake with increasing ethanol concentration, while their male counterparts are cued to titrate consumption.[113,115–117] Female rats also acquire self-administration of cannabinoid agonists, methamphetamine, and nicotine faster than male rats.[118] Once substance dependent, females show increased vulnerability to drug reinstatement or relapse compared to males.[114,115] The reproductive hormones, estrogen, progesterone, and its metabolite allopregnanolone, play a significant role in regulating reproduction and may influence disordered substance consumption.

ESTROGEN

Estrogen's relationship to substance use is modulated by its influence on GABA, dopamine, and glutamate.[115,119] Estrogen increases dopamine both directly and indirectly by:
1. Inducing dopamine gene transcription
2. Decreasing inhibitory GABA firing and GABA-B receptor stimulation
3. Downregulating D2 auto-receptors with consequential dopamine enhancement.[115]

Estrogen is the reproductive hormone primarily responsible for increased drug seeking and relapse found preferentially in females.[113,115,118–120] Through its alpha receptor, estrogen is associated with the glutamatergic system in the striatum and the prefrontal cortex, both known to play a role in craving.[120,121]

ESTROGEN AND STIMULANTS

Estrogen's role in stimulant acquisition has been explored in several preclinical studies. Estradiol has been found to increase the initial binge length and amount of cocaine animals self-administer.[119,122] Data suggests that ovariectomized (OVX) female rats receiving estrogen responded more robustly to cocaine acquisition than those OVX rats who did not receive estrogen.[115,123] In addition, rats receiving tamoxifen, a specific estrogen receptor modulator, showed less stimulant response.[115,123] Another analysis demonstrated that antagonizing the metabotropic glutamate receptor 5 (mGluR5) that is coupled to estrogen prevented cocaine-induced sensitization.[120,121] Hence, there may be a role for exploiting the relationship between estrogen and glutamate receptors to target substance use disorders.

PROGESTERONE

If estrogen can be thought of as the hormonal "gas pedal" for disordered substance use, then progesterone serves as a homeostatic "break." On a neurobiological level, progesterone and its metabolites demonstrate prostriatal GABA activity and dopamine reduction.[118,124] Decreased dopamine potentiation leads to decreased drug acquisition. Progesterone interacts with GABA-A, glycine, sigma1, kainite, serotonin 3, and nicotinic cholinergic receptors and may facilitate synaptic plasticity and cognition by influencing spine density in the hippocampus.[125]

PROGESTERONE AND NICOTINE

Clinically, progesterone appears to influence nicotine reward and craving. Females reported less pleasure from smoking when they had higher plasma progesterone.[113,126] Nicotine craving reports have also shown an inverse correlation with plasma progesterone levels.[113,127] It is perhaps unsurprising then that favorable outcomes for smoking cessation have been linked to women quitting during the luteal phase of their menstrual cycle when progesterone is at its peak.[128] Randomized control trials (RCT) with micronized progesterone herald a significant potential for this hormone in treating nicotine use disorders, as doses of 400 mg per day reduced urges to smoke in males and females.[129]

PROGESTERONE AND STIMULANTS

Preclinical investigations of progesterone treatment for stimulant use disorders seem promising. In rats, progesterone counteracted estradiol's effects on cocaine acquisition.[125,130] Progesterone also appears to reduce relapse or reinstatement by inhibiting the stress response during the estrous cycle in rats and monkeys.[113,131] Clinically, progesterone dampens reward. Subjective stimulant effects have been negatively correlated with female salivary progesterone levels,[119,132] as have cravings for cocaine.[113,133] In an RCT, a week of progesterone at 400 mg per day significantly attenuated cue-induced craving in cocaine-dependent men and women. Cognitive performance was improved and women reported less negative mood states and higher relaxation compared to placebo.[120,134,135]

ALLOPREGNANOLONE (ALLO)

A progesterone metabolite, allopregnanolone is a neuroactive steroid and GABA-A receptor modulator.[136] The effects of neuroactive steroids are much swifter than steroids since they do not require intracellular binding and gene transcription.[123] Evidence suggests that ALLO may play a pivotal role in substance consumption, withdrawal, and reinstatement.

ALLO AND STIMULANTS

Allopregnanolone may affect stimulant craving and subsequent relapse. In a preclinical examination, ALLO blocked cocaine reinstatement in female rats.[118] This was reversed by inhibiting progesterone's conversion to ALLO with finasteride administration.[137] A recent clinical trial showed that men and women with elevated ALLO levels who received 400 mg per day of progesterone had decreased cocaine craving, improved cognition, higher mood, and normalized cortisol response to stress.[138]

ALLO AND ALCOHOL

There may be utility in ALLO therapy for alcohol withdrawal. ALLO's anticonvulsant and neuroprotective properties may be responsible for the diminished kindling response and withdrawal symptoms observed in female versus male animal models.[113,118,139,140] Clinically, an inverse relationship between ALLO plasma levels and alcohol withdrawal symptoms has been demonstrated. As ALLO levels declined in early withdrawal, subjects reported increased ratings of anxiety and depression.[141] Interestingly, ALLO administration has been found to reduce alcohol consumption in alcohol dependent rats.[136,142] It was hypothesized that ALLO may counteract the reinforcing anxiolytic effects of alcohol.[136]

BIOMARKERS

Neuroactive steroids may prove useful as potential biomarkers. Severe alcohol use disorder is associated with polymorphisms in the enzymes 5 alpha and 3 alpha hydroxysteroid dehydrogenase, which are required to make neurosteroids like ALLO.[143] Protective polymorphisms are associated with higher neuroactive steroid levels and greater sedative effects when consuming alcohol.[144] Tolerance to the sedative effects of alcohol may lead to the development of an AUD and may be facilitated by risk allele C homozygotes.[144] Of note, naltrexone was found to selectively elevate ALLO levels by 49.4% relative to placebo among individuals with the Asp40 allele of the OPRM1 gene. It was suggested that naltrexone may influence subjective alcohol effects through ALLO production; adjunct ALLO therapy could potentially help naltrexone nonresponders achieve sobriety.[145]

OREXIN

Orexin (also known as hypocretin) is a neuropeptide implicated in appetite, arousal, and reward, among other things.[146] Increasing evidence suggests that it may have a significant role to play in future treatment for substance use disorders. Orexin-A and orexin-B neurons are situated in the hypothalamus with numerous projections including the adrenergic locus coeruleus, serotonergic raphe nuclei, histaminergic tuberomammilary nucleus, dopaminergic substantia nigra, and ventral tegmental area.[146,147] While orexin neurons may be found in the perifornical area and dorsomedial hypothalamic nucleus, reward function has most commonly been associated with orexin neurons located in the lateral hypothalamus.[148] There are 2G protein receptors for orexin, orexin receptor-1 (OX1R), and orexin receptor-2 (OX2R).[148] Orexin-A can bind to either receptor, while orexin-B binds to OX2R.[148,149] Most preclinical data implicates orexin-A via OX1R, in modulating substance use and reward, while orexin-B is thought to mitigate arousal and alertness through OX2R.[150]

OREXIN AND ALCOHOL

Orexin-A has a demonstrated association with alcohol use. For instance, injecting orexin-A into the hypothalamus results in a significant increase in rat alcohol intake.[2] Comparatively, reduced alcohol consumption was significantly associated with reduced orexin-A in the plasma of pregnant rats.[147] In a clinical correlate, orexin-A mRNA plasma levels were lower in alcoholics who were 90 days abstinent compared to those undergoing acute alcohol withdrawal.[148,151]

Orexin-A inhibition through OX1R antagonism has been associated with reducing positive reinforcement of alcohol.[148] Orexin-A antagonism blunted binge ethanol use in male rats[152] and absolute ethanol consumption in C57BL/6 mice.[153] In another very recent study,[154] it was concluded that OX1R antagonism may be particularly helpful for individuals with severe alcohol use disorders as rats exhibiting high levels of motivation for alcohol consumption were significantly affected by selective orexin-1 receptor blockade.

OREXIN AND CANNABIS

OX1R has also demonstrated use as a novel target to modulate cannabinoid reward.[155] Only 29% of mice receiving OX1R antagonists were able to acquire cannabis agonist self-administration compared to 75% of controls with uninhibited orexin transmission.[155] Furthermore, mice who did not have the gene for OX1R did not demonstrate increased dopamine levels in the nucleus accumbens following THC administration.[155] Given that there are no medications currently FDA approved for the treatment of cannabis use disorder, OX1R antagonism could represent a unique way to target this problem.

OREXIN AND OPIOIDS

Orexin has also been linked to substance withdrawal, including opioid withdrawal. When physiological dependence to a drug develops, antistress peptide-like neuropeptide Y are downregulated and dynorphin, orexin and substance P are recruited.[156] Orexin neurons situated in the lateral hypothalamus are interconnected with the extended amygdala, the center commonly associated with withdrawal.[148,149,156] In a study evaluating morphine dependence, orexin activation and gene induction was demonstrated during opioid withdrawal.[157] Immunofluorescence revealed that nearly 50% of orexin cells display mu opioid receptors.[157] The same study demonstrated that mice lacking orexin genes (orexin knock outs) exhibited attenuated morphine withdrawal[157] suggesting that orexin may facilitate physical dependence on opioids. Withdrawal may be mitigated by the antireward neuropeptide dynorphin, which is also expressed by a majority of orexin neurons.[157,158] Orexin's dynamic involvement with the opioid network may have profound implications for the treatment of this serious use disorder going forward.

In fact, there may be a potential role for OX2R antagonists in targeting neuroadaptive changes that may mediate negative reinforcement and opioid dependence.[149] A recent study demonstrated that rats with extended access to heroin selectively decreased drug self-administration with the use of a selective OX2R antagonist.[149] mRNA levels of OX2R receptor expression were increased specifically in the amygdala of such rats, which is the area implicated in opioid withdrawal.[149]

OREXIN AND STIMULANTS

Preclinical data demonstrating orexin's consistent association with stimulant locomotor sensitization and conditioned place preference[148] provided the groundwork for further investigations with medicines on the current market. Suvorexant, an antagonist of both OX1R and OX2R, has been found to attenuate motivational cocaine properties in rat models.[159] The drug was recently approved by the FDA for the treatment of primary insomnia.[150] Given its dual receptor antagonism, the sedation associated with OX2R was exploited to treat sleep disorders. It is still too early to tell if this medication may prove effective for comorbid treatment of substance use disorders and insomnia, a common dual diagnosis.[160]

Another dual orexin antagonist (DORA), almorexant, was tested clinically before it was taken off the market due to tolerability concerns.[150] In a crossover study aimed at evaluating abuse potential, recreational drug users preferred zolpidem over almorexant.[161] Low abuse potential makes orexin antagonists attractive options for targeting substance use disorders.

BIOMARKERS

Orexin polymorphisms may be associated with a vulnerability to substance use disorders.[162] A recent genome-wide and subsequent association study found that carriers of the A/G genotype of an SNP (single-nucleotide polymorphism) for OX2R had more severe levels of nicotine dependence.[162] In addition, there was suggestion that the polymorphism may lead to a higher risk of initiating methamphetamine use at younger ages.[162] The stimulating properties of nicotine and methamphetamine and OX2R's relationship with arousal may help explain this potentially toxic interdependence.

OXYTOCIN

Oxytocin is a neuropeptide consisting of nine amino acids[163] and is synthesized in the paraventricular nucleus (PVN) and the supraoptic nucleus (SON) of the hypothalamus.[164] Oxytocin's receptors can be found in regions associated with mood, social affiliation and addiction, including the amygdala, nucleus accumbens, and ventral pallidum.[165] While some of its more commonly known functions involve parturition and lactation, the neuropeptide has also been linked to reducing anxiety, diminishing stress response, stimulating the immune system, and reducing drug reward while promoting social reward.[163] In fact, the utility of oxytocin may just be its unique ability to reorient the hedonistic hijacking from disordered substance use back to healthy, affiliative prosocial processes. It has been the subject of several clinical and preclinical studies investigating novel ways of treating substance use disorders.

In the absence of oxytocin, excess dopamine can elicit perseverative object-oriented behaviors such as the stereotypy induced by stimulant use, dopamine agonism, or mechanistic compulsions characterizing autism.[164] Breaking the object-oriented loops of isolation may be possible with oxytocin[164,166] and may have profound implications for substance use disorder treatment. Intra-amygdala administration of oxytocin has been shown to reverse social isolation precipitated by subchronic PCP exposure.[164,167] In prairie voles, affiliation by pair bonding reduced the rewarding properties of stimulants.[163,164,168,169] Oxytocin's potential to shift people toward supportive social relationships for reward and away from solitary substance use could account for the success of 12-step models. Though not yet tested, there may be therapeutic utility for oxytocin in addressing gambling disorder or behavioral compulsions such as sexual- or technology-related dysfunction with object-oriented foci.

The relationship between oxytocin and substance use disorders is most likely reciprocal. As a result of chronic drug use, the endogenous oxytocin system is downregulated, impacting tolerance and motivation for social exchange.[163,163a] However, deficiencies in oxytocin may have contributed to the development of disordered substance use in the first place. Early experiences and adverse childhood events are known to impact and predict long-term oxytocin adaptation.[170] Childhood trauma victims have reduced CSF, plasma and urine oxytocin levels.[170] Diminished oxytocin receptors are considered to be the result of disrupted attachment and subsequent epigenetic alterations involving DNA methylation.[170]

OXYTOCIN AND STIMULANTS

Oxytocin may have maximal efficacy in stress primed situations for substance using individuals with early stressor neuroadaptation. In one of the first clinical trials evaluating the therapeutic benefits of intranasal oxytocin, cocaine-dependent subjects with a history of childhood maltreatment were significantly more likely to have an attenuated cortisol response and exhibit decreased stress reactivity when utilizing oxytocin.[171] Oxytocin may also disrupt the relationship between anger and cue reactivity according to another study of chronic cocaine-dependent individuals with prolonged abstinence in a controlled environment.[172] While individuals reported increased baseline desire to use in response to drug cues, evidence suggested that there may be benefit in patients self-administering oxytocin prior to contexts with high risk for anger relapse.[172] Positive therapeutic benefit for oxytocin may therefore be related to higher acuity situations.[173]

OXYTOCIN AND CANNABIS

Oxytocin was also found to mitigate stress cues for cannabis. Another positive clinical study utilizing intranasal oxytocin involved the stress response of individuals with cannabis use disorder.[174] Pretreatment with intranasal oxytocin at doses of 40 IU reduced stress-induced reactivity and craving in cannabis-dependent individuals.[174]

OXYTOCIN AND ALCOHOL

Physiologic and psychological stress associated with alcohol withdrawal was also positively impacted by intranasal oxytocin use. A randomized double-blind, placebo-controlled trial demonstrated that subjects receiving a 24 IU dose of oxytocin required nearly five times less total lorazepam to complete detoxification than controls.[175] Mean withdrawal and craving scores on days 1 and 2 were almost 3 times lower with oxytocin treatment.[175] It has been suggested that oxytocin may be able to block alcohol withdrawal by rapidly reversing alcohol tolerance.[175]

Substance self-administration is significantly reduced with oxytocin intervention for most drugs of abuse in animal models.[173] Recently, it was shown that voluntary ethanol consumption was inhibited by oxytocin and that oxytocin completely blocked alcohol-induced dopamine release in the nucleus accumbens following acute and chronic alcohol exposure.[176] This builds upon earlier preclinical work that demonstrated a single administration of oxytocin resulted in a 6-week decline in preference for alcohol.[164] Additional preclinical studies have demonstrated oxytocin's role in altering substance-induced changes in dopamine, glutamate, and Fos expression in cortical and basal ganglia sites to prevent stress and priming-induced drug relapse.[164] Tolerance to alcohol and opioids may be prevented by oxytocin,[164] and withdrawal phenomena may be similarly affected.[164,177]

OXYTOCIN AND OPIOIDS
Withdrawal was one of the concerns in a recent pilot investigation looking at the effects of intranasal oxytocin in subjects with OUD. In that study, subjects receiving either maintenance methadone or buprenorphine tolerated oxytocin treatment without precipitated withdrawal or adverse effect. However, oxytocin did not diminish opioid craving as hoped.[178]

BIOMARKERS
As clinical studies with oxytocin continue to evolve, an important variable to keep in mind is genetic variability. Single-nucleotide polymorphisms of the oxytocin receptor gene have been associated with very different phenotypes. In a study assessing subjective response to the drug MDMA, individuals with the A/A genotype of rs53576 did not report increased sociability while G allele carriers did.[179] Additionally, another study found that males homozygous for the A allele were more frequent alcohol consumers at ages 15 and 18 and were more likely to have had an alcohol use disorder by age 25 compared to male G allele carriers.[165] Interestingly, the relationship between alcohol use disorders and A allele carriers may have been moderated by poor social interactions.[165] Previous reports have suggested that carriers of the A allele show deficits in social processing, may be less likely to receive psychological benefit from social support, and altogether implies that the genotype may affect sensitivity to exogenously administered oxytocin.[179] Future clinical studies utilizing exogenous oxytocin therapy to target substance use disorders should consider genotype as well as sex differences at play in treatment response.

CONCLUSION
A new population of individuals with substance use disorders demands new ways of managing this problem. Currently available treatments rely on modulating various neurotransmitters that are known players in the addictions reward pathway. Our goal is to encourage exploration of new ways to treat a very old problem utilizing safe and effective interventions. By harnessing the body's own homeostatic systems involved in stress, volume, appetite, sleep, reproduction and parturition regulation, we may be able to restore wellness.

REFERENCES
1. Landgren S, Engel JA, Hyytia P, Zetterberg H, Blennow K, Jerlhag E. Expression of the gene encoding the ghrelin receptor in rats selected for differential alcohol preference. *Behav Brain Res.* 2011;221(1):182—188. https://doi.org/10.1016/j.bbr.2011.03.003.
2. Schneider ER, Rada P, Darby RD, Leibowitz SF, Hoebel BG. Orexigenic peptides and alcohol intake: differential effects of orexin, galanin, and ghrelin. *Alcohol Clin Exp Res.* 2007;31(11):1858—1865.
3. Cepko LC, Selva JA, Merfeld EB, Fimmel AI, Goldberg SA, Currie PJ. Ghrelin alters the stimulatory effect of cocaine on ethanol intake following mesolimbic or systemic administration. *Neuropharmacology.* 2014;85:224—231. https://doi.org/10.1016/j.neuropharm.2014.05.030.
4. Jerlhag E, Egecioglu E, Landgren S, et al. Requirement of central ghrelin signaling for alcohol reward. *Proc Natl Acad Sci USA.* 2009;106(27):11318—11323. https://doi.org/10.1073/pnas.0812809106.
5. Cruz MT, Herman MA, Cote DM, Ryabinin AE, Roberto M. Ghrelin increases GABAergic transmission and interacts with ethanol actions in the rat central nucleus of the amygdala. *Neuropsychopharmacology.* 2013;38(2):364—375. https://doi.org/10.1038/npp.2012.190.
6. Hansson C, Alvarez-Crespo M, Taube M, et al. Influence of ghrelin on the central serotonergic signaling system in mice. *Neuropharmacology.* 2014;79:498—505. https://doi.org/10.1016/j.neuropharm.2013.12.012.
7. Calissendorff J, Gustafsson T, Holst JJ, Brismar K, Rojdmark S. Alcohol intake and its effect on some appetite-regulating hormones in man: influence of gastroprotection with sucralfate. *Endocr Res.* 2012;37(3):154—162. https://doi.org/10.3109/07435800.2012.662662.
8. Leggio L, Schwandt ML, Oot EN, Dias AA, Ramchandani VA. Fasting induced increase in plasma ghrelin is blunted by intravenous alcohol administration: a within-subject placebo-controlled study. *Psychoneuroendocrinology.* 2013;38(12):3085—3091. https://doi.org/10.1016/j.psyneuen.2013.09.005.
9. Kim JH, Kim SJ, Lee WY, et al. The effects of alcohol abstinence on BDNF, ghrelin, and leptin secretions in alcohol-dependent patients with glucose intolerance. *Alcohol Clin Exp Res.* 2013;37(suppl 1):E52—E58. https://doi.org/10.1111/j.1530-0277.2012.01921.x.
10. Leggio L, Ferrulli A, Cardone S, et al. Ghrelin system in alcohol-dependent subjects: role of plasma ghrelin levels in alcohol drinking and craving. *Addict Biol.* 2012;17(2):452—464. https://doi.org/10.1111/j.1369-1600.2010.00308.x.

11. Kim DJ, Yoon SJ, Choi B, et al. Increased fasting plasma ghrelin levels during alcohol abstinence. *Alcohol Alcohol.* 2005;40(1):76—79. https://doi.org/10.1093/alcalc/agh108.

12. Addolorato G, Capristo E, Leggio L, et al. Relationship between ghrelin levels, alcohol craving, and nutritional status in current alcoholic patients. *Alcohol Clin Exp Res.* 2006;30(11):1933—1937. https://doi.org/10.1111/j.1530-0277.2006.00238.x.

13. Akkisi Kumsar N, Dilbaz N. Relationship between craving and ghrelin, adiponectin, and resistin levels in patients with alcoholism. *Alcohol Clin Exp Res.* 2015;39(4):702—709. https://doi.org/10.1111/acer.12689.

14. Leggio L, Zywiak WH, Fricchione SR, et al. Intravenous ghrelin administration increases alcohol craving in alcohol-dependent heavy drinkers: a preliminary investigation. *Biol Psychiatry.* 2014;76(9):734—741. https://doi.org/10.1016/j.biopsych.2014.03.019.

15. Suchankova P, Yan J, Schwandt ML, et al. The Leu72Met polymorphism of the prepro-ghrelin gene is associated with alcohol consumption and subjective responses to alcohol: preliminary findings. *Alcohol Alcohol.* 2017;52(4):425—430. https://doi.org/10.1093/alcalc/agx021.

16. Gomez JL, Cunningham CL, Finn DA, et al. Differential effects of ghrelin antagonists on alcohol drinking and reinforcement in mouse and rat models of alcohol dependence. *Neuropharmacology.* 2015;97:182—193. https://doi.org/10.1016/j.neuropharm.2015.05.026.

17. Stevenson JR, Buirkle JM, Buckley LE, Young KA, Albertini KM, Bohidar AE. GHS-R1a antagonism reduces alcohol but not sucrose preference in prairie voles. *Physiol Behav.* 2015;147:23—29. https://doi.org/10.1016/j.physbeh.2015.04.001.

18. Stevenson JR, Francomacaro LM, Bohidar AE, et al. Ghrelin receptor (GHS-R1a) antagonism alters preference for ethanol and sucrose in a concentration-dependent manner in prairie voles. *Physiol Behav.* 2016;155:231—236.

19. Bahi A, Tolle V, Fehrentz JA, et al. Ghrelin knockout mice show decreased voluntary alcohol consumption and reduced ethanol-induced conditioned place preference. *Peptides.* 2013;43:48—55. https://doi.org/10.1016/j.peptides.2013.02.008.

20. Crowley WR, Ramoz G, Keefe KA, Torto R, Kalra SP, Hanson GR. Differential effects of methamphetamine on expression of neuropeptide Y mRNA in hypothalamus and on serum leptin and ghrelin concentrations in ad libitum-fed and schedule-fed rats. *Neuroscience.* 2005;132(1):167—173. https://doi.org/10.1016/j.neuroscience.2004.11.037.

21. Kobeissy FH, Jeung JA, Warren MW, Geier JE, Gold MS. Changes in leptin, ghrelin, growth hormone and neuropeptide-y after an acute model of MDMA and methamphetamine exposure in rats. *Addict Biol.* 2008;13(1):15—25. https://doi.org/10.1111/j.1369-1600.2007.00083.x.

22. Tessari M, Catalano A, Pellitteri M, et al. Correlation between serum ghrelin levels and cocaine-seeking behavior triggered by cocaine-associated conditioned stimuli in rats. *Addict Biol.* 2007;12(1):22—29.

23. Schuette LM, Gray CC, Currie PJ. Microinjection of ghrelin into the ventral tegmental area potentiates cocaine-induced conditioned place preference. *J Behav Brain Sci.* 2013;3(8):576—580.

24. Wellman PJ, Davis KW, Nation JR. Augmentation of cocaine hyperactivity in rats by systemic ghrelin. *Regul Pept.* 2005;125(1—3):151—154. https://doi.org/10.1016/j.regpep.2004.08.013.

25. Jang JK, Kim WY, Cho BR, Lee JW, Kim JH. Microinjection of ghrelin in the nucleus accumbens core enhances locomotor activity induced by cocaine. *Behav Brain Res.* 2013;248:7—11. https://doi.org/10.1016/j.bbr.2013.03.049.

26. Suchankova P, Jerlhag E, Jayaram-Lindstr€om N, et al. Genetic variation of the ghrelin signalling system in individuals with amphetamine dependence. *PLoS One.* 2013;8(4):e61242.

27. Jerlhag E, Egecioglu E, Dickson SL, Engel JA. Ghrelin receptor antagonism attenuates cocaine- and amphetamine-induced locomotor stimulation, accumbal dopamine release, and conditioned place preference. *Psychopharmacology.* 2010;211(4):415—422. https://doi.org/10.1007/s00213-010-1907-7.

28. Suchankova P, Engel JA, Jerlhag E. Sub-chronic ghrelin receptor blockade attenuates alcohol- and amphetamine-induced locomotor stimulation in mice. *Alcohol Alcohol.* 2016;51(2):121—127. https://doi.org/10.1093/alcalc/agv100.

29. Palotai M, Bagosi Z, Jaszberenyi M, et al. Ghrelin amplifies the nicotine-induced dopamine release in the rat striatum. *Neurochem Int.* 2013;63(4):239—243. https://doi.org/10.1016/j.neuint.2013.06.014.

30. Tomoda K, Kubo K, Nishii Y, Yamamoto Y, Yoshikawa M, Kimura H. Changes of ghrelin and leptin levels in plasma by cigarette smoke in rats. *J Toxicol Sci.* 2012;37(1):131—138.

31. Ali SS, Hamed EA, Ayuob NN, Shaker Ali A, Suliman MI. Effects of different routes of nicotine administration on gastric morphology and hormonal secretion in rats. *Exp Physiol.* 2015;100(8):881—895. https://doi.org/10.1113/ep085015.

32. Bouros D, Tzouvelekis A, Anevlavis S, et al. Smoking acutely increases plasma ghrelin concentrations. *Clin Chem.* 2006;52(4):777—778. https://doi.org/10.1373/clinchem.2005.065243.

33. Al'Absi M, Lemieux A, Nakajima M. Peptide YY and ghrelin predict craving and risk for relapse in abstinent smokers. *Psychoneuroendocrinology.* 2014;49:253—259. https://doi.org/10.1016/j.psyneuen.2014.07.018.

34. Lemieux AM, Al'Absi M. Changes in circulating peptide YY and ghrelin are associated with early smoking relapse. *Biol Psychol.* 2018;131:43—48.

35. Jerlhag E, Engel JA. Ghrelin receptor antagonism attenuates nicotine-induced locomotor stimulation, accumbal dopamine release and conditioned place preference in mice. *Drug Alcohol Depend.* 2011;117(2—3):126—131. https://doi.org/10.1016/j.drugalcdep.2011.01.010.

36. Wellman PJ, Clifford PS, Rodriguez J, et al. Pharmacologic antagonism of ghrelin receptors attenuates development of nicotine induced locomotor sensitization in rats. *Regul Pept.* 2011;172(1−3):77−80. https://doi.org/10.1016/j.regpep.2011.08.014.

37. Maric T, Sedki F, Ronfard B, Chafetz D, Shalev U. A limited role for ghrelin in heroin self-administration and food deprivation-induced reinstatement of heroin seeking in rats. *Addict Biol.* 2012;17(3):613−622. https://doi.org/10.1111/j.1369-1600.2011.00396.x.

38. Engel JA, Nylander I, Jerlhag E. A ghrelin receptor (GHS-R1a) antagonist attenuates the rewarding properties of morphine and increases opioid peptide levels in reward areas in mice. *Eur Neuropsychopharmacol.* 2015;25(12):2364−2371. https://doi.org/10.1016/j.euroneuro.2015.10.004.

39. Sustkova-Fiserova M, Jerabek P, Havlickova T, Syslova K, Kacer P. Ghrelin and endocannabinoids participation in morphine-induced effects in the rat nucleus accumbens. *Psychopharmacology.* 2016;233(3):469−484. https://doi.org/10.1007/s00213-015-4119-3.

40. Mazidi M, Baghban Taraghdari S, Rezaee P, et al. The effect of hydroalcoholic extract of Cannabis sativa on appetite hormone in rat. *J Complement Integr Med.* 2014;11(4):253−257. https://doi.org/10.1515/jcim-2014-0006.

41. Riggs PK, Vaida F, Rossi SS, et al. A pilot study of the effects of cannabis on appetite hormones in HIV-infected adult men. *Brain Res.* 2012;1431:46−52. https://doi.org/10.1016/j.brainres.2011.11.001.

42. Inui A. Feeding and body-weight regulation by hypothalamic neuropeptides—mediation of the actions of leptin. *Trends Neurosci.* 1999;2:62−67.

43. Hillemacher T, Bleich S, Frieling H, et al. Evidence of an association of leptin serum levels and craving in alcohol dependence. *Psychoneuroendocrinology.* 2007;32:87−90.

44. Kiefer F, Jahn H, Jaschinski M, et al. Leptin: a modulator of alcohol craving? *Biol Psychiatry.* 2001;49:782−787.

45. Nicolas JM, Fernandez-Sola J, Fatjo F, et al. Increased circulating leptin levels in chronic alcoholism. *Alcohol Clin Exp Res.* 2001;1:83−88.

46. Kraus T, Reulbach U, Bayerlein K, et al. Leptin is associated with craving in females with alcoholism. *Addict Biol.* 2004;3−4:213−219.

47. Haass-Koffler CL, Aoun EG, Swift RM, de la Monte SM, Kenna GA, Leggio L. Leptin levels are reduced by intravenous ghrelin administration and correlated with cue-induced alcohol craving. *Transl Psychiatry.* 2015:e646. https://doi.org/10.1038/tp.2015.140.

48. Figlewicz DP, Evans SB, Murphy J, Hoen M, Baskin DG. Expression of receptors for insulin and leptin in the ventral tegmental area/substantia nigra (VTA/SN) of the rat. *Brain Res.* 2003;964:107−115.

49. Shen M, Jiang C, Liu P, Wang F, Ma L. Mesolimbic leptin signaling negatively regulates cocaine-conditioned reward. *Transl Psychiatry.* 2016;6:e972. https://doi.org/10.1038/tp.2016.223.

50. You Z-B, Wang B, Liu Q-R, Wu Y, Otvos L, Wise RA. Reciprocal inhibitory interactions between the reward-Related effects of leptin and cocaine. *Neuropsychopharmacology.* 2016;41:1024−1033. https://doi.org/10.1038/npp.2015.230.

51. Martinotti G, Montemitro C, Baroni G, et al. Relationship between craving and plasma leptin concentrations in patients with cocaine addiction. *Psychoneuroendocrinology.* 2017;85:35−41.

52. Ypsilantis P, Politou M, Anagnostopoulos C, et al. Effects of cigarette smoke exposure and its cessation on body weight, food intake and circulating leptin, and ghrelin levels in the rat. *Nicotine Tob Res.* 2013;15(1):206−212. https://doi.org/10.1093/ntr/nts113.

53. Kroemer NB, Wuttig F, Bidlingmaier M, Zimmermann US, Smolka MN. Nicotine enhances modulation of food-cue reactivity by leptin and ghrelin in the ventromedial prefrontal cortex. *Addict Biol.* 2015;20(4):832−844. https://doi.org/10.1111/adb.12167.

54. Lee H, Joe KH, Kim W, et al. Increased leptin and decreased ghrelin level after smoking cessation. *Neurosci Lett.* 2006;409(1):47−51. https://doi.org/10.1016/j.neulet.2006.09.013.

55. Al'Absi M, Hooker S, Fujiwara K, et al. Circulating leptin levels are associated with increased craving to smoke in abstinent smokers. *Pharmacol Biochem Behav.* 2011;97:509−513. https://doi.org/10.1016/j.pbb.2010.10.004.

56. Housova J, Wilczek H, Haluzik MM, Kremen J, Krizova J, Haluzik M. Adipocyte derived hormones in heroin addicts: the influence of methadone maintenance treatment. *Physiol Res.* 2005;54:73−78.

57. Engel JA, Jerlhag E. Role of appetite-regulating peptides in the pathophysiology of addiction: implications for pharmacotherapy. *CNS Drugs.* 2014;28:875−886. https://doi.org/10.1007/s40263-014-0178-y.

58. Egecioglu E, Steensland P, Fredriksson I, et al. The glucagon-like peptide 1 analogue exendin-4 attenuates alcohol mediated behaviors in rodents. *Psychoneuroendocrinology.* 2013;38(8):1259−1270, 113.

59. Shirazi RH, Dickson SL, Skibicka KP. Gut peptide GLP-1 and its analogue, exendin-4, decrease alcohol intake and reward. *PLoS One.* 2013;8(4):e61965.

60. Sorensen G, Caine SB, Thomsen M. Effects of the GLP-1 agonist Exendin-4 on intravenous ethanol self-administration in mice. *Alcohol Clin Exp Res.* 2016;40(10):2247−2252. https://doi.org/10.1111/acer.13199 [Epub 2016 Aug 31].

61. Vallöf D, Maccioni P, Colombo G, et al. The glucagon-like peptide 1 receptor agonist liraglutide attenuates the reinforcing properties of alcohol in rodents. *Addict Biol.* 2016;21:422−437.

62. Thomsen M, Dencker D, Wörtwein G, et al. The glucagon-like peptide 1 receptor agonist Exendin-4 decreases relapse-like drinking in socially housed mice Pharmacology. *Biochem Behav.* 2017;160:14−20.

63. Davis JF, Schurdak JD, Magrisso IJ, et al. Gastric bypass surgery attenuates ethanol consumption in ethanol-preferring rats. *Biol Psychiatry.* 2012;72(5):354−360.

64. Suchankova P, Yan J, Schwandt ML, et al. The glucagon-like peptide-1 receptor as a potential treatment target in alcohol use disorder: evidence from human genetic association studies and a mouse model of alcohol dependence. *Transl Psychiatry*. 2015;5:e583. https://doi.org/10.1038/tp.2015.68.

65. Graham DL, Erreger K, Galli A, et al. GLP-1 analog attenuates cocaine reward. *Mol Psychiatry*. 2013;18(9):961–962.

66. Erreger K, Davis AR, Poe AM, et al. Exendin-4 decreases amphetamine-induced locomotor activity. *Physiol Behav*. 2012;106(4):574–578.

67. Egecioglu E, Engel JA, Jerlhag E. The glucagon-like peptide 1 analogue, exendin-4, attenuates the rewarding properties of psychostimulant drugs in mice. *PLoS One*. 2013;8(7):e69010.

68. Sorensen G, Reddy IA, Weikop P, et al. A. The glucagon-like peptide 1 (GLP-1) receptor agonist exendin-4 reduces cocaine self-administration in mice. *Physiol Behav*. 2015;149:262–268.

69. Bouhlal S, Ellefsen KN, Sheskier MB, et al. Acute effects of intravenous cocaine administration on serum concentrations of ghrelin, amylin, glucagon-like peptide-1, insulin, leptin and peptide YY and relationships with cardiorespiratory and subjective responses. *Drug Alcohol Depend*. 2017;180:68–75.

70. Egecioglu E, Engel JA, Jerlhag E. The glucagon-like peptide 1 analogue exendin-4 attenuates the nicotine-induced locomotor stimulation, accumbal dopamine release, conditioned place preference as well as the expression of locomotor sensitization in mice. *PLoS One*. 2013;8(10):e77284.

71. Edwards S, Koob GF. Neurobiology of dysregulated motivational systems in drug addiction. *Future Neurol*. 2010;5:393–401.

72. Kovács GL. The role of atrial natriuretic peptide in alcohol withdrawal: a peripheral indicator and central modulator? *Eur J Pharmacol*. 2000;405:103–112.

73. Doring WKH, Herzenstiel M-N, Krampe H, et al. Persistent alterations of vasopressin and N-terminal proatrial natriuretic peptide plasma levels in long-term abstinent alcoholics. *Alcohol Clin Exp Res*. 2003;27:849–861.

74. Leggio L, Ferrulli A, Cardone S, et al. Renin and aldosterone but not the natriuretic peptide correlate with obsessive craving in medium-term abstinent alcohol-dependent patients: a longitudinal study. *Alcohol*. 2008;42:375–381.

75. Bezzegh A, Nyuli L, Kovács GL. α-Atrial natriuretic peptide, aldosterone secretion and plasma renin activity during ethanol withdrawal: a correlation with the onset of delirium tremens? *Alcohol*. 1991;8:333–336.

76. Hillemacher T. Volume intake and craving in alcohol withdrawal. *Alcohol Alcohol*. 2006;41:61–65.

77. Aoun EG, Jimenez VA, Vendruscolo LF, et al. A relationship between the aldosterone-mineralocorticoid receptor pathway and alcohol drinking: preliminary translational findings across rats, monkeys and humans. *Mol Psychiatry*. May 2, 2017. https://doi.org/10.1038/mp.2017.97 [Epub ahead of print].

78. Kiefer F, Wiedemann K. Neuroendocrine pathways of addictive behaviour. *Addict Biol*. 2004;9(3–4):205–212.

79. Fox HC, et al. Stress-induced and alcohol cue-induced craving in recently abstinent alcohol dependent individuals. *Alcohol Clin Exp Res*. 2007;31:395–403.

80. Hyman SM, et al. Stress and drug-cue-induced craving in opioid-dependent individuals in naltrexone treatment. *Exp Clin Psychopharmacol*. 2007;15:134–143 [PubMed: 17469937].

81. Sinha R. Chronic stress, drug use, and vulnerability to addiction. *Ann NY Acad Sci*. 2008;1141:105–130. https://doi.org/10.1196/annals.1441.030.

82. Lemieux AM, Al'Absi M. Stress psychobiology in the context of addiction medicine: from drugs of abuse to behavioral addictions. *Prog Brain Res*. 2016;223:43–62. https://doi.org/10.1016/bs.pbr.2015.08.001. Epub 2015 Nov 24.

83. Boyson CO, Holly EN, Shimamoto A, et al. Social stress and CRF-dopamine interactions in the VTA: role in long-term escalation of cocaine self-administration. *J Neurosci*. 2014;34:6659–6667.

84. Higley AE, Crane NA, Spadoni AD, Quello SB, Goodell V, Mason BJ. Craving in response to stress induction in a human laboratory paradigm predicts treatment outcome in alcohol-dependent individuals. *Psychopharmacol Berl*. 2011;218:121–129.

85. Ehrenreich H, et al. Endocrine and hemodynamic effects of stress versus systemic CRF in alcoholics during early and medium term abstinence. *Alcohol Clin Exp Res*. 1997;21:1285–1293.

86. Adinoff B, et al. Hypothalamic-pituitary-adrenal axis functioning and cerebrospinal fluid corticotropin releasing hormone and corticotropin levels in alcoholics after recent and long-term abstinence. *Arch Gen Psychiatry*. 1990;47:325–330.

87. Ingjaldsson JT, Laberg JC, Thayer JF. Reduced heart rate variability in chronic alcohol abuse: relationship with negative mood, chronic thought suppression, and compulsive drinking. *Biol Psychiatry*. 2003;54:1427–1436.

88. Adinoff B, et al. Suppression of the HPA axis stress-response: implications for relapse. *Alcohol Clin Exp Res*. 2005;29:1351–1355.

89. Lovallo WR, et al. Blunted stress cortisol response in abstinent alcoholic and polysubstance abusing men. *Alcohol Clin Exp Res*. 2000;24:651–658.

90. Sinha R, et al. Enhanced negative emotion and alcohol craving, and altered physiological responses following stress and cue exposure in alcohol dependent individuals. *Neuropsychophamacol*. 2008.

91. Junghanns K, Backhaus J, Tietz U. Impaired serum cortisol stress response is a predictor of early relapse. *Alcohol Alcohol*. 2003;38:189–193.

92. Brady KT, et al. Cold pressor task reactivity: predictors of alcohol use among alcohol-dependent individuals with and without comorbid posttraumatic stress disorder. *Alcohol Clin Exp Res*. 2006;30:938–946 [PubMed: 16737451].

93. Breese GR, et al. Stress enhancement of craving during sobriety and the risk of relapse. *Alcohol Clin Exp Res.* 2005;29:185–195.

94. Cooney NL, et al. Alcohol cue reactivity, negative-mood reactivity, and relapse in treated alcoholic men. *J Abnorm Psychol.* 1997;106:243–250 [PubMed: 9131844].

95. Marinelli M, et al. Corticosterone circadian secretion differentially facilitates dopamine-mediated psychomotor effect of cocaine and morphine. *J Neurosci.* 1994;14: 2724–2731.

96. Deroche-Gamonet V, et al. The glucocorticoid receptor as a potential target to reduce cocaine abuse. *J Neurosci.* 2003;23:4785–4790.

97. Hamidovic A, Childs E, Conrad M, King A, de Wit H. Stress-induced changes in mood and cortisol release predict mood effects of amphetamine. *Drug Alcohol Depend.* 2010;109:175–180.

98. Wand GS, et al. Association of amphetamine-induced striatal dopamine release and cortisol responses to psychological stress. *Neuropsychopharmacology.* 2007;32: 2310–2320.

99. Mantsch JR, et al. Daily cocaine self-administration under long-access conditions augments restraint-induced increases in plasma corticosterone and impairs glucocorticoid receptor-mediated negative feedback in rats. *Brain Res.* 2007;1167:101–111.

100. Mello NK, Mendelson JH. Cocaine's effects on neuroendocrine systems: clinical and preclinical studies. *Pharmacol Biochem Behav.* 1997;57:571–599.

101. Vescovi PP, et al. Diurnal variations in plasma ACTH, cortisol and beta-endorphin levels in cocaine addicts. *Horm Res.* 1992;37:221–224.

102. Sinha R, et al. Stress-induced cocaine craving and hypothalamic-pituitary-adrenal responses are predictive of cocaine relapse outcomes. *Arch Gen Psychiatry.* 2006; 63:324–331.

103. Mendelson JH, et al. Effects of low- and high-nicotine cigarette smoking on mood states and the HPA axis in men. *Neuropsychopharmacology.* 2005;30:1751–1763.

104. Tsuda A, et al. Cigarette smoking and psychophysiological stress responsiveness: effects of recent smoking and temporary abstinence. *Psychopharmacology.* 1996;126: 226–233.

105. Al'absi M, Hatsukami DK, Davis G. Attenuated adrenocorticotropic responses to Psychological stress are associated with early smoking relapse. *Psychopharmacol (Berl).* 2005;181:107–117.

106. Badrick E, Kirschbaum C, Kumari M. The relationship between smoking status and cortisol secretion. *J Clin Endocrinol Metab.* 2007;92:819–824.

107. Marinelli M, et al. Dopamine-dependent responses to morphine depend on glucocorticoid receptors. *Proc Natl Acad Sci USA.* 1998;95:7742–7747.

108. Fatseas M, Denis C, Massida Z, Verger M, Franques-Reneric P, Auriacombe M. Cue-induced reactivity, cortisol response and substance use outcome in treated heroin dependent individuals. *Biol Psychiatr.* 2011; 70(8):720–727.

109. Ho WKK, et al. Comparison of plasma hormonal levels between heroin-addicted and normal subjects. *Clin Chim Acta.* 1977;75:415–419.

110. Facchinetti F, et al. Hypothalamic-pituitary-adrenal axis of heroin addicts. *Drug Alcohol Depend.* 1985;15: 361–366.

111. Schluger JH, et al. Altered HPA axis responsivity to metyrapone testing in methadone maintained former heroin addicts with ongoing cocaine addiction. *Neuropsychopharmacology.* 2001;24:568–575.

112. Fox HC, Tuit KL, Sinha R. Stress system changes associated with marijuana dependence may increase craving for alcohol and cocaine. *Hum Psychopharmacol.* 2013;28: 40–53.

113. Becker JB, Koob GF. Sex differences in animal models: focus on addiction. *Pharmacol Rev.* 2016;68:242–263.

114. Lynch WJ, Taylor JR. Sex differences in the behavioral effects of 24-h access to cocaine under a discrete trial procedure. *Neuropsychopharmacology.* 2004;29:943–951.

115. Roth ME, Cosgrove KP, Carroll ME. Sex differences in the vulnerability to drug abuse: a review of preclinical studies. *Neurosci Biobehav Rev.* 2004;28:533–546.

116. Lancaster FE, Spiegel KS. Sex differences in pattern drinking. *Alcohol.* 1992;9:415–420.

117. Torres OV, Walker EM, Beas BS, O'Dell LE. Female rats display enhanced rewarding effects of ethanol that are hormone dependent. *Alcohol Clin Exp Res.* 2014;38: 108–115.

118. Carroll ME, Anker JJ. Sex differences and ovarian hormones in animal models of drug dependence. *Horm Behav.* 2010:44–56.

119. Becker JB, Hu M. Sex differences in drug abuse. *Front Neuroendocrinol.* 2008:36–47.

120. Moran-Santa Maria MM, Flanagan J, Brady K. Ovarian hormones and drug abuse. *Curr Psychiatry Rep.* 2014; 16(11):511.

121. Martinez LA, et al. Estradiol facilitation of cocaine-induced locomotor sensitization in female rats requires activation of mGluR5. *Behav Brain Res.* 2014;271:39–42.

122. Lynch WJ, Taylor JR. Decreased motivation following cocaine self-administration under extended access conditions: effects of sex and ovarian hormones. *Neuropsychopharmacology.* 2005;30:927–935.

123. Lynch WJ, Roth ME, Mickelberg JL, Carroll ME. Role of estrogen in the acquisition of intravenously self-administered cocaine in female rats. *Pharmacol Biochem Behav.* 2001;68:641–646.

124. Mermelstein PG, Becker DJ. Estradiol reduces calcium currents in rat neostriatal neurons through a membrane receptor. *J Neurosci.* 1996;16:595–604.

125. Lynch WJ, Sofuoglu M. Role of progesterone in nicotine addiction: evidence from initiation to relapse. *Exp Clin Psychopharmacol.* 2010;18(6):451–461.

126. Goletiani NV, Siegel AJ, Lukas SE, Hudson JI. The effects of smoked nicotine on measures of subjective states and hypothalamic-pituitary-adrenal axis hormones in women during the follicular and luteal phases of the menstrual cycle. *J Addict Med.* 2015;9:195–203.

127. Allen AM, Lunos S, Heishman SJ, al'Absi M, Hatsukami D, Allen SS. Subjective response to nicotine by menstrual phase. *Addict Behav.* 2015;43:50−53.

128. Allen SS, Bade T, Center B, Finstad D, Hatsukami D. Menstrual phase effects on smoking relapse. *Addiction.* 2008; 103:809−821.

129. Sofuoglu M, Mouratidis M, Mooney M. Progesterone improves cognitive performance and attenuates smoking urges in abstinent smokers. *Psychoneuroendocrinology.* 2011;36(1):123−132.

130. Jackson LR, Robinson TE, Becker JB. Sex differences and hormonal influences on acquisition of cocaine self-administration in rats. *Neuropsychopharmacology.* 2006; 31:129−138.

131. Kennedy AP, Epstein DH, Phillips KA, Preston KL. Sex differences in cocaine/heroin users: drug use triggers and carving in daily life. *Drug Alcohol Depend.* 2013;132: 29−37.

132. White FJ. A behavioral/systems approach to the neuroscience of drug addiction. *J Neurosci.* 2002;22: 3303−3305.

133. Sinha R, Folx H, Hong KI, Sofuoglu M, Morgan PT, Berquist KT. Sex steroid hormones, stress response, and drug carving in cocaine-dependent women: implications for relapse susceptibility. *Exp Clin Psychopharmacol.* 2007; 15:445−452.

134. Fox HC, et al. The effects of exogenous progesterone on drug craving and stress arousal in cocaine dependence: impact of gender and cue type. *Psychoneuroendocrinology.* 2013;38(9):1532−1544.

135. Sofuoglu M, et al. Progesterone effects on cocaine use in male cocaine users maintained on methadone: a randomized, double blind, pilot study. *Exp Clin Psychopharmacol.* 2007;15(5):453−460.

136. Sharma AN, Chopde AT, Hirani K, Kokare DM, Ugage RR. Chronic progesterone treatment augments while dehydroepiandrosterone sulphate prevents tolerance to ethanol anxiolysis and withdrawal anxiety in rats. *Eur J Pharmacol.* 2007;567:211−212.

137. Anker JJ, Holtz NA, Zlebnik N, Carroll ME. Effects of allopregnanolone on the reinstatement of cocaine-seeking behavior in male and female rats. *Psychopharmacology.* 2009;203:63−72.

138. Milivojevic V, Fox HC, Sofuoglu M, Covault J, Sinha R. Effects of progesterone stimulated allopregnanolone on craving and stress response in cocaine dependent men and women. *Psychoneuroendocrinology.* 2016;65:44−53.

139. Frye CA. The neurosteroid 3alpha,5alpha-THP has anti-seizure and possible neuroprotective effects in an animal model of epilepsy. *Brain Res.* 1995;696:113−120.

140. Tanchuck-Nipper MA, Ford MM, Hertzberg A, Beadles-Bohling A, Cozzoli DK, Finn DA. Sex differences in ethanol's anxiolytic effect and chronic ethanol withdrawal sensitivity in mice with a null mutation of the 5alpha-reductase type 1 gene. *Behav Genet.* 2015;45:354−367.

141. Finn DA, Beadles-Bohling AS, Beckley EH, et al. A new look at the 5alpha-reductase inhibitor finasteride. *CNS Drug Rev.* 2006;12(1):53−76.

142. Morrow AL, VanDoren MJ, Penland SN, Matthews DB. The role of GABAergic neuroactive steroids in ethanol action, tolerance and dependence. *Brain Res Rev.* 2001; 37:98−109.

143. Milivojevic V, Kranzler HR, Gelernter J, Burian L, Covault J. Variation in genes encoding the neuroactive steroid synthetic enzymes 5alpha-reductase type 1 and 3alpha-reductase type 2 is associated with alcohol dependence. *Alcohol Clin Exp Res.* 2011;35(5):946−952.

144. Milivojevic V, Feinn R, Kranzler HR, Covault J. Variation in AKR1C3, which encodes the neuroactive steroid synthetic enzyme 3alpha-HSD Type 2 (17beta-HSD Type 5), moderates the subjective effects of alcohol. *Psychopharmacol (Berl).* 2014;231(17):3597−3608.

145. Ray LA, Hutchinson KE, Ashenhurst JR, Morrow AL. Naltrexone selectively elevates GABAergic neuroactive steroid levels in heavy drinkers with the ASP40 Allele of the OPRM1 gene: a pilot investigation. *Alcohol Clin Exp Res.* 2010;34(8):1479−1487.

146. Nishino S. The hypocretin/orexin system in health and disease. *Biol Psychiatry.* 2003;54:87−95.

147. Schmidt KA, Ho A, Frye MA, Choi DS. Association of plasma orexin A and ethanol-drinking behaviors in pregnant rats. *J Alcohol Drug Depend.* 2016;4(5):1−6.

148. Mahler SV, Smith RJ, Moorman DE, Sartor GC, Aston-Jones G. Multiple roles for orexin/hypocretin in addiction. *Prog Brain Res.* 2012;198:79−121.

149. Schmeichel BE, Barbier E, Misra KK, et al. Hypocretin receptor 2 antagonism dose-dependently reduces escalated heroin self administration in rats. *Neuropsychopharmacology.* 2015;40(5):1123−1129.

150. Ubaldi M, Cannella N, Ciccocioppo R. Emerging targets for addiction neuropharmacology; from mechanisms to therapeutics. *Prog Brain Res.* 2016;224:251−284.

151. Bayerlein K, Kraus T, Leinonen I, et al. Orexin A expression and promoter methylation in patients with alcohol dependence comparing acute and protracted withdrawal. *Alcohol.* 2011;45:541−547.

152. Olney JJ, Navarro M, Thiele TE. Binge-like consumption of ethanol and other salient reinforcers is blocked by orexin-1 receptor inhibition and leads to a reduction of hypothalamic orexin immunoreactivity. *Alcohol Clin Exp Res.* 2015;39:21−29.

153. Carvajal F, Alcaraz-Iborra M, Lerma-Cabrera JM, Valor LM, de la Fuente L, et al. Orexin receptor 1 signaling contributes to ethanol binge-like drinking: pharmacological and molecular evidence. *Behav Brain Res.* 2015;287: 230−237.

154. Moorman DE, James MH, Kilroy EA, Aston-Jones G. Orexin/hypocretin-1 receptor antagonism reduces ethanol self-administration and reinstatement selectively in highly-motivated rats. *Brain Res.* 2017;1654:34−42.

155. Flores A, Maldonado R, Berrendero F. The hypocretin/orexin receptor-1 as a novel target to modulate cannabinoid reward. *Biol Psychiatry.* 2014;75:499−507.

156. Koob GF, Mason BJ. Existing and future drugs for the treatment of the dark side of addiction. *Annu Rev Pharmacol Toxicol.* 2016;56:299−322.

157. Georgescu D, Zachariou V, Barrot M, et al. Involvement of the lateral hypothalamic peptide orexin in morphine dependence and withdrawal. *J Neurosci*. 2003;23(8): 3106−3111.

158. Chou TC, Lee CE, Lu J, et al. Orexin (hypocretin) neurons contain dynorphin. *J Neurosci*. 2001:RC168, 1−6.

159. Gentile TA, Simmons SJ, Barker DJ, Shaw JK, Espana RA, Muschamp JW. Suvorexant, an orexin/hypocretin receptor antagonist, attenuates motivational and hedonic properties of cocaine. *Addict Biol*. 2017:1−9.

160. Schmidt KA, Kolla BP. Understanding and addressing sleep disruptions in alcohol use disorders. *Psychiatr Times*. 2017:1−3.

161. Cruz HG, Hoever P, Chakraborty B, Schoedel K, Sellers EM, Dingemanse J. Assessment of the abuse liability of a dual orexin receptor antagonist: a crossover study of almorexant and zolpidem in recreational drug users. *CNS Drugs*. 2014;28:361−372.

162. Nishiwaza D, Kasai S, Hasegawa J, et al. Associations between the orexin (hypocretin) receptor 2 gene polymorphism Val3081le and nicotine dependence in genome-wide and subsequent association studies. *Mol Brain*. 2015;8(50):1−17.

163. Buisman-Pijlman FT, Sumracki NM, Gordon JJ, Hull PR, Carter CS, Tops M. Individual differences underlying susceptibility to addiction: role for the endogenous oxytocin system. *Pharmacol Biochem Behav*. 2014;119:22−38.

163a. McGregor IS, Callaghan PD, Hunt GE. From ultrasocial to antisocial: a role for oxytocin in the acute reinforcing effects and long-term adverse consequences of drug use? *Br J Pharmacol*. 2008;154(2):358−368.

164. McGregor IS, Bowen MT. Breaking the loop: oxytocin as a potential treatment for drug addiction. *Horm Behav*. 2012;61:331−339.

165. Vaht M, Kurrikoff T, Laas K, Veidebaum T, Harro J. Oxytocin receptor gene variation rs53576 and alcohol abuse in a longitudinal population representative study. *Psychoneuroendocrinology*. 2016;74:333−341.

166. Sala M, Braida D, Lentini D, et al. Pharmacologic rescue of impaired cognitive flexibility, social deficits, increased aggression, and seizure susceptibility in oxytocin receptor null mice: a neurobehavioral model of autism. *Biol Psychiatry*. 2011;69:875−882.

167. Lee PR, Brady DL, Shapiro RA, dorsa DM, Koenig JI. Social interaction deficits caused by chronic phencyclidine administration are reversed by oxytocin. *Neuropsychopharmacology*. 2005;30:1883−1894.

168. Liu Y, Young KA, Curtis JT, Aragona BJ, Wang Z. Social bonding decreases the rewarding properties of amphetamine through a dopamine D1 receptor mechanism. *J Neurosci*. 2011;31:7960−7966.

169. Young KA, Liu Y, Wang Z. The neurobiology of social attachment: a comparative approach to behavioral, neuroanatomical, and neurochemical studies. *Comp Biochem Physiol C Toxicol Pharmacol*. 2008;148(4): 401−410.

170. Kim S, Kwok S, Mayes LC, Potenza MN, Rutherford HJ, Strathearn L. Early adverse experience and substance addiction: dopamine, oxytocin, and glucocorticoid pathways. *Ann NY Acad Sci*. 2017;1394:74−91.

171. Flanagan JC, Baker NL, McRae-Clark AL, Brady KT, Moran-Santa Maria MM. Effects of adverse childhood experiences on the association between intranasal oxytocin and social stress reactivity among individuals with cocaine dependence. *Psychiatry Res*. 2015;229(0): 94−100.

172. Lee MR, Glassman M, King-Casas B, et al. Complexity of oxytocin's effects in a chronic cocaine dependent population. *Eur Neuropsychopharmacol*. 2014;24(9): 1483−1491.

173. Bowen MT, Neumann ID. The multidimensional therapeutic potential of targeting the brain oxytocin system for the treatment of substance use disorders. *Curr Top Behav Neurosci*. 2017:1−19.

174. McRae-Clark AL, Baker NL, Moran-Santa Maria M, Brady KT. Effect of oxytocin on craving and stress response in marijuana-dependent individuals: a pilot study. *Psychopharmacol Berl*. 2013;228(4):623−631.

175. Pedersen CA, Smedley KL, Leserman J, et al. Intranasal oxytocin blocks alcohol withdrawal in human subjects. *Alcohol Clin Exp Res*. 2013;37(3):484−489.

176. Peters ST, Bowen MT, Bohrer K, McGregor IS, Neumann ID. Oxytocin inhibits ethanol consumption and ethanol-induced dopamine release in the nucleus accumbens. *Addict Biol*. 2016;22:702−711.

177. Kovacs GL, Sarnyai Z, Szabo G. Oxytocin and addiction: a review. *Psychoneuroendocrinology*. 1998;23:945−962.

178. Woolley JD, Arcuni PA, Stauffer CS, et al. The effects of intranasal oxytocin in opioid-dependent individuals and healthy control subjects: a pilot study. *Psychopharmacology*. 2016;233:2571−2580.

179. Bershad AK, Weafer JJ, Kirkpatrick MG, Wardle MC, Miller MA, de Wit H. Oxytocin receptor gene variation predicts subjective responses to MDMA. *Soc Neurosci*. 2016;11(6):592−599.

FURTHER READING

1. Reddy DS, Kulkarni SK. Chronic neurosteroid treatment prevents the development of morphine tolerance and attenuates abstinence behavior in mice. *Eur J Pharmacol*. 1997; 337:19−25.

2. Reddy DS, Kulkarni SK. Neurosteroid coadministration prevents development of tolerance and augments recovery from benzodiazepine withdrawal anxiety and hyperactivity in mice. *Meth Find Exp Clin Pharmacol*. 1997;19: 395−405.

CHAPTER 5

Technological Innovations in Addiction Treatment

ALAN J. BUDNEY, PHD • JACOB T. BORODOVSKY, PHD • LISA A. MARSCH, PHD • SARAH E. LORD, PHD

Just for fun, check out the last five to ten years of *"10 Breakthrough Technologies"* published in the MIT Technology Review.[1] In most years, well over half of the discoveries in each list have clear relevance to health and health care or are communication, connectivity, and computational advances. If you allow yourself to imagine how some of these technological advances might be applied to advance the health of persons suffering from various medical conditions, including addictions and other mental disorders, the possibilities abound, and exponential progress toward reducing harm from these conditions may seem within reach. A large number of innovative applications of digital technology are now permeating the world of healthcare with the goals of improving health, extending the reach of health care, and reducing the cost of providing care.

So, why is this so important and why should this excite you? Don't we already have effective ways to identify and treat substance use disorders (SUDs) and systems designed to provide such care? Yes, we have pharmacological and behavioral interventions, and health care providers to deliver them; however, there are substantial limitations. Controlled studies show that the short- and long-term response rates for the most efficacious interventions remain well under 50% and are even lower for many SUDs.[2,3] This may be because evidence-based interventions are either not readily available, not being used by providers or are not of interest to individuals with SUDs. Only 10%–20% of those with substance-use-related problems report receiving any treatment in the past year.[4] Each of these issues must be better addressed to effectively confront the problems associated with SUDs.

Over the last 25 years, scientists in the field of addiction science have studied how to enhance outcomes, how to improve the dissemination and implementation of efficacious treatments, and how to reach a greater proportion of the population experiencing SUD.

Barriers have included substandard screening for and identification of cases, limited trained personnel, the burden associated with training, poor fidelity and integrity of treatment delivery, low pay for providers, high cost to deliver the most effective interventions, difficulty in self-identifying as a person with an SUD, stigma and burden associated with seeking treatment, and lack of individualization and personalization of treatment.

The healthcare field has integrated advances in digital technology at an escalating pace to improve health behavior, healthcare delivery, and cost-effectiveness. This new area of science is often referred to as "digital health"[5,6] and includes advancements in the ways mobile communications and sensing devices, software development, cloud computing, and data analytics enhance the patient experience. The progress being made in digital health offers multiple pathways that can help overcome the existing limitations to providing optimal care to patients with SUDs. This chapter will illustrate the ways in which principles and practices from this exciting new field are being tested and applied to enhance treatment for SUD. This chapter will also explore several issues that we expect will need to be addressed to maximize the opportunities offered by digital health, some of which are similar to the barriers that have impeded dissemination and implementation of evidence-based, novel interventions for behavioral health care throughout the years (Table 5.1).

HOW CAN DIGITAL TECHNOLOGY ENHANCE CARE FOR SUDS?

Global access to digital technology has grown exponentially over the past 10 years, with some estimates suggesting that 90% of the world's population will have a mobile device by the 2020s.[7] Of great importance to health care—and to SUD and psychiatric care in particular—is that even the most vulnerable,

The Assessment and Treatment of Addiction. https://doi.org/10.1016/B978-0-323-54856-4.00005-5

TABLE 5.1
Putative Benefits of Digital Health Applications for Substance Use Disorders (SUD)

1. Facilitate greater and easier access to treatment
   a. not dependent on therapist availability
   b. can reach people with difficulties accessing in-person treatment
   c. can readily provide treatment in non-SUD specialty-care settings (e.g., Primary Care)
2. Increase access to therapeutic materials
   a. anytime/anywhere, on-demand availability via the internet
3. Enhance learning of therapeutic information and coping skills
   a. engage effective learning technologies
4. Facilitate monitoring of target behavior
   a. promote self-awareness and progress
   b. facilitate contingency management interventions
5. Improve integrity and fidelity of treatment delivery of evidence-based treatment
   a. digital delivery of active components eliminates human variability in delivery of interventions
   b. can be used in the format under which it was scientifically evaluated
6. Promote easier and more rapid dissemination of evidence-based treatments
7. Reduce cost and efficiency of treatment delivery in clinic settings
   a. reduce therapist time by digitally delivering some treatment components
   b. optimize clinical resource allocation by better utilizing unique therapist skills
   c. ease the burden and time associated with therapist training
   d. provide care to more people in need
8. Prompt use of therapeutic skills between clinic visits and post-treatment
9. Increase access to social support through various social media platforms
10. Enhance motivation through automated or scheduled text messaging
11. More easily personalize interventions to meet the individuals' needs
12. Empower individuals to take charge of their care
    a. to pursue change on their own
    b. to control when and how one chooses to work on their problems
    c. provide increased control over the content of the care received

Adapted from Budney AJ, Stanger C, Tilford JM, et al. Computer-assisted behavioral therapy and contingency management for cannabis use disorder. *Psychol Addict Behav*. 2015;29(3):501–511. https://doi.org/10.1037/adb0000078.

disadvantaged and underserved populations have high rates of access to personal digital technology devices.[8–12] If effective health care can be delivered via digital health applications, such ubiquitous availability of these devices can facilitate access to care that is potentially much less burdensome to obtain (e.g., access from home), more available (e.g., received at any time of day), and less costly (e.g., provider costs reduced). Moreover, digital health tools can offer methods for engaging individuals more fully in their own health care through interactive monitoring and prompting of health behaviors in real time throughout the day when many of the most important health-related choices are made (e.g., food and drink consumption, exercise activities, medication adherence, stress management, alcohol or drug use). Individualized and daily engagement with intervention plans and actions holds promise for enhanced outcomes. Some data even suggest that interaction with a digital health device rather than with a healthcare worker may increase willingness to identify and address highly sensitive issues such as substance use, risky sexual behaviors or diseases, and other mental disorders.[13–15] Digital tools could be readily available to all persons with access to digital devices and could effectively address the tremendous health disparities disadvantaged populations face worldwide with regard to access to quality care.

Digital health offers multiple potential benefits not only for the individual, but for the healthcare provider as well. Digital interventions offer greater availability of and access to evidence-based interventions in the clinic or the patient's home. For clinicians, digital screening and electronic health record (EHR) systems can provide more effective and efficient means for identifying problems, communicating within and across provider systems, and coordinating care. Moreover, digital delivery holds promise for addressing potential diminished efficacy of treatments due to the use of nonevidence-based interventions or failure to deliver evidence-based interventions with high fidelity.[16,17] Utilizing digital health interventions could also greatly lower the cost of SUD treatment by reducing the time and costs associated with training personnel and delivery of effective care (e.g., Refs. 18, 19). Furthermore, technology-delivered treatment models may facilitate and expedite integration of scientific discoveries and treatment innovations, resulting in continuous enhancement of health outcomes (i.e., quality improvement).

Several articles and book chapters have explored actual and conceivable benefits of digital health and reviewed outcomes from pilot studies and controlled trials of specific digital interventions.[19–23] Below, we first expound on the potential benefits of digital technology for SUD care and the multitude of clinical settings that can benefit. This discussion is followed by a brief synthesis of what the research to date has revealed about the efficacy of digital health applications in this area. We then provide examples of a few select types of digital interventions for SUDs to illustrate the progress being made and the breadth of their potential future impact. Last, we discuss challenges and barriers to adoption and implementation of the digital health applications in the SUD field.

Advantages and Value of Digital Health Technologies for SUDs

Perhaps the most obvious and important impact of digital technology on SUD is its potential to greatly extend access to evidence-based interventions. The availability of SUD treatment, state-of-the-art science-based interventions in particular, is generally poor across all segments of society and even more so in rural or disadvantaged populations and developing countries.[16,24,25] However, mobile phone and internet access is ubiquitous even among some of the most disadvantaged and remote populations.[9,10,12,26] The ability to deliver efficacious SUD interventions remotely could decrease the number of persons in need of SUD services and sharply reduce health disparities.

In addition to increased access, digital interventions hold promise for enhancing the quality of care that is delivered. Removing the human element should theoretically improve the fidelity and integrity of delivery of evidence-based care, as treatment delivered in community settings may not align closely with how the intervention was designed and thus may lose efficacy. In contrast, a digital program that has been tested in a controlled setting could be installed and made available to the patient in a format that better maintains the fidelity of the intervention.

Digital interventions allow patients the flexibility to engage with an intervention (receive care) at their convenience, potentially increasing their engagement with and commitment to their own care. Anytime access to digital interventions could facilitate opportunities for patients to expedite or enhance the learning and practice of the coping skills often involved in SUD interventions. Additionally, empirically based learning methods (e.g., fluency learning) that can be programmed into such interventions could further enhance mastery of coping skills.[27,28] Offering patients the option to access care in the home environment may reduce inconsistencies in service delivery stemming from factors such as missed appointments, clinic closures, lack of transportation, or stigma.

Much attention has recently turned to the potential for "just-in-time" interventions using digital therapeutics.[29] Research on what is being called just-in-time adaptive interventions (JITAI) is beginning to provide data on how this exciting new area of innovation in digital health may enhance treatment outcomes for SUD.[29] JITAI models aim to leverage personal sensing technology in addition to digital mobile devices and programming to provide the right type of therapeutic assistance at the time it is most needed. Automated information about an individual's personal environment obtained via mobile sensors (e.g., from a watch or phone) or automated self-reported assessments via programmed ecological momentary assessment programs are being used to identify emotional states and environmental contexts that are high risk for substance use or relapse.[27,30] The assessment then triggers an automated digital intervention or prompts the user to engage a coping skill.

Digital therapeutics have the potential to foster highly individualized or personalized care that can respond to an individual's profile of needs, preferences, culture, cognitive functioning, stage of recovery, and clinical trajectory over time. Individuals can control the pace of their treatment, and programming can readily facilitate patient choice of intervention topics, amount of practice, repetition or return to a desired topic, self-monitoring and assessment, re-examination and modification of goals, and ignoring of irrelevant topics or exercises.

Digital technology can enhance screening processes, standardization of assessment, accuracy of personal data collection, and potentially enhance assessment by extending it to the individual's environment. Most recently, digital screening models have proven helpful in increasing the efficiency and accuracy of identifying those who might benefit from SUD interventions when employed in primary care, emergency departments, pediatrics, and other non-SUD healthcare settings.[31-35] Many of these systems have also used technology to more efficiently communicate screening results to providers. Systematic assessment of SUDs conducted on mobile devices or personal computers that are either patient-administered or used to guide healthcare workers can increase the probability of an SUD assessment being performed, and improve reliability and accuracy of the identification of SUDs. Digital assessment of substance use, behavior, and personal functioning in the patient's environment over time can improve accuracy and self-awareness of important treatment process variables such as identification of emotional or environmental triggers for use, or temporal relationships between substance use and positive and negative mood or consequences.

By reducing the need for SUD specialists, digital interventions and assessment platforms can extend the possibility and probability of offering care in non-SUD specialty settings such as primary care, schools, the emergency room, and pediatrics. Stand-alone, self-help SUD digital interventions can further extend care by allowing access to anyone at any time via the internet. Evidence-based self-help may be a good alternative for those who are reluctant to seek out professional help due to stigma, cost, or logistical challenges.

Finally, digital interventions may also be combined with traditional clinician-delivered care to enhance outcomes, increase efficiency, provide clinician training, and increase treatment capacity in community SUD specialty clinics. When combined with standard psychosocial approaches, digital interventions can contribute to improved outcomes by delivering essential treatment components, such as coping skills.[36,37] These interventions can also address the large shortage of SUD and mental health clinicians in multiple ways.[38] Digital therapeutics can effectively function as a partial substitute for clinician-based interventions and thus free up therapist time to devote to issues that cannot be addressed digitally. Such combination treatment models for SUD can be cost-effective[39,40] and increase the availability of treatment slots.

EVIDENCE SUPPORTING THE POSITIVE POTENTIAL OF DIGITAL HEALTH FOR SUDS

A relatively large body of data illustrates and supports the potential of applying various types of technological devices and platforms to effectively treat SUDs. This accumulation of data and knowledge progressed to the extent that a "review of reviews" was published in 2013 identifying nine meta-analytic and 13 qualitative reviews of technology-based interventions for SUDs.[20] Much of this literature comprised examples of studies using web-based intervention programs accessed via a desktop or laptop computer to provide computerized versions of behavioral treatments that had been previously manualized for delivery by a therapist. This review of reviews concluded that *"technology-based interventions for substance use problems are efficacious, effect sizes are generally small to medium, and treatment mechanisms remain largely unknown."*[20] One could argue that such a conclusion closely parallels the status of clinical research on much of traditional evidence-based, therapist-delivered interventions.

Several reviews have evaluated treatments delivered via mobile technologies such as smartphones and tablets,[41] while others have focused on technology-based interventions designed to treat specific types of SUDs, such as tobacco,[42] cannabis,[43] or alcohol use disorders.[19,21,41,44-46] Other reviews have synthesized data on interventions designed to address multiple types of substances. Collectively, this body of work has consistently concluded that technology-delivered treatments can be highly useful and acceptable to diverse populations; have a meaningful impact on health behavior and outcomes; produce outcomes comparable to, or better than clinicians in some settings; increase quality, reach, and personalization of care; improve cost-effectiveness; and respond to individuals' health behavior over time.

EXAMPLES OF DIGITAL HEALTH APPLICATIONS

No consensus definition exists for what comprises the increasingly broad range of technology-delivered health interventions, and the types of applications being tested and utilized to assist in SUD treatment continue to escalate. Perhaps the most developed and evaluated of these applications are software programs that "deliver" therapy via a desktop or laptop computer, tablet, or mobile phone, either through web-based connections to servers or applications housed directly on the device's hard drive. Examples of these clinical tools include: self-assessments, skills training or psychoeducation modules, automated ecological momentary assessment or intervention programs used to self-monitor target behaviors and prompt use of coping skills, text-based motivational and coping programs, and integration of social media-type support groups. In the sections below, we provide snapshots of a few of the more well-developed and tested digital health applications.

DIGITAL SCREENING AND ASSESSMENT

A chronic challenge facing the SUD treatment field is how to effectively identify individuals with or at-risk for developing an SUD, and once identified, how to engage them in effective interventions. Screening, brief intervention, and referral to treatment (SBIRT) models were developed to address this problem and have existed for over 20 years. While such models provide positive steps in addressing this issue, statistics indicate that 85%–90% of persons who might benefit from an SUD intervention do not receive the appropriate services, which suggests that much more progress is needed. Technology-based innovations have the potential to close this gap.

Utilization of digital self-screening and assessment tools in primary care or emergency department waiting rooms has resulted in increased rates of screening and subsequently identifying patients with SUD problems.[47–49] Integrating the digital screening with a healthcare system's electronic health records (EHR) has been proposed to enhance real-time communication regarding substance use screening results to the health provider scheduled to meet with the patient.[50] Screening results can automatically populate EHRs and clinical protocols built into EHRs can prompt provider adherence with engagement and delivery of an intervention.[49,51] Such interventions could be delivered either by a provider (e.g., physician, nurse, mental health therapist, etc.) or via a digital health tool.[52,53] Such models have been tested in part, and current studies that evaluate these types of models of care in primary care settings, emergency departments, and school systems are ongoing.

Digital Treatment Interventions

Much of the digital health intervention literature on SUDs has focused on translating existing evidenced-based, manualized behavioral therapies for delivery via a technology-based platform. These interventions have been developed primarily for (1) people already engaged in SUD treatment or (2) people who are not being treated for SUD, but who seek a stand-alone, self-help intervention via the web or a mobile application. Three well-researched digital interventions designed and tested for use within clinical settings in addition to several prominent stand-alone interventions provide useful examples of these innovations.

Digital interventions within clinical settings

The Therapeutic Education System (TES) is a complex web-based, SUD treatment digital therapeutic that facilitates self-directed behavior therapy.[28] Its development was guided by two major SUD treatments with established efficacy: the Community Reinforcement Approach (CRA)[54,55] and Cognitive Behavioral Therapy (CBT).[56,57] The therapeutic content comprises over 65 interactive, multimedia modules focused on basic CBT for SUD coping skills, coping skills to increase psychosocial functioning drawn from CRA (e.g., employment, social relations, financial management, communication, decision-making, negative moods, time management, and recreation), and additional coping skills and psychoeducation to assist in the prevention of HIV and other sexually transmitted infections. TES uniquely uses a variety of informational technologies to assist with learning and practicing the targeted skills. A fluency-based teaching method assesses participants' comprehension of the psychoeducational material and the coping skill components by administering interactive quizzes, then adjusts the pace and level of training to optimize learning and mastery of the skills. Experiential learning is conveyed through interactive videos of actors modeling coping skills. Interactive exercises further enhance learning and personalize content. TES was also developed to assist in the implementation of incentive-based or contingency management programs, via a system for tracking and rewarding treatment targets (e.g., substance abstinence). TES can provide summaries of patient TES activity and progress, which therapists can use to monitor progress and integrate into sessions.

TES has been tested in multiple controlled studies and has demonstrated positive treatment outcomes for opioid, cannabis, and methamphetamine use disorders, and reduction in HIV risk behavior that were comparable to that produced by clinicians delivering evidence-based behavior therapy. A few brief summaries of example TES studies follow. In an initial controlled trial testing TES for treating individuals with opioid and cocaine use disorders, TES sessions combined with supportive counselor contact produced superior abstinence outcomes compared to standard drug counseling and performed equally well to a completely therapist-delivered CRA/CBT treatment condition.[18]

A large multisite trial conducted as part of the National Institute on Drug Abuse Clinical Trials Network (CTN) assigned individuals seeking outpatient treatment for SUD to a standard intensive outpatient intervention or to a model in which TES replaced 2 h per week of counseling time.[36] Those who received

TES were less likely to drop out and achieved a higher drug abstinence rate. This effect was most robust among the subset of outpatients who initially tested positive for substance use at study intake.

Several other studies support the potential breadth of impact of digital health interventions like TES. A controlled multisite study compared prison inmates with SUDs who received either therapist-delivered behavior therapy or TES delivered as a stand-alone treatment. Inmates rated the TES more favorably than the therapist delivered treatment, though no differences between treatment conditions were observed in drug relapse or reductions in HIV risk behavior or criminality.[58,59] In the context of primary care, TES has also been evaluated in combination with a larger digital health recovery support program to increase access to evidence-based SUD interventions.[52,60] Two studies evaluating the HIV/STD prevention modules of TES observed no differences in outcomes between TES-delivered and prevention specialist-delivered interventions.[61,62] TES has been redesigned several times and a rebranded mobile version of TES (called reSET) is approved by the FDA as an intervention that healthcare professionals can prescribe for SUDs.

A second example of a well-researched, efficacious technology-based SUD treatment intervention is CBT4CBT.[37] CBT4CBT engages graphics, video, text, interactive assessments, and practice exercises based on standard CBT SUD treatment principles and practices. Patients learn to identify patterns of substance use and develop coping skills through six modules. Video demonstrations and homework assignments foster development of coping skills and reinforce their use. Originally developed as an adjunct to therapist-delivered CBT or standard drug counseling, CBT4CBT is delivered via personal computers or tablets.[37] Randomized controlled trials evaluating diverse samples of SUD patients have demonstrated that CBT4CBT can engender and maintain drug abstinence and fosters effective use of the coping skills targeted in treatment.[37,63] More recently, a small clinical trial for alcohol use disorder tested CBT4CBT as a stand-alone intervention delivered in a clinic setting.[64] This stand alone CBT4CBT produced alcohol abstinence outcomes that did not differ from standard weekly alcohol counseling or from standard counseling plus CBT4CBT; however, the combined treatment did produce outcomes superior to standard counseling alone.

Motivation enhancement system (MES) is another brief digital health intervention that has undergone considerable evaluation in controlled trials. MES is an example of a class of digital health interventions

sometimes referred to as Computer-based Brief Interventions. MES was originally developed to address substance use among perinatal and postpartum women. This software program primarily employs principles of motivational interviewing to engage women to actively change of their substance use behaviors.[65] Three primary components are delivered during a single MES session: (1) assessment and personalized feedback; (2) evaluation of pros and cons of substance use and change; and (3) goal setting. The program includes a narrator who engages the participant by asking questions, reflecting back answers, reading back normative feedback reports, and prompting the development of pros and cons lists for using substances, and the setting of goals.[65] Multiple pilot and controlled trials have demonstrated modest outcomes on motivation to change and reductions in alcohol, illicit substances or tobacco use with perinatal women, but with little evidence to date of sustained effects.[53,65–67] Nonetheless, cost-effectiveness, increased access, and good patient acceptance suggest that these types of brief interventions can be an important part of healthcare delivery for substance use and SUDs and warrant additional development and testing.

Self-help Internet-Based Applications

Many digital health interventions have been designed for use outside of traditional healthcare systems to putatively meet the needs of the vast number of individuals with problematic substance use who do not engage in formal treatment due to concerns related to stigma, finances, distrust, lack of treatment availability, or other reasons. These stand-alone interventions provide a potentially powerful and important opportunity for those experiencing problems related to substance use or SUDs. A growing body of literature documents the potential efficacy of a small minority of these interventions that can be accessed via the web or mobile applications.[68–71] Tobacco, alcohol, and cannabis use has been the most common target of these web-based interventions. As with the clinic-based interventions described above, many of these programs incorporate principles and practices of well-established behavioral approaches to SUD (i.e., motivational enhancement, cognitive behavior therapy).

Interventions such as the web-based *RealU* and *Stoptabac* have been evaluated in randomized controlled trials for smoking reduction or cessation, with outcomes demonstrating significant, although modest reductions in tobacco cigarette use.[72–74] The *Drinkers Check Up*—a program for problems with alcohol use—was first evaluated in the context of a clinic setting.[75] The efficacy of

Drinkers Check-Up was observed in subsequent trials in which it was delivered in the home environment of military veterans and college students.[76,77] More recently, a web-based, self-guided alcohol intervention program developed and tested in Germany showed positive effects on alcohol outcomes that were maintained out to 6 months.[78] Observed reductions in alcohol outcomes were comparable to a condition that added an e-counseling component to the self-guided intervention. Several recent tests of internet-based interventions targeting cannabis use have been conducted in Australia, Germany, and Switzerland.[79–83] These self-help programs incorporated treatment components from evidence-based behavioral approaches and were compared with waitlist control or psychoeducational conditions, chat-based counseling over the web, or combinations of the self-help and chat-based programs. Outcomes across studies suggest that the self-help programs for cannabis can produce significant, albeit modest reductions in cannabis use and associated problems; in some cases, further benefit was gained by including web-based guidance or counseling sessions with the self-help program.

Because teens and young adults are high-risk populations for problematic substance use and are high end-users of technological devices, a notable amount of effort has been directed at the development of and research on self-guided digital health interventions targeting reduction of youth substance use and related problems. The bulk of this effort has focused on college or university students.[84–87] The proliferation of assessment and intervention digital tools to identify and address substance use problems on college campuses has been remarkable. In addition to the usual motivational and behavioral concepts embedded in digital tools for SUD, many of these interventions utilize normative feedback strategies to correct students' inflated perceptions of the prevalence of alcohol or cannabis use among their peers.[21] Here, we discuss just a few of tools that have been tested in controlled trials.

AlcoholEdu is an internet-delivered course containing modules that are tailored to meet the needs different genders and alcohol use risk profiles. Students are provided with normative feedback and exercises in which they are challenged to reevaluate their beliefs and choices around alcohol use. In one study, 30 universities were randomly assigned to either the "Alcohol Edu for College" intervention or control.[88] Universities that implemented AlcoholEdu demonstrated significantly greater reductions in alcohol use and binge drinking among their students. The Electronic

CHECKUP TO GO (e-CHUG) intervention utilizes assessment and normative feedback and enables students to monitor changes in drinking patterns to alert them to potentially dangerous drinking habits. Controlled studies have demonstrated that students who received e-CHUG showed reduced alcohol consumption and experienced fewer consequences related to risky alcohol use compared with those who only receive an initial assessment.[89–91]

Similarly, web-based interventions for cannabis, such as the Marijuana E-Checkup (E-Toke) have leveraged personalized normative feedback to alter college students' descriptive norms. Studies have observed reductions in perceived norms related to cannabis use among peers; however, rates of cannabis initiation and use did not differ from students in control conditions.[92,93]

Overall, data suggests that standalone self-help digital health programs are beneficial. Individuals seeking help for substance use are advised to inquire about the applications that they are considering and to ensure that there is a robust evidence base backing the efficacy of the chosen application. While stand-alone interventions delivered in nonclinical settings are not extremely effective, such interventions can reach individuals who might not otherwise engage in traditional treatment settings.

FDA and Digital Health

The U.S. Food and Drug Administration (FDA) recently launched an initiative to incorporate digital health into mainstream medical practice.[94] This significant step acknowledges the potential of and the growing evidence for digital health interventions. Many technology-delivered SUD treatments are largely based on previously validated and manualized psychotherapies delivered via innovative software or mobile applications. The FDA now classifies "software as a medical device" (SaMD) if the *software in and of itself* is intended to be therapeutic or repurposes hardware to perform a new therapeutic function.[94,95] This is distinct from software designed only to allow a piece of hardware to perform an intended therapeutic function. A class of digital therapeutics that falls within the definition of SaMD is what the FDA has referred to as "mobile medical applications" (MMAs). The FDA defines MMAs as *"a software application that meets the definition of a medical device"*. An example of an MMA is a mobile app that is *"performing patient-specific analysis and providing patient-specific diagnosis, or treatment recommendations."*[94] In 2017, *reSET* was the first MMA permitted for marketing by the FDA for the treatment of SUDs. *reSET* is a mobile digital therapeutic[96,97] based almost entirely on the previously validated and empirically tested TES program. The *reSet* device is indicated as a prescription-only adjunct treatment for patients with SUD who are not currently on opioid replacement therapy, who do not abuse alcohol solely, or whose primary substance problem is not with opioids—an opioid use disorder version of *reSET* is currently under development and testing.

CAVEATS TO TRANSLATION, UPTAKE, AND EFFICACY

Digital health holds promise for enhancing public health by expanding treatment access and options and improving treatment outcomes for those suffering from addictions. That said, realizing this promise in a way that is truly in the best interest of those in need will require a clear focus and strong effort to address implementation challenges and barriers. Many of these challenges will be similar to those that handicap the current health care system, while others will be novel to digital health. Identifying these issues and developing strategies to address them is imperative and some such work has been initiated (Table 5.2).

Adoption by Community Clinics

Dissemination and implementation of science-based interventions for SUD and other mental disorders to community practice has been a topic of ongoing frustration and controversy for decades. Some of the hurdles to widespread translation from research and development to practice will be similar to those faced by innovative, evidence-based, clinician-delivered treatments, and others will be unique to digital technology approaches. Current implementation science frameworks can help identify areas to focus solutions to overcome barriers to adoption and sustainable implementation of evidence-based digital health approaches.[98,99]

Characteristics of Clinicians and Providers

Resistance to adoption can be anticipated from frontline providers. Many clinicians trained to provide psychosocial treatments for SUD might naturally be hesitant to accept alternative intervention models, particularly those that remove the human element.[100–102] The suggestion that a digital program can replace or substitute for what clinicians have been trained to do and have been practicing for years will likely be met with skepticism and resistance to

change. Such opposition may occur not only among those delivering care, but also among administrative staff and leadership who many times hold strong beliefs about what optimal care should look like. Acceptance and integration of digital approaches within community SUD clinics is predicated on demonstrating that these approaches can enhance patient outcomes when used as alternatives or supplements to existing practices. Note that these concerns may be less of an issue when trying to integrate digital health into nonspecialty clinics where there is less commitment and investment in traditional models of care for SUDs.

Organization Characteristics

Agency or administrative system-related hurdles can be anticipated and must be addressed. A number of factors can lower enthusiasm for embracing and including digital health interventions in a community setting, including change in distribution of workloads and responsibilities, levels and type of expertise needed across the agency, time required and the disruption associated with learning how to use and implement technology-based tools. Finance-related concerns may also be pervasive. Billing systems and reimbursement structures for digital health interventions have not been developed. Moreover, in capitated systems, digital health interventions may not be an accepted modality of care. Actual or perceived affordability of technology-based tools and infrastructure and about how it will impact overall budget and internal or external program funding are also of concern. Another point of concern is the current state of many SUD treatment systems, which may have outdated, unreliable, or inadequate technological infrastructure to support some digital interventions.

External Contexts

Agencies also are wary of the degree with which digital health applications can protect patient health information and prevent HIPAA violations. Such concerns are also of obvious importance to patients. Moreover, current organizational regulations, restrictions, and ethical considerations may not be compatible with digital intervention delivery.

Although access to mobile devices is generally ubiquitous, the access necessary to support some digital interventions or components may be lacking for some participants. This could be due to cost of the device or service, type of device required by the intervention, or inadequate internet service providers in their area.

TABLE 5.2
Potential or Perceived Barriers to Implementation

Challenge Areas	Example Concerns
Funding/cost	• High initial cost of technology-based tools. • Budget constraints and potential impact on budget if adopted. • Lack of internal or external funding prioritization or investment.
Billing/reimbursement	• Inability to charge a fee for service, bill, or otherwise be reimbursed for digital health services.
Privacy/security/regulations/ethics	• Patient health information: privacy, security, confidentiality, HIPAA violations. • Organizational regulations, restrictions, and ethical considerations related to technology-based care delivery.
Need for knowledge/skill building	• Lack of necessary provider knowledge, skills, or abilities. • Perceived need for skills training and other professional development.
Equipment/infrastructure	• Old, outdated, unreliable, or inadequate equipment, technology systems, or IT infrastructure to support digital health interventions.
Negative impact/bad experiences	• Detrimental impact of digital treatment delivery on the provider-client relationship, quality of care, and treatment outcomes. • History of negative experiences related to technology; patient complaints.
Client access to and maintenance of tools	• Patients inability to access, obtain, understand, maintain, or properly use digital health tools.
Provider/agency openness and buy-in	• Resistance or lack of openness or acceptance to using digital tools among clinicians or other health care providers, administrators, and general staff.
Demands/time	• Will add to the current excess work demands and a lack of time to meet obligations and performance goals.
Staffing/support	• Lack of trained staff or information technology (IT) support persons to accommodate digital health implementation effectively.
Client internet connectivity/service	• Patient inability to connect to the Internet or receive mobile service due to lack of service coverage, inadequate service providers, or resistance to use because of personal cost.

Adapted from Ramsey A, Lord S, Torrey J, Marsch L, Lardiere M. Paving the way to successful implementation: identifying key barriers to use of technology-based therapeutic tools for behavioral health care. *J Natl Behav Health Serv Res.* 2014. https://doi.org/10.1007/s11414-014-9436-5.

Obsolescence, Quality Control, and Adherence

Technological obsolescence can also impact motivation and acceptance of digital health interventions, as many interventions are designed using specific software operating systems and hardware (devices). However, because technology evolves rapidly, an intervention may already be incompatible with newer technologies being used by individuals or healthcare systems by the time the intervention is validated in controlled studies. Conversely, interventions may be developed using the most recent innovative technology that end-users have not yet adopted. Electronic health record systems that are not compatible or not flexible enough to take advantage of digital health intervention innovations are an example of a common frustration experienced by healthcare systems and innovators seeking to implement or test new applications.

For stand-alone or self-help digital interventions—particularly mobile apps that can be easily downloaded from the internet either free of charge or at a relatively low cost—there is growing concern about how to provide consumers with empirical support for their quality or efficacy. There now likely exist over 200,000 apps marketed to help quit tobacco, cannabis/marijuana or alcohol, or for other mental or behavioral problems;

however, there is little to no oversight of their content or clear ways to assess their quality. Very few of these apps (less than 0.01%) have been tested in controlled trials. Organizations like the American Psychiatric Association have engaged a task force charged with providing guidance to providers, patients, and the general public on how to evaluate an app, with an eventual goal of coming up with a rating system.[103] Although many digital interventions may be helpful, consumer protection is certainly warranted in this new frontier, as there are a number of potential harms that can occur (e.g., selling of personal information, lack of efficacy leading to worsening of a condition that could benefit from established intervention modalities, misleading or detrimental advice or intervention that can cause adverse effects).

Adherence

Digital interventions (e.g., text-messaging, automated prompting via mobile devices) have been proposed as methods for increasing adherence to prescribed health behaviors of many kinds, including pharmacotherapies and behavioral interventions for SUDs. Ironically, as with traditional interventions for health behavior problems, getting people to engage and adequately adhere or comply with the active components of digital health interventions for SUD is difficult, but essential for one to reap the benefits of the application. Several studies of persons with SUDs or risky substance use patterns have demonstrated that while many are initially motivated to engage with a mobile application or web-based intervention to treat their substance use, a large portion disengage and cease using the digital intervention within a short timeframe.[104–106] Although mobile apps and web-based treatments are much easier to access than traditional modalities of SUD care, finding ways to promote ongoing engagement so that an adequate dose of the intervention is received still presents a formidable challenge for digital health interventions.

In summary, as with most innovations in health care, gaining acceptance and integrating digital health applications for SUD into current healthcare systems will face many challenges. Recent perspectives on sustainability support consideration of implementation throughout digital intervention development phases, with a focus on dynamic processes and adaptation to optimize intervention fit with person and environment contexts.[102,107] Fortunately, models to study and address implementation barriers at the designer, organization, provider, and patient levels of SUD health care have been developed and are being applied.[108–111]

IT IS JUST THE BEGINNING

There is great optimism for the potential and opportunity afforded by digital technology applications to advance and improve public health and health care, including care for those at risk for or suffering from SUDs. An overwhelmed and undertrained system and the individual burdens associated with accessing care have resulted in only a small minority of those in need of SUD treatment receiving it, and the quality of the care provided to those who do engage the system has not been uniformly evidence-based or of high quality. This chapter has reviewed some of the many ways that digital technology can and has been applied to help address this chronic public health problem. We also highlighted the barriers and challenges of implementing these digital health applications in the community. Of note, we were only able to discuss and illustrate a fraction of the multitude of exciting innovations currently under development and testing. We also did not delve into some of the ongoing and critical work that addresses how we might best address the challenges of quality control, dissemination, and uptake of digital therapeutics for SUDs. The digital health world is expanding rapidly and keeping pace with the newest developments requires constant vigilance. We hope that this introduction generates increased awareness, interest, the pursuit of knowledge, and the willingness to explore the use of digital applications to combat the public health problem of addiction.

With that in mind, we offer a few final comments. Others have discussed what has become known as the "5000-h problem" related to those with chronic health problems.[112,113] That is, people with chronic disorders spend only a few hours a year with their healthcare provider and are otherwise unsupervised during their 5000 plus waking hours. As a result, the provider does not know how the patient is managing their health and usually does not have the tools necessary to help them. SUDs are an example of such chronic problems. However, mobile digital therapeutics can provide ways to (1) continuously monitor target problems or warning signs, (2) digitally communicate patient information passively or actively to providers, and (3) prompt the patient to engage in coping behaviors at any time. One can easily envision how leveraging technology in this way could advance care for SUD and many other health conditions.

That said, it is imperative that those seeking to develop, test, and implement digital therapeutics for SUD seek out and learn from technological applications that are advancing within other areas of clinical medicine. Researchers and clinicians in all areas of health care are on similar quests to find ways to utilize digital technology to optimize care. Recent discoveries and recognition of transdisease processes and interventions illustrate a number of common mechanisms that operate in disease states and health behavior problems, including SUDs.[114–116] It follows that common intervention approaches that target such processes may positively impact change across disorders. Also, digital technologies that can extend access to care, improve assessment of problems and progress, or facilitate better communication between providers would share obvious benefits across many health conditions.

Future development and research must continue to seek innovative digital applications that are more potent and yield larger effects. To date, outcomes demonstrated with digital interventions for SUDs generally show the same small to medium effects sizes as traditional SUD treatments. The potential for digital therapeutics to escalate progress toward *personalized*, or *precision*, medicine approaches that optimize care and increase the probability of achieving positive outcomes must remain a high priority.

Leveraging increasingly powerful analytic methodologies that can utilize the rich data sets captured by mobile devices—including data acquired with passive sensing and from social media sources—may inform more effective interventions. For example, applications of machine learning and associated novel analytic strategies provide innovative ways to continuously learn from patterns and predictions identified within the data. The collection and analysis of such extensive, multimodal data may provide new insights into a person's behavior, health, and environment that can inform highly personalized interventions and perhaps predict and characterize a person's needs and health outcomes over time.[29]

It is imperative for digital health technologies to safeguard protected personal health information. A research agenda and the development of quality assurance standards will be necessary to not only guarantee people's privacy but to reassure consumers that their privacy is secure so that they are willing to engage in digital health programs.

Finally, it is important to determine how to best scale up access to science-based digital therapeutics in real-world settings. Advancing the field of digital health for SUDs will require a program of research that emphasizes the following: (1) efficacy (developing the most potent interventions); (2) scientific rigor (e.g., obtaining definitive evidence of the effects of interventions); (3) relevance (e.g., creating digital tools that are readily accepted by consumers and healthcare systems);

(4) integration (establishing guidelines for how to motivate use in healthcare settings); and (5) economics (understanding and communicating the costs, cost-benefit, and cost-effectiveness to healthcare systems and policymakers).

REFERENCES

1. MIT Technology Review. *10 Breakthrough Technologies 2017*. 2017. Retrieved from: https://www.technologyreview.com/lists/technologies/2017/. Archived at: http://www.webcitation.org/6wT5nYt37.
2. Dutra L, Stathopoulou G, Basden SL, Leyro TM, Powers MB, Otto MW. A meta-analytic review of psychosocial interventions for substance use disorders. *Am J Psychiatry*. 2008;165(2):179–187. https://doi.org/10.1176/appi.ajp.2007.06111851.
3. McLellan AT, Lewis DC, O'Brien CP, Kleber HD. Drug dependence, a chronic medical illness: implications for treatment, insurance, and outcomes evaluations. *JAMA*. 2000;284:1689–1695.
4. Substance Abuse and Mental Health Services Administration. Key substance use and mental health indicators in the United States: results from the 2016 national survey on drug use and health. In: *Center for Behavioral Health Statistics and Quality*. 2017. Rockville, M.D.
5. Bhavnani SP, Narula J, Sengupta PP. Mobile technology and the digitization of healthcare. *Eur Heart J*. 2016;37(18): 1428–1438. https://doi.org/10.1093/eurheartj/ehv770.
6. Dallery J, Kurti A, Erb P. A new frontier: integrating behavioral and digital technology to promote health behavior. *Behav Anal*. 2015;38(1):19–49. https://doi.org/10.1007/s40614-014-0017-y.
7. Ericsson. *Ericsson Mobility Report*; 2016. Retrieved from: www.ericsson.com/mobility-report.
8. Antoine D, Heffernan S, Chaudhry A, King V, Strain EC. Age and gender considerations for technology-assisted delivery of therapy for substance use disorder treatment: a patient survey of access to electronic devices. *Addict Disord Their Treat*. 2016;15(4):149–156. https://doi.org/10.1097/ADT.0000000000000088.
9. Dahne J, Lejuez CW. Smartphone and mobile application utilization prior to and following treatment among individuals enrolled in residential substance use treatment. *J Subst Abuse Treat*. 2015;58:95–99. https://doi.org/10.1016/j.jsat.2015.06.017.
10. McClure EA, Acquavita SP, Harding E, Stitzer ML. Utilization of communication technology by patients enrolled in substance abuse treatment. *Drug Alcohol Depend*. 2013;129(1–2):145–150. https://doi.org/10.1016/j.drugalcdep.2012.10.003.
11. Tofighi B, Campbell AN, Pavlicova M, Hu MC, Lee JD, Nunes EV. Recent internet use and associations with clinical outcomes among patients entering addiction treatment involved in a web-delivered psychosocial intervention study. *J Urban Health*. 2016;93(5): 871–883. https://doi.org/10.1007/s11524-016-0077-2.

12. Tofighi B, Grossman E, Buirkle E, McNeely J, Gourevitch M, Lee JD. Mobile phone use patterns and preferences in safety net office-based buprenorphine patients. *J Addict Med*. 2015;9(3):217–221. https://doi.org/10.1097/ADM.0000000000000121.

13. Butler SF, Villapiano A, Malinow A. The effect of computer-mediated administration on self-disclosure of problems on the addiction severity index. *J Addict Med*. 2009;3(4):194–203. https://doi.org/10.1097/ADM.0b013e3181902844.

14. Kobak KA, Greist JH, Jefferson JW, Katzelnick DJ. Computer-administered clinical rating scales. A review. *Psychopharmacol Berl*. 1996;127(4):291–301.

15. Marsch LA, Bickel WK. Efficacy of computer-based HIV/AIDS education for injection drug users. *Am J Health Behav*. 2004;28(4):316–327.

16. McLellan AT, Meyers K. Contemporary addiction treatment: a review of systems problems for adults and adolescents. *Biol Psychiatry*. 2004;56(10):764–770. https://doi.org/10.1016/j.biopsych.2004.06.018.

17. Miller W, Rollnick S. The effectiveness and ineffectiveness of complex behavioral interventions: impact of treatment fidelity. *Contemp Clin Trials*. 2014;37(2):234–241. https://doi.org/10.1016/j.cct.2014.01.005.

18. Bickel WK, Marsch LA, Buchhalter AR, Badger GJ. Computerized behavior therapy for opioid-dependent outpatients: a randomized controlled trial. *Exp Clin Psychopharmacol*. 2008;16(2):132–143. https://doi.org/10.1037/1064-1297.16.2.132.

19. Budney AJ, Stanger C, Tilford JM, et al. Computer-assisted behavioral therapy and contingency management for cannabis use disorder. *Psychol Addict Behav*. 2015a;29(3):501–511. https://doi.org/10.1037/adb0000078.

20. Litvin EB, Abrantes AM, Brown RA. Computer and mobile technology-based interventions for substance use disorders: an organizing framework. *Addict Behav*. 2013;38(3):1747–1756. https://doi.org/10.1016/j.addbeh.2012.09.003.

21. Marsch LA, Borodovsky JT. Technology-based interventions for preventing and treating substance use among youth. *Child Adolesc Psychiatr Clin N Am*. 2016;25(4):755. https://doi.org/10.1016/j.chc.2016.06.005.

22. Marsch LA, Guarino H, Grabinski MJ, et al. Comparative effectiveness of web-based vs. educator-delivered HIV prevention for adolescent substance users: a randomized, controlled trial. *J Subst Abuse Treat*. 2015;59:30–37. https://doi.org/10.1016/j.jsat.2015.07.003.

23. Wood SK, Eckley L, Hughes K, et al. Computer-based programmes for the prevention and management of illicit recreational drug use: a systematic review. *Addict Behav*. 2014;39(1):30–38. https://doi.org/10.1016/j.addbeh.2013.09.010.

24. Capoccia VA, Cotter F, Gustafson DH, et al. Making "stone soup": improvements in clinic access and retention in addiction treatment. *Jt Comm J Qual Patient Saf*. 2007;33(2):95–103.

25. Lundgren L, Chassler D, Amodeo M, D'Ippolito M, Sullivan L. Barriers to implementation of evidence-based addiction treatment: a national study. *J Subst Abuse Treat*. 2012;42(3):231–238. https://doi.org/10.1016/j.jsat.2011.08.003.

26. Milward J, Day E, Wadsworth E, Strang J, Lynskey M. Mobile phone ownership, usage and readiness to use by patients in drug treatment. *Drug Alcohol Depend*. 2015;146:111–115. https://doi.org/10.1016/j.drugalcdep.2014.11.001.

27. Gustafson DH, McTavish FM, Chih MY, et al. A smartphone application to support recovery from alcoholism: a randomized clinical trial. *JAMA Psychiatry*. 2014;71(5):566–572. https://doi.org/10.1001/jamapsychiatry.2013.4642.

28. Marsch LA, Dallery J. Advances in the psychosocial treatment of addiction: the role of technology in the delivery of evidence-based psychosocial treatment. *Psychiat Clin N Am*. 2012;35(2):481–493. https://doi.org/10.1016/j.psc.2012.03.009. Epub 2012 Apr 11.

29. Nahum-Shani I, Smith SN, Spring BJ, et al. Just-in-time adaptive interventions (JITAIs) in mobile health: key components and design principles for ongoing health behavior support. *Ann Behav Med*. 2016. https://doi.org/10.1007/s12160-016-9830-8.

30. Dennis ML, Scott CK, Funk RR, Nicholson L. A pilot study to examine the feasibility and potential effectiveness of using smartphones to provide recovery support for adolescents. *Subst Abus*. 2015;36(4):486–492. https://doi.org/10.1080/08897077.2014.970323.

31. Gadomski AM, Fothergill KE, Larson S, et al. Integrating mental health into adolescent annual visits: impact of previsit comprehensive screening on within-visit processes. *J Adolesc Health*. 2015;56(3):267–273. https://doi.org/10.1016/j.jadohealth.2014.11.011.

32. Harris SK, Knight JR. Putting the screen in screening: technology-based alcohol screening and brief interventions in medical settings. *Alcohol Res*. 2014;36(1):63–79.

33. Harris SK, Knight JR, Van Hook S, et al. Adolescent substance use screening in primary care: validity of computer self-administered versus clinician-administered screening. *Subst Abus*. 2016;37(1):197–203. https://doi.org/10.1080/08897077.2015.1014615.

34. Johnson JA, Woychek A, Vaughan D, Seale JP. Screening for at-risk alcohol use and drug use in an emergency department: integration of screening questions into electronic triage forms achieves high screening rates. *Ann Emerg Med*. 2013;62(3):262–266. https://doi.org/10.1016/j.annemergmed.2013.04.011.

35. McNeely J, Strauss SM, Rotrosen J, Ramautar A, Gourevitch MN. Validation of an audio computer-assisted self-interview (ACASI) version of the alcohol, smoking and substance involvement screening test (ASSIST) in primary care patients. *Addiction*. 2016;111(2):233–244. https://doi.org/10.1111/add.13165.

36. Campbell AN, Nunes EV, Matthews AG, et al. Internet-delivered treatment for substance abuse: a multisite randomized controlled trial. *Am J Psychiatry*. 2014; 171(6):683−690. https://doi.org/10.1176/appi.ajp.2014. 13081055.

37. Carroll KM, Ball SA, Martino S, et al. Computer-assisted delivery of cognitive-behavioral therapy for addiction: a randomized trial of CBT4CBT. *Am J Psychiatry*. 2008;165(7):881−888. https://doi.org/10.1176/appi. ajp.2008.07111835. Epub 2008 May 1.

38. Hoge MA, Stuart GW, Morris J, Flaherty MT, Paris Jr M, Goplerud E. Mental health and addiction workforce development: federal leadership is needed to address the growing crisis. *Health Aff (Millwood)*. 2013;32(11): 2005−2012. https://doi.org/10.1377/hlthaff.2013.0541.

39. Chen YF, Madan J, Welton N, et al. Effectiveness and cost-effectiveness of computer and other electronic aids for smoking cessation: a systematic review and network meta-analysis. *Health Technol Assess*. 2012;16(38): 1−205. https://doi.org/10.3310/hta16380.

40. Olmstead TA, Ostrow CD, Carroll KM. Cost-effectiveness of computer-assisted training in cognitive-behavioral therapy as an adjunct to standard care for addiction. *Drug Alcohol Depend*. 2010;110(3):200−207. https:// doi.org/10.1016/j.drugalcdep.2010.02.022.

41. Fowler LA, Holt SL, Joshi D. Mobile technology-based interventions for adult users of alcohol: a systematic review of the literature. *Addict Behav*. 2016;62(supplement C): 25−34. https://doi.org/10.1016/j.addbeh.2016.06.008. Epub 2016 Jun 7.

42. Crocamo C, Carretta D, Ferri M, Dias S, Bartoli F, Carrá G. Web- and text-based interventions for smoking cessation: meta-analysis and meta-regression. *Drugs Educ Prev Policy*. 2017:1−10. https://doi.org/10.1080/ 09687637.2017.1285867.

43. Hoch E, Preuss UW, Ferri M, Simon R. Digital interventions for problematic cannabis users in non-clinical settings: findings from a systematic review and meta-analysis. *Eur Addict Res*. 2016;22(5):233−242. https:// doi.org/10.1159/000445716. Epub 2016 May 4.

44. Dedert EA, McDuffie JR, Stein R, et al. Electronic interventions for alcohol misuse and alcohol use disorders: a systematic review. *Ann Intern Med*. 2015;163(3):205−214. https://doi.org/10.7326/M15-0285.

45. Quanbeck AR, Chih MY, Isham A, Johnson R, Gustafson D. Mobile delivery of treatment for alcohol use disorders a review of the literature. *Alcohol Res Curr Rev*. 2014;36(1):111−122.

46. Resko SM, Brown S, Lister JJ, Ondersma SJ, Cunningham RM, Walton MA. Technology-based interventions and trainings to reduce the escalation and impact of alcohol problems. *J Social Work Pract Addict*. 2017; 17(1−2):114−134. https://doi.org/10.1080/1533256x. 2017.1304948.

47. McNeely J, Wu LT, Subramaniam G, et al. Performance of the tobacco, alcohol, prescription medication, and other substance use (TAPS) tool for substance use screening in primary care patients. *Ann Intern Med*. 2016;165(10): 690−699. https://doi.org/10.7326/M16-0317.

48. Spirito A, Bromberg JR, Casper TC, et al. Reliability and validity of a two-question alcohol screen in the pediatric emergency department. *Pediatrics*. 2016;138(6). https:// doi.org/10.1542/peds.2016-0691.

49. Tai B, McLellan AT. Integrating information on substance use disorders into electronic health record systems. *J Subst Abuse Treat*. 2012;43(1):12−19. https://doi.org/10.1016/ j.jsat.2011.10.010. Epub 2011 Dec 7.

50. Keyhani S, Vali M, Cohen B, et al. A search algorithm for identifying likely users and non-users of marijuana from the free text of the electronic medical record. *PLoS One*. 2018;13(3):e0193706. https://doi.org/ 10.1371/journal.pone.0193706.

51. Tai B, Wu LT, Clark HW. Electronic health records: essential tools in integrating substance abuse treatment with primary care. *Subst Abuse Rehabil*. 2012;3:1−8. https:// doi.org/10.2147/SAR.S22575.

52. Mares ML, Gustafson DH, Glass JE, et al. Implementing an mHealth system for substance use disorders in primary care: a mixed methods study of clinicians' initial expectations and first year experiences. *BMC Med Inf Decis Mak*. 2016;16(1):126. https://doi.org/10.1186/s12911-016-0365-5.

53. Ondersma SJ, Svikis DS, Schuster CR. Computer-based brief intervention a randomized trial with postpartum women. *Am J Prev Med*. 2007;32(3):231−238. https:// doi.org/10.1016/j.amepre.2006.11.003. Epub 2007 Jan 22.

54. Budney AJ, Higgins ST. *A Community Reinforcement Plus Vouchers Approach: Treating Cocaine Addiction*. Bethesda, MD: National Institute on Drug Abuse; 1998.

55. Meyers RJ, Villanueva M, Smith JE. Community reinforcement approach: history and new directions. *J Cognit Psychotherapy*. 2005;19(3):247−260.

56. Carroll KM, Rounsaville BJ. A vision of the next generation of behavioral therapies research in the addictions. *Addiction*. 2007;102(6):850−862.

57. Monti P, Abrams D, Kadden R, Cooney N. *Treating Alcohol Dependence*. New York, NY: The Guilford Press; 1989.

58. Chaple M, Sacks S, McKendrick K, et al. Feasibility of a computerized intervention for offenders with substance use disorders: a research note. *J Exp Criminol*. 2014;10:105−127. https://doi.org/10.1007/s11292-013-9187-y.

59. Chaple M, Sacks S, McKendrick K, et al. A comparative study of the therapeutic education system for incarcerated substance-abusing offenders. *Prison J*. 2016;96(3): 485−508. https://doi.org/10.1177/0032885516636858.

60. Quanbeck AR, Gustafson DH, Marsch LA, et al. Integrating addiction treatment into primary care using mobile health technology: protocol for an implementation research study. *Implement Sci.* 2014;9:65. https://doi.org/10.1186/1748-5908-9-65.

61. Marsch LA, Grabinski MJ, Bickel WK, et al. Computer-assisted HIV prevention for youth with substance use disorders. *Subst Use Misuse.* 2011;46(1):46–56. https://doi.org/10.3109/10826084.2011.521088.

62. Marsch LA, Lord SE, Dallery J. *Behavioral Healthcare and Technology: Using Science-based Innovations to Transform Practice.* Oxford; New York: Oxford University Press; 2015.

63. Carroll KM, Kiluk BD, Nich C, et al. Computer-assisted delivery of cognitive-behavioral therapy: efficacy and durability of CBT4CBT among cocaine-dependent individuals maintained on methadone. *Am J Psychiatry.* 2014;171(4):436–444. https://doi.org/10.1176/appi.ajp.2013.13070987.

64. Kiluk BD, Devore KA, Buck MB, et al. Randomized trial of computerized cognitive behavioral therapy for alcohol use disorders: efficacy as a virtual stand-alone and treatment add-on compared with standard outpatient treatment. *Alcohol Clin Exp Res.* 2016;40(9):1991–2000. https://doi.org/10.1111/acer.13162. Epub 2016 Aug 4.

65. Ondersma SJ, Chase SK, Svikis DS, Schuster CR. Computer-based brief motivational intervention for perinatal drug use. *J Subst Abuse Treat.* 2005;28(4):305–312. https://doi.org/10.1016/j.jsat.2005.02.004 10.

66. Martino S, Ondersma SJ, Forray A, et al. A randomized controlled trial of screening and brief interventions for substance misuse in reproductive health. *Am J Obstet Gynecol.* 2017. https://doi.org/10.1016/j.ajog.2017.12.005.

67. Ondersma SJ, Svikis DS, Thacker LR, Beatty JR, Lockhart N. A randomised trial of a computer-delivered screening and brief intervention for postpartum alcohol use. *Drug Alcohol Rev.* 2016;35(6):710–718. https://doi.org/10.1111/dar.12389. Epub 2016 Mar 23.

68. Powell AC, Torous J, Chan S, et al. Interrater reliability of mHealth app rating measures: analysis of top depression and smoking cessation apps. *JMIR Mhealth Uhealth.* 2016;4(1):e15. https://doi.org/10.2196/mhealth.5176.

69. Riper H, Blankers M, Hadiwijaya H, et al. Effectiveness of guided and unguided low-intensity internet interventions for adult alcohol misuse: a meta-analysis. *PLoS One.* 2014;9(6):e99912. https://doi.org/10.1371/journal.pone.0099912.

70. Riper H, Spek V, Boon B, et al. Effectiveness of E-self-help interventions for curbing adult problem drinking: a meta-analysis. *J Med Internet Res.* 2011;13(2):e42. https://doi.org/10.2196/jmir.1691.

71. White A, Kavanagh D, Stallman H, et al. Online alcohol interventions: a systematic review. *J Med Internet Res.* 2010;12(5):e62. https://doi.org/10.2196/jmir.1479.

72. An LC, Demers MR, Kirch MA, et al. A randomized trial of an avatar-hosted multiple behavior change intervention for young adult smokers. *J Natl Cancer Inst Monogr.* 2013;2013(47):209–215. https://doi.org/10.1093/jncimonographs/lgt021.

73. An LC, Klatt C, Perry CL, et al. The RealU online cessation intervention for college smokers: a randomized controlled trial. *Prev Med.* 2008;47(2):194–199. https://doi.org/10.1016/j.ypmed.2008.04.011.

74. Etter JF. Comparing the efficacy of two Internet-based, computer-tailored smoking cessation programs: a randomized trial. *J Med Internet Res.* 2005;7(1):e2. https://doi.org/10.2196/jmir.7.1.e2.

75. Hester RK, Squires DD, Delaney HD. The drinker's check-up: 12-month outcomes of a controlled clinical trial of a stand-alone software program for problem drinkers. *J Subst Abuse Treat.* 2005;28(2):159–169. https://doi.org/10.1016/j.jsat.2004.12.002.

76. Hester RK, Delaney HD, Campbell W. The college drinker's check-up: outcomes of two randomized clinical trials of a computer-delivered intervention. *Psychol Addict Behav.* 2012;26(1):1–12. https://doi.org/10.1037/a0024753.

77. Williams J, Herman-Stahl M, Calvin SL, Pemberton M, Bradshaw M. Mediating mechanisms of a military Web-based alcohol intervention. *Drug Alcohol Depend.* 2009;100(3):248–257. https://doi.org/10.1016/j.drugalcdep.2008.10.007. Epub 2008 Dec 9.

78. Bob L, Lehr D, Schaub MP, et al. Efficacy of a web-based intervention with and without guidance for employees with risky drinking: results of a three-arm randomized controlled trial. *Addiction.* 2017. https://doi.org/10.1111/add.14085.

79. Monney G, Penzenstadler L, Dupraz O, Etter JF, Khazaal Y. mHealth app for cannabis users: satisfaction and perceived usefulness. *Front Psychiatry.* 2015;6:120. https://doi.org/10.3389/fpsyt.2015.00120.

80. Rooke S, Copeland J, Norberg M, Hine D, McCambridge J. Effectiveness of a self-guided web-based cannabis treatment program: randomized controlled trial. *J Med Internet Res.* 2013;15(2):e26. https://doi.org/10.2196/jmir.2256.

81. Schaub MP, Haug S, Wenger A, et al. Can reduce—the effects of chat-counseling and web-based self-help, web-based self-help alone and a waiting list control program on cannabis use in problematic cannabis users: a randomized controlled trial. *BMC Psychiatry.* 2013;13(1):305. https://doi.org/10.1186/1471-244X-13-305.

82. Schaub MP, Wenger A, Berg O, et al. A web-based self-help intervention with and without chat counseling to reduce cannabis use in problematic cannabis users: three-arm randomized controlled trial. *J Med Internet Res.* 2015;17(10):e232. https://doi.org/10.2196/jmir.4860.

83. Tossmann HP, Jonas B, Tensil MD, Lang P, Struber E. A controlled trial of an internet-based intervention program for cannabis users. *Cyberpsychol Behav Soc Netw.* 2011;14(11):673−679. https://doi.org/10.1089/cyber.2010.0506. Epub 2011 Jun 8.

84. Carey KB, Scott-Sheldon LA, Elliott JC, Bolles JR, Carey MP. Computer-delivered interventions to reduce college student drinking: a meta-analysis. *Addiction.* 2009;104(11):1807−1819. https://doi.org/10.1111/j.1360-0443.2009.02691.x. Epub 2009 Sep. 10.

85. Dotson KB, Dunn ME, Bowers CA. Stand-alone personalized normative feedback for college student drinkers: a meta-analytic review, 2004 to 2014. *PLoS One.* 2015; 10(10):e0139518. https://doi.org/10.1371/journal.pone.0139518. eCollection 2015.

86. Leeman RF, Perez E, Nogueira C, DeMartini KS. Very-brief, web-based interventions for reducing alcohol use and related problems among college students: a review. *Front Psychiatry.* 2015;6:129. https://doi.org/10.3389/fpsyt.2015.00129. eCollection 2015.

87. O'Rourke L, Humphris G, Baldacchino A. Electronic communication based interventions for hazardous young drinkers: a systematic review. *Neurosci Biobehav Rev.* 2016;68(supplement C):880−890. https://doi.org/10.1016/j.neubiorev.2016.07.021 10. Epub 2016 Jul 22.

88. Paschall MJ, Antin T, Ringwalt CL, Saltz RF. Evaluation of an internet-based alcohol misuse prevention course for college freshmen: findings of a randomized multicampus trial. *Am J Prev Med.* 2011;41(3):300−308. https://doi.org/10.1016/j.amepre.2011.03.021.

89. Doumas DM, McKinley LL, Book P. Evaluation of two Web-based alcohol interventions for mandated college students. *J Subst Abuse Treat.* 2009;36(1):65−74. https://doi.org/10.1016/j.jsat.2008.05.009.

90. Doumas DM, Workman C, Smith D, Navarro A. Reducing high-risk drinking in mandated college students: evaluation of two personalized normative feedback interventions. *J Subst Abuse Treat.* 2011;40(4):376−385. https://doi.org/10.1016/j.jsat.2010.12.006.

91. Walters ST, Vader AM, Harris TR. A controlled trial of web-based feedback for heavy drinking college students. *Prev Sci.* 2007;8(1):83−88. https://doi.org/10.1007/s11121-006-0059-9.

92. Elliott JC, Carey KB. Correcting exaggerated marijuana use norms among college abstainers: a preliminary test of a preventive intervention. *J Stud Alcohol Drugs.* 2012; 73(6):976−980.

93. Palfai TP, Saitz R, Winter M, et al. Web-based screening and brief intervention for student marijuana use in a university health center: pilot study to examine the implementation of eCHECKUP TO GO in different contexts. *Addict Behav.* 2014;39(9):1346−1352. https://doi.org/10.1016/j.addbeh.2014.04.025.

94. U.S. Food and Drug Administration. *Digital Health Criteria.* 2017a. Retrieved from: https://www.fda.gov/MedicalDevices/DigitalHealth/ucm575766.htm. Archived at: http://www.webcitation.org/6wQFwrU6g.

95. U.S. Food and Drug Administration. *Digital Health Software Precertification (Pre-cert) Program.* 2017b. Retrieved from: https://www.fda.gov/MedicalDevices/DigitalHealth/DigitalHealthPreCertProgram/default.htm. Archived at: http://www.webcitation.org/6wQGHE27Z.

96. Pear Therapeutics Inc. *reSET for Substance Use Disorder.* 2018. Retrieved from: https://peartherapeutics.com/reset/. Archived at: http://www.webcitation.org/6wQGbeE2q.

97. U.S. Food and Drug Administration. *FDA Permits Marketing of Mobile Medical Application for Substance Use Disorder.* 2017c. Retrieved from: https://www.fda.gov/NewsEvents/Newsroom/PressAnnouncements/ucm576087.htm. Archived at: http://www.webcitation.org/6wQGvAAxn.

98. Damschroder LJ, Hagedorn HJ. A guiding framework and approach for implementation research in substance use disorders. *Psychol Addict Behav.* 2011;25(2): 194−205.

99. Mohr DC, Lyon AR, Lattie EG, Reddy M, Schueller SM. Accelerating digital mental health research from early design and creation to successful implementation and sustainment. *J Med Internet Res.* 2017;19(5):e153. https://doi.org/10.2196/jmir.7725.

100. Buti AL, Eakins D, Fussell H, Kunkel LE, Kudura A, McCarty D. Clinician attitudes, social norms and intentions to use a computer-assisted intervention. *J Subst Abuse Treat.* 2013;44(4):433−437. https://doi.org/10.1016/j.jsat.2012.08.220.

101. Mohr DC, Burns MN, Schueller SM, Clarke G, Klinkman M. Behavioral intervention technologies: evidence review and recommendations for future research in mental health. *Gen Hosp Psychiatry.* 2013;35(4):332−338. https://doi.org/10.1016/j.genhosppsych.2013.03.008.

102. Mohr DC, Schueller SM, Montague E, Burns MN, Rashidi P. The behavioral intervention technology model: an integrated conceptual and technological framework for eHealth and mHealth interventions. *J Med Internet Res.* 2014;16(6):e146. https://doi.org/10.2196/jmir.3077.

103. American Psychiatric Association. *App Evaluation Model.* 2018. Retrieved from: https://www.psychiatry.org/psychiatrists/practice/mental-health-apps/app-evaluation-model. Archived at: http://www.webcitation.org/6wQH7bzmT.

104. Attwood S, Parke H, Larsen J, Morton KL. Using a mobile health application to reduce alcohol consumption: a mixed-methods evaluation of the drinkaware track & calculate units application. *BMC Public Health.* 2017; 17(1):394. https://doi.org/10.1186/s12889-017-4358-9.

105. Balmford J, Borland R, Benda P. Patterns of use of an automated interactive personalized coaching program for smoking cessation. *J Med Internet Res.* 2008;10(5): e54. https://doi.org/10.2196/jmir.1016.

106. Strecher VJ, McClure J, Alexander G, et al. The role of engagement in a tailored web-based smoking cessation program: randomized controlled trial. *J Med Internet Res.* 2008;10(5):e36. https://doi.org/10.2196/jmir.1002.

107. Chambers D, Glasgow R, Stange K. The dynamic sustainability framework: addressing the paradox of sustainment amid ongoing change. *Implement Sci.* 2013;8(1). https://doi.org/10.1186/1748-5908-8-117.

108. Kelders MS, Kok NR, Ossebaard CH, Van Gemert-Pijnen EWCJ. Persuasive system design does matter: a systematic review of adherence to web-based interventions. *J Med Internet Res.* 2012;14(6):e152. https://doi.org/10.2196/jmir.2104.

109. Lord S, Moore SK, Ramsey A, Dinauer S, Johnson K. Implementation of a substance use recovery support mobile phone app in community settings: qualitative study of clinician and staff perspectives of facilitators and barriers. *JMIR Ment Health.* 2016;3(2):e24. https://doi.org/10.2196/mental.4927.

110. McGovern MP, Saunders EC, Kim E. Substance abuse treatment implementation research. *J Subst Abuse Treat.* 2013;44(1):1–3. https://doi.org/10.1016/j.jsat.2012.09.006.

111. Ramsey A, Lord S, Torrey J, Marsch L, Lardiere M. Paving the way to successful implementation: identifying key barriers to use of technology-based therapeutic tools for behavioral health care. *J Natl Behav Health Serv Res.* 2014. https://doi.org/10.1007/s11414-014-9436-5.

112. Asch DA, Muller RW, Volpp KG. Automated hovering in health care—watching over the 5000 hours. *N Engl J Med.* 2012;367(1):1–3. https://doi.org/10.1056/NEJMp1203869.

113. Patel MS, Asch DA, Volpp KG. Wearable devices as facilitators, not drivers, of health behavior change. *JAMA.* 2015;313(5).

114. Bickel WK, Johnson MW, Koffarnus MN, MacKillop J, Murphy JG. The behavioral economics of substance use disorders: reinforcement pathologies and their repair. *Annu Rev Clin Psychol.* 2014;10:641–677. https://doi.org/10.1146/annurev-clinpsy-032813-153724.

115. Bickel WK, Moody L, Higgins ST. Some current dimensions of the behavioral economics of health-related behavior change. *Prev Med.* 2016. https://doi.org/10.1016/j.ypmed.2016.06.002.

116. Otto MW, Eastman A, Lo S, et al. Anxiety sensitivity and working memory capacity: risk factors and targets for health behavior promotion. *Clin Psychol Rev.* 2016;49:67–78. https://doi.org/10.1016/j.cpr.2016.07.003.

CHAPTER 6

State-of-The-Art Treatment of Opioid Use Disorder

LARISSA J. MOONEY, MD • ANDREW SAXON, MD

INTRODUCTION

Definition and Epidemiology of Opioid Use Disorder. Opioid use disorder is a chronic, relapsing disease marked by loss of control over opioid use (e.g., heroin or prescription opioids such as oxycodone or hydrocodone) despite social, psychological, or medical consequences related to use. Per the Diagnostic and Statistical Manual-5 (DSM-5), additional clinical criteria for OUD may include cravings, failed role obligations, use in physically hazardous situations, tolerance, and withdrawal symptoms upon attempts at cessation of opioid use in the past 12 months. OUD may be classified as mild (2–3 criteria), moderate (4–5 criteria), or severe (6 or more criteria).[1] Increasing rates of opioid use disorder (OUD), treatment admissions related to OUD, and opioid overdose deaths in the United States are clear indications of OUD as a public health crisis. Deaths associated with prescription opioid and heroin use were more than five times higher in 2016 than in 1999.[2,3]

Pharmacotherapy for Opioid Use Disorder. Pharmacotherapy represents a central component of treatment for OUD, with behavioral interventions serving as an adjunct. Attempts to manage patients with moderate to severe (i.e. "attempts to manage patients with moderate to severe OUD") OUD without medications typically fail, with 80%–90% relapse rates.[4,5] Three medications have FDA approval for the treatment of OUD: **methadone**, a full μ-opioid agonist; **buprenorphine**, a μ-opioid partial agonist and κ-opioid antagonist; and **naltrexone**, an opioid antagonist.

The focus of this chapter is on pharmacologic treatment of OUD with the three FDA-approved medications: methadone, buprenorphine, and naltrexone. The chapter also describes behavioral interventions for OUD, which typically work best in concert with pharmacologic interventions rather than as stand-alone modalities. Additional topics include common co-occurring substance use disorders, psychiatric disorders, and medical disorders that may require attention during treatment for OUD.

METHADONE FOR OPIOID USE DISORDER

In the United States, methadone for OUD can only be dispensed from federally licensed clinics. Some countries (e.g., Canada, United Kingdom) allow physicians to prescribe methadone for OUD from their practices. Methadone clinics in the United States are highly regulated. Doses are initially dispensed under daily observation; eventually some take-home doses for self-administration are permitted based upon continuous time in treatment and patient stability. Regulations also specify that counseling, vocational, and other treatment services be provided.

Characteristics of Methadone

Methadone Pharmacology. Methadone has a unique and complex pharmacology. It has good oral bioavailability, a gradual onset of action, and is generally long-acting. These characteristics contribute to its efficacy, but its long half-life may also lead to medication build-up and unintended toxicity. Methadone has many possible drug–drug interactions and effects on cardiac conduction; as a result, it has an FDA black box warning concerning respiratory depression and prolongation of the cardiac QT interval. Oral methadone is supplied as a solid tablet, a rapidly dissolving wafer, and a premixed liquid; these formulations are essentially bioequivalent. Methadone consists of a racemic mixture of two stereoisomers, *levo*(L)-methadone and *dextro* (D)-methadone. The L-methadone enantiomer provides the majority of pharmacologic activity, and the D-methadone may contribute to side effects.

Methadone Pharmacokinetics and Pharmacodynamics: There is significant variability in methadone absorption,

The Assessment and Treatment of Addiction. https://doi.org/10.1016/B978-0-323-54856-4.00006-7

metabolism, and clearance both across individuals and within a given individual over time. Methadone has an average bioavailability of about 80%, but interindividual variation ranges from 41% to 95%.[6] Absorption occurs rapidly after oral ingestion of methadone[7]; initial effects appear within 30 min after ingestion, but peak effects and plasma levels are achieved after approximately 4 h, with a range of 1—6 h.[8] The average half-life of methadone is 22 h, with a wide potential range of 5—130 h.[9] The metabolism of methadone is complex, and wide interindividual variation in enzyme activity occurs. Most available data suggests that methadone is mainly catalyzed by the liver enzyme CYP 450 3A4,[10] but there is evidence that other enzymes including CYP2B6, CYP2D6, CYP1A2, CYP2C9, and CYP2C19 also contribute.[9,11] Questions have been raised about the primary role of 3A4,[12] with data suggesting that 2B6 may be the main enzyme responsible for methadone metabolism.[13] Methadone has the ability to induce its own metabolism, particularly during the first month of treatment, causing reduced serum levels.[9] The primary route of methadone elimination is renal with some eliminated in the feces. Methadone primarily acts as an agonist at the μ-opioid receptor, but, unlike most other opioids, it also antagonizes the N-methyl, D-aspartate (NMDA) receptor[8] and blocks serotonin and norepinephrine transporters.[14] Methadone also blocks the cardiac potassium channel, hERG, which can cause a prolonged QT interval on the ECG.[15] Typical μ-opioid agonist effects of methadone include miosis, analgesia, sedation, possible euphoria, decrease in gut motility, and respiratory depression; like other opioids, tolerance may develop to some of these effects.

Clinical Use of Methadone

Given the complex pharmacology of methadone elucidated above, the potential for individualized responses to any given dose of methadone warrants personalized attention to clinical management. Dose conversion calculators are often inaccurate when switching patients from other opioids to methadone or vice versa. Because of methadone's long half-life, a steady-state level on a given dose is not attained for several days; dose escalation that is too rapid can lead to unanticipated medication accumulation causing adverse effects, including potentially fatal respiratory depression. The greatest risk period for overdose death occurs during the first few weeks of treatment and during periods of dose adjustments.[16]

Though the long half-life of methadone is associated with potential adverse intoxication effects, it also makes methadone a highly effective pharmacologic intervention for OUD. For the vast majority of individuals, once-daily dosing alleviates opioid withdrawal symptoms and cravings, which are common drivers of ongoing illicit opioid use. Preclinical evidence indicates that methadone antagonism of excitatory NMDA receptors could decrease opioid tolerance, mitigating the need for repeated dose escalation over time to obtain the same effect.[17,18]

Methadone Induction. The induction period after initial dosing of methadone is about two to 4 weeks to achieve a stable dose. Determination of initial induction dose, which can range from 5 to 30 mg, is partly based on knowledge of the patient's opioid use history, including recent use patterns, tolerance, and withdrawal. Thirty milligrams is the maximum allowable initial dose per federal regulations. For individuals not exposed to any opioids for three or more days prior to induction, 5—10 mg represents the most appropriate initial dose range. Age must also be considered since older individuals generally metabolize methadone less rapidly. For patients with extensive recent use of heroin or other opioids, a 30 mg initial dose typically successfully ameliorates withdrawal symptoms.

If signs or symptoms of withdrawal persist after clinical assessment two to 4 h following the initial methadone dose, additional doses of methadone to a maximum of 40 mg total on day one may be administered. If for any reason a dose higher than 40 mg on day one is considered, it must be clearly documented that additional dosing was essential to manage opioid withdrawal. If sedation or intoxication effects are observed after initial dosing, observation is warranted until effects have resolved, or, if necessary, additional measures such as naloxone administration may be initiated.

Achieving a stable dose of methadone. Given the 22-h average half-life of methadone, upward titration of methadone dosage in 5—10 mg increments every four to 5 days will yield dosages of 60—80 mg per day within 4 weeks of initiation. Induction period goals are to achieve dose stabilization such that opioid cravings and withdrawal symptoms over the 24 h following dose administration are eliminated. Additional goals include production of adequate tolerance to preclude euphoria caused by illicit opioid use, elimination of illicit opioid use as evidenced by self-report and urine drug screen, and minimization of adverse effects and intoxication symptoms that impair daily functioning. Upward titration of methadone doses in increments of 5—10 mg every five to seven days should be continued until induction goals are achieved. After the daily dose exceeds 40 mg, 10 mg dose increments are usually safe and appropriate. Evidence from clinical trials has demonstrated that daily methadone doses of 80–100 mg have significant advantages over lower doses in reducing illicit opioid use and retaining patients in treatment[19]; given individual variation some patients will stabilize on lower doses and others will require doses higher than 100 mg per day.

Methadone interactions with other medications. Multiple drug–drug interactions are possible with methadone given its complex metabolic pathways. Synergistic or additive effects can occur between methadone and other central nervous system depressants, such as opioids or other sedatives, including suppression of respiratory drive leading to toxicity or overdose. Methadone has a boxed warning for QT interval prolongation, so coadministration of methadone with medications that also prolong the QT interval may have additive QT prolongation effects.

Clinically significant medication interactions may occur with coadministration of medications that induce enzymes that catalyze the metabolism of methadone. Decreases in methadone serum level may trigger opioid withdrawal. Medications known to induce methadone metabolism include certain anticonvulsants, such as phenytoin and carbamazepine, the antibiotic rifampin, and antiretroviral medications including lopinavir, efavirenz, and nevirapine.[20] Concurrent use of antiretrovirals may require substantial increases in methadone dose to manage withdrawal symptoms. Inhibitors of enzymes that catalyze methadone metabolism have the potential to elevate methadone serum levels and increase opioid effects.[21,22]

Methadone-related cardiac effects: A corrected QT interval longer than 500 msec may increase the risk of a serious cardiac ventricular arrhythmia, torsades de pointes.[23] In individuals treated with methadone, this arrhythmia has almost always been reported to occur in the context of other risk factors in addition to methadone treatment[24] and likely occurs very rarely.[25,26] Some recommendations encourage routine ECG screening for all patients on methadone, whereas others suggest ECG screening only in the presence of other risk factors,[25,27] such as known structural heart disease or family history of sudden cardiac death.[28] For patients treated with methadone with a corrected QT interval above 500 ms, consideration should be given to discontinuing other medications with QT interval prolongation effects, correcting electrolyte imbalances, or reducing the methadone dose if clinically appropriate.

Interim Methadone Maintenance. In areas of the United States where methadone treatment services are not easily accessible, interim methadone maintenance provides medication-only treatment in place of wait-lists for comprehensive treatment including ancillary services. Interim methadone provides methadone induction followed by daily dosing with no take-home doses and no services except emergency counseling. Although comprehensive methadone treatment has demonstrated superior outcomes to medication-only treatment, interim methadone compared to a wait-list control in at least three randomized controlled trials demonstrated reduced substance use and higher rates of subsequent entry into full methadone treatment services.[29]

BUPRENORPHINE FOR OPIOID USE DISORDER

In contrast to methadone, buprenorphine for OUD can be prescribed by appropriately qualified medical clinicians (e.g., physicians, nurse practitioners, physician assistants) in any office-based medical setting. To qualify as buprenorphine prescribers, clinicians must complete waiver training provided by several different medical specialty organizations. Upon satisfactory completion of training, applicants must request a waiver and a special number from the Drug Enforcement Agency (DEA). During the first year after obtaining the waiver, clinicians are limited to a total of 30 patients to whom they can prescribe buprenorphine at any given time. After the first year, clinicians can request to increase the total number to 100 or to 275 if certain criteria are met. Buprenorphine can also be administered and dispensed in federally licensed Opioid Treatment Programs, which typically provide methadone, where the clinician is not required to have a waiver as long as all federal regulations for these clinics are followed. The regulations for take-home doses of buprenorphine are different from the regulations for take-home doses of methadone, in that once patients on buprenorphine demonstrate adequate stability, there are no requirements for continuous time in treatment to receive the number of take-home doses (up to a maximum of 30) that are clinically indicated.

Characteristics of Buprenorphine

Buprenorphine Pharmacology: Buprenorphine has a unique pharmacology that confers a greater safety profile than methadone. Buprenorphine has extremely poor oral/gastric bioavailability, so several of the currently FDA approved formulations for treatment of OUD are taken by the sublingual or buccal route and absorbed via mucosa. As with methadone, buprenorphine has a gradual onset of action and generally long half-life. Buprenorphine is a partial μ-opioid agonist, rather than a full agonist (e.g., methadone), so its activity has a ceiling effect such that at some point increased doses do not lead to markedly (i.e. "lead to markedly increased effects") increased effects. Thus, the risk of respiratory depression and overdose on buprenorphine, in the absence of concurrent central nervous system depressants, (i.e. "...and overdose on buprenoprphine, is low in healthy adults.") is low in healthy (i.e. "in healthy adults.") adults.[30,31] Buprenorphine has fewer clinically meaningful medication interactions than does methadone, and buprenorphine appears to have smaller and fewer effects on cardiac conduction.[32]

Buprenorphine/Naloxone: There are three transmucosal formulations of buprenorphine marketed for OUD: (1) buprenorphine sublingual tablets; (2) buprenorphine/naloxone sublingual tablets; and (3) buprenorphine/naloxone as a film for sublingual or buccal absorption. The buprenorphine/naloxone formulation is intended to deter parenteral misuse of the medication. Naloxone, a μ-opioid receptor antagonist, has minimal sublingual bioavailability; when taken by the sublingual route, insufficient naloxone is absorbed to have any clinically significant effect. However, since naloxone has very good parenteral bioavailability, attempts to crush and inject buprenorphine/naloxone result in naloxone blunting parenteral effects of buprenorphine and possibly precipitating opioid withdrawal if full agonist opioids are present.[33] Buprenorphine/naloxone is the predominant formulation prescribed in the nation, with few problems related to parental misuse of buprenorphine.

Other buprenorphine formulations. Buprenorphine is also available as a subdermal implant that consistently releases active medication over 6 months.[34,35] Implants must be surgically inserted in a brief office procedure and surgically removed after the treatment period. FDA approval was obtained in 2015[36] for individuals already stabilized on 8 mg or less of transmucosal buprenorphine per day. A newer monthly extended release (i.e. "monthly extended-release injectable formulation") injectable formulation of buprenoprhine was approved in 2017[37] for the treatment of moderate to severe OUD in individuals who have initiated a transmucosal buprenorphine-containing product and have been stabilized on treatment for at least 7 days. The product is administered subcutaneously and deposits buprenorphine dissolved in a biodegradable delivery system (depot) that releases buprenorphine steadily as it biodegrades over time. In one study supporting its approval, the proportion of patients (N = 504) achieving treatment success (≥80% opioid-free weeks) was significantly higher in both 300 and 100 mg groups versus placebo (28.4%, 29.1%, and 2%, respectively).[38] The approved dosing regimen is 300 mg administered subcutaneously for the first 2 months, followed by maintenance doses of 100 mg/month. It must be prescribed as part of a Risk Evaluation and Mitigation Strategy to ensure that the product is not distributed directly to patients.

Buprenorphine Pharmacokinetics and Pharmacodynamics: Absorption of buprenorphine occurs rapidly after sublingual administration. Bioavailability shows large interindividual variability but is generally around 35% for the tablet.[39,40] Initial effects appear within 30 min with peak plasma levels occurring an average of 1 h after ingestion.[39,41,42] Buprenorphine has an estimated average half-life of 32 h,[39] although there is wide variation across studies and individuals.[43] Most available data suggest that metabolism is primarily catalyzed by the liver enzyme CYP 450 3A4. The product of N-dealkylation is an active metabolite, norbuprenorphine.[39,42] The main route of buprenorphine clearance is fecal with lesser amounts excreted by the kidneys.[39]

Buprenorphine serves as a partial agonist with high affinity at the μ-opioid receptor and slow dissociation and acts as an antagonist at the κ-opioid receptor.[44,45] It also has agonist properties at the nociceptin/orphanin FQ (NOP) receptor (formerly known as ORL1 receptor).[46] Buprenorphine has typical clinically observable μ-opioid agonist effects including analgesia, sedation, possible euphoria, decrease in gut motility, and respiratory depression with a ceiling on the latter effect given its partial agonist activity.[44]

Clinical Use of Buprenorphine

With its excellent safety profile as a partial μ-opioid receptor agonist, buprenorphine poses virtually no risk from rapid dose escalation. However, given its high affinity for the receptor, it may precipitate opioid withdrawal if administered in the presence of full agonists because it can displace them from the receptors.[47] As with methadone, buprenorphine's long half-life permits once-daily dosing.

Buprenorphine Induction: Induction onto a stable dose of buprenorphine may typically be achieved within a few days. To avoid the risk of precipitated opioid withdrawal, patients must abstain from short-acting opioids for approximately 12−24 h and enter a state of moderate opioid withdrawal prior to the administration of the initial dose of buprenorphine. If an individual has recently taken methadone, which has a long half-life, abstinence for at least 48−72 h is recommended for opioid withdrawal to commence and to avoid precipitated withdrawal. A standardized assessment to measure opioid withdrawal severity, such as the Clinical Opiate Withdrawal Scale (COWS)[48] may be used.

Once objective signs of withdrawal are observed, induction can begin with a low buprenorphine dosage of 2 or 4 mg which is likely to alleviate withdrawal signs and symptoms within 30−60 min. Additional 2 mg doses may be administered every 1−2 h until withdrawal symptoms are eliminated, usually within one or 2 days at doses up to 24 mg total per day.

Managing Precipitated Opioid Withdrawal during Buprenorphine Induction. If buprenorphine is administered prior to the development of sufficient opioid withdrawal symptoms, precipitated withdrawal may occur. Since buprenorphine is occupying the μ-opioid receptors and has strong affinity, full-agonist opioids will not relieve this precipitated withdrawal. Management options are as follows: (1) stop the induction and treat the withdrawal symptomatically using clonidine or lofexidine (recently approved in the United States[37]) for autonomic nervous system signs and symptoms, muscle relaxants for muscle cramping, benzodiazepines for anxiety, and antiemetics and antidiarrheals for gastrointestinal symptoms. When withdrawal symptoms have subsided, buprenorphine induction may be restarted; (2) continue buprenorphine induction dosing every 1−2 h knowing that withdrawal symptoms will resolve within 24 h. Medications for symptomatic management described above may also be used as needed.

Maintenance Buprenorphine Dosing. Stabilization of buprenorphine dose after induction may involve additional adjustments until the optimal dose is attained that is sufficient to eliminate opioid craving, withdrawal symptoms, and illicit opioid use as evidenced by self-report and urine drug screen. The daily maintenance dose can range from a minimum of 2 mg to a maximum of 32 mg per day, although most individuals stabilize on a dose between 12 and 24 mg per day. Even after stability is achieved, adjustments up or down over time may be needed. For many individuals after a period of time, the dose can be gradually reduced without compromising clinical stability.

Buprenorphine Interactions with other Medications. Additive or synergistic effects may occur between buprenorphine and other central nervous system depressants that suppress respiratory drive leading to sedation or overdose. Rare cases of fatal overdoses have been reported from the combination of benzodiazepines and buprenorphine,[49] but the combination is not contraindicated as long as the benzodiazepine doses are moderate and the patient is under close clinical supervision. Although buprenorphine metabolism is catalyzed by the same CYP 450 3A4 enzyme system as methadone, combining medications that induce or inhibit CYP 450 3A4 with buprenorphine do not typically cause

clinically significant adverse effects.[20] The proposed explanation is that, given its strong affinity for the μ-opioid receptor, changes in plasma levels of buprenorphine do not rapidly affect receptor occupancy of buprenorphine. If buprenorphine is initiated when other opioids are occupying the μ-opioid receptor, it can precipitate withdrawal. If other opioids are administered in the presence of buprenorphine, effects are likely to be greatly diminished given that buprenorphine is already occupying the majority of μ-opioid receptors.

MANAGING SIDE EFFECTS OF METHADONE AND BUPRENORPHINE

Methadone and buprenorphine can produce many of the adverse effects commonly associated with other opioid medications. Side effects can often be managed by incremental dose reductions of methadone 5−10 mg or of buprenorphine 2−4 mg every 5−7 days until side effects are resolved or until withdrawal symptoms occur. If dose reductions are not possible because they compromise clinical stability on the medication, other interventions can be attempted to manage side effects.

Constipation is common when taking methadone or buprenorphine and can be managed by encouraging patients to consume more water, increasing fiber in the diet, and if needed, taking bulk-forming laxatives (e.g., psyllium) or emollient laxatives such as docusate. If necessary, stimulant laxatives (bisacodyl) or osmotic laxatives (lactulose) may be prescribed. Edema can be associated with methadone use[50] but occurs much less often with buprenorphine. It usually does not improve with sodium restriction but sometimes improves with a decrease in methadone dosage. If severe, diuretics such as furosemide may be prescribed, but potassium levels should be checked to monitor for potassium depletion.

Excessive sweating is commonly reported by patients on methadone[51] and may respond to dose reduction or changes in other medications that may also induce sweating (e.g., cholinesterase inhibitors, selective serotonin reuptake inhibitors, or tricyclic antidepressants). Headache is more commonly reported by patients taking buprenorphine; it is usually mild and may spontaneously resolve. If needed, dose reduction or use of acetaminophen or nonsteroidal anti-inflammatory medications may be considered.

Both methadone and buprenorphine may cause hormonal alterations related to sexual functioning, but these alterations seem to be more common with methadone.[52] All opioids act at the hypothalamus and alter the release of gonadotropin releasing hormone, leading to subsequent suppression of testosterone levels or estrogen levels. Side effects include erectile dysfunction or decreased sexual desire and may respond to dose reduction.

Alternately, phosphodiesterase type 5 inhibitors may be prescribed for erectile dysfunction, or testosterone replacement may improve sexual functioning if low serum testosterone levels are present. Women on methadone have also reported oligomenorrhea or amenorrhea; conversely, in other cases, regular menses resume after stabilizing on medication treatment.

Methadone is associated with hyperprolactinemia in some individuals.[53] Problems related to hyperprolactinemia may include galactorrhea, menstrual disturbance, erectile dysfunction, and bone density loss. Higher rates of low bone mineral density have been reported in methadone maintained individuals.[54,55] Hormonal effects of buprenorphine have been less well studied, but lower rates of testosterone deficiency and sexual dysfunction have been observed relative to methadone.[56]

WITHDRAWAL FROM METHADONE OR BUPRENORPHINE UNDER MEDICAL SUPERVISION

Medically supervised withdrawal or tapering from methadone or buprenorphine requires a careful assessment of risks and benefits because of high rates of relapse to opioid use.[5,57] When taper is necessary or desired, evidence indicates that for methadone gradual tapers promote better outcomes,[57] whereas for buprenorphine, rapid tapers (~7 days) may be tolerated by some, but not all, patients.[58,59] In general, the rate of taper should be adjusted based on the patient's preferences, expectations, and tolerability. For methadone, a decrease of 5–10 mg every one to two weeks might be initially attempted; as the daily dosage drops below 40–60 mg per day, the rate of taper should typically be decreased. Buprenorphine tapers may be conducted by reducing the daily dosage in increments of 2 or 4 mg over an extended period, though outcomes are not necessarily improved by prolonging the taper. To mitigate opioid withdrawal symptoms, the use of α_2-adrenergic agonists such as clonidine or lofexidine may be considered.[60,61] A maximum of 1.2 mg of clonidine or a maximum of 3.2 mg of lofexidine per 24 h in divided doses may be given, and the dosage is usually tapered over 5–14 days.[61–63]

NALTREXONE FOR OPIOID USE DISORDER

Naltrexone is a μ-opioid receptor antagonist and blocks the effects of exogenously administered opioids. In order to start naltrexone, individuals must be fully abstinent from opioids to avoid the risk of precipitated opioid withdrawal. The state of being opioid free is typically determined by self-report, urine drug screen, and ideally a naloxone challenge test.[64]

Naltrexone Pharmacology. Naltrexone is available in two formulations, 50 mg oral tablets or a 380 mg extended-release intramuscular injection. The tablets were initially approved for treatment of opioid dependence in 1984, and the extended-release injection received FDA approval for treatment of opioid use disorder in 2010 after a double-blind, placebo-controlled trial in Russia demonstrated reduction in opioid relapse, reduced opioid cravings, and improved treatment retention.[65] In the injectable formulation, naltrexone microspheres are encapsulated in a biodegradable polylactide-co-glycolid polymer that slowly degrades and releases naltrexone into the surrounding tissue.[66]

Naltrexone Pharmacokinetics and Pharmacodynamics. The clinical effects of naltrexone result primarily from its activity as a μ-opioid receptor antagonist, but naltrexone has some capacity to also block δ- and κ-opioid receptors.[67,68] Absorption of naltrexone occurs rapidly, and peak plasma levels are reached approximately 1 h after ingestion.[66,69] Oral naltrexone has a half-life of 4-h.[66,69] After injection of the extended-release formulation, naltrexone located near the surface of the microspheres is quickly released, causing an initial peak in plasma concentrations 1–2 h after administration; after a subsequent decline, naltrexone embedded deeper in the microspheres is released, resulting in a second and higher peak approximately 2 days after administration. Plasma levels of injectable naltrexone are measurable for longer than 35 days.[66]

Naltrexone metabolism. The metabolism of naltrexone is catalyzed by aldo-keto reductase enzymes AKR1C1, AKR1C2, and AKR1C4 rather than CYP 450 enzymes.[70] Naltrexone undergoes reduction via these enzymes to its major active metabolite 6-β-naltrexol.[71] The primary route of elimination is renal, with minor amounts in the feces. After oral dosing, the ratio of 6-β-naltrexol to naltrexone plasma levels is 10:1, and for injection it is 1:1 because of reduced first pass metabolism with the injection.[66]

Naltrexone Interactions with Other Medications. Because naltrexone is not metabolized by the CYP

450 system, it does not affect the metabolism of other medications. As an opioid antagonist, naltrexone blocks the effects of other opioids, so if an individual on naltrexone requires treatment with opioid analgesics to manage pain from physical trauma or surgery, he or she must be treated in a medically monitored setting using high intravenous doses of a potent opioid such as fentanyl in order to overcome the blockade. Patients also need to be warned of the theoretical risks of overdose from using large quantities of intravenous opioids to overcome the blockade or from using opioids after stopping naltrexone; since opioid tolerance decreases during the time, individuals are on naltrexone.[72]

Clinical Use of Naltrexone

In order to initiate naltrexone, individuals must not have opioids in the system and be free of signs and symptoms of opioid withdrawal. Acute withdrawal typically resolves approximately 5–7 days after last dose of short-acting opioids and up to 10 days for methadone or buprenorphine. Various induction strategies using low ascending doses of oral naltrexone, tapering doses of buprenorphine, and ancillary medications to facilitate comfortable transition onto extended-release naltrexone are under investigation (e.g., [73–75]). If any opioids remain on the receptor at the time of initial dosing of naltrexone, severe opioid withdrawal will be precipitated. Therefore, it is important to verify opioid-negative status by self-report and urine drug screen. A procedure called a "naloxone challenge" test may also be performed to verify the absence of opioids; since naloxone is a short-acting opioid antagonist, any precipitated withdrawal will be very brief relative to that precipitated by naltrexone.[64] Naloxone may be administered via subcutaneous, intramuscular, or intravenous route up to a total dose of 0.8 mg. If any indication of even mild withdrawal is observed, induction onto naltrexone should be postponed at least 24 h, followed by a repeat naloxone challenge test. Once the absence of opioids is verified, 25–50 mg of oral naltrexone may be given, followed by administration of the extended-release injection if tolerated. If precipitated withdrawal occurs from naloxone or naltrexone, α_2 agonists and ancillary medications may be administered to ameliorate symptoms.

The usual oral naltrexone dose is 50 mg daily. However, given poor adherence to the oral formulation observed in individuals with opioid use disorder,[76] use of the extended-release preparation is recommended. Extended-release naltrexone is administered as a deep intramuscular gluteal injection of 380 mg every 28 or 30 days using alternating sides of the buttocks each month. Therapeutic blood levels will be maintained for more than 30 days.

Naltrexone Side Effects. Common side effects of naltrexone include nausea, diarrhea, headache, dizziness, and insomnia. Typically, these effects are transient and dissipate early in treatment. If necessary, ancillary medications, such as antiemetics, can be prescribed. Though oral naltrexone has a boxed warning for hepatic injury, no serious or lethal hepatic toxicity has been observed when prescribed at recommended doses. Depression and suicidal ideation have also been reported in association with naltrexone treatment. The extended-release preparation has the additional potential side effect of injection site reactions, such as redness, tenderness, or induration. Mild reactions can usually be managed with palliative measures such as warm compresses and use of over-the-counter analgesics. In rare severe cases, antibiotics or minor surgical intervention might be necessary.

EFFICACY AND CLINICAL UTILITY OF THE THREE MEDICATIONS FOR OPIOID USE DISORDER

Research over the past several decades has documented that the three approved medications are effective for OUD, especially compared to placebo or to other non-medication interventions such as mutual-support groups, behavioral interventions, or abstinence-based residential treatment, after which relapse is common. While on medication, patients are far more likely to cease or greatly reduce their use of opioids, reduce behaviors associated with infectious disease transmission, improve overall health, and engage in more prosocial behaviors.

Methadone and Buprenorphine. Multiple randomized clinical trials have directly compared buprenorphine treatment to methadone treatment on the outcomes of illicit opioid use and treatment retention. A meta-analysis of 31 studies found both treatments equally efficacious at reducing illicit opioid use but found methadone slightly better at retaining patients in treatment, particularly when prescribed in flexible dose regimens. When prescribed at fixed medium to high doses, no differences in treatment retention were observed between buprenorphine and methadone. However, results of flexible dose studies are likely more clinically relevant because dose adjustment based on individual need occurs.[77]

Naltrexone. Adherence to oral naltrexone for opioid use disorder is generally poor, with early dropout commonly observed. When studies that compared oral naltrexone versus placebo combined with psychosocial treatment were pooled with studies comparing naltrexone and placebo without psychosocial treatment, oral naltrexone had a slight statistically significant edge over placebo in reducing illicit opioid use when participants remained in treatment but no advantage in treatment retention.[76] The placebo-controlled randomized trials done so far with extended-release naltrexone suggest that the active medication improves both treatment retention and illicit opioid use and reduces opioid cravings.[65,78] In the criminal justice population, treatment for OUD with extended release naltrexone has also been found to be more effective in reducing relapse to opioids than usual treatment (e.g., counseling, referrals).[79]

Extended-release Naltrexone and Buprenorphine. Two clinical trials have compared monthly extended-release naltrexone with daily sublingual buprenorphine in individuals with OUD and found little difference in opioid relapse rates between the two groups; however, initial induction on buprenorphine may be easier to accomplish than naltrexone. A 12-week open-label trial comparing monthly extended-release naltrexone and daily sublingual buprenorphine (4−24 mg/day) found the two medications to be similarly effective in reducing opioid use in 159 adult participants.[80] At the end of the trial, naltrexone was noninferior to buprenorphine in the proportion of opioid-negative urine drug tests and in days of illicit opioid use. The trial did not adequately assess the efficacy of buprenorphine because the mean daily dose of buprenorphine was 11.2 mg/day, below what would typically be considered its therapeutic range (12−16 mg/day). Another open-label trial randomly assigned 570 individuals with OUD to receive monthly injectable naltrexone or daily sublingual buprenorphine (mean maintenance dose 16 mg/day) for 24 weeks.[79] Participants had entered inpatient programs for planned withdrawal from opioids, but had not necessarily completed withdrawal at the time of enrollment. Induction onto monthly naltrexone was successful in a smaller proportion of participants than buprenorphine (72% vs. 94%). However, among participants successfully inducted onto either medication, relapse rates were equivalent between both groups.

NALOXONE FOR OVERDOSE PREVENTION

Naloxone is a short-acting opioid receptor antagonist that rapidly reverses symptoms of opioid overdose including sedation and respiratory depression. It may be administered intravenously, intramuscularly, or subcutaneously in cases of suspected overdose, with recent formulations offering easy-to-administer intranasal administration. It has been increasingly prescribed or dispensed to opioid users and their friends or family members for take-home use in many countries across the world. Naloxone was added to the World Health Organization list of essential medications in 2013,[81] and the US Surgeon General issued an advisory in 2017 that more Americans should be familiar with naloxone and how to use it.[82] Consideration should be given to prescribing naloxone for individuals with risk factors for opioid overdose, including those who (1) have a history of OUD, (2) have a history of prescription opioid misuse or illicit opioid use, (3) have been discharged from medical care after opioid overdose, (4) are taking long-term prescription opioids for chronic pain, particularly at higher doses or in combination with alcohol or other sedatives, or (5) who have been recently released from incarcerated settings and have a history of OUD.[82]

Available formulations of naloxone for take-home use include intramuscular injection, intranasal, and auto-injector products. Brief education focused on overdose prevention and recognition of signs of opioid overdose are given in conjunction with take-home naloxone, and individuals are instructed to call emergency services for medical evaluation together with use. Research to date supports the relative benefits and minimal risks of naloxone administration and overdose education as demonstrated by reductions in overdose deaths in communities in which naloxone is available for use.[81,83]

BEHAVIORAL INTERVENTIONS FOR OPIOID USE DISORDER

Studies to date largely favor the use of behavioral interventions as an adjunct to pharmacotherapy to improve treatment retention and reduce substance use in individuals with OUD. Behavioral treatments may also be combined with other forms of support, such as 12-step mutual help groups. However, the incremental benefit and utility of behavioral treatments vary widely across interventions, outcomes, and medications, and studies do not demonstrate superiority of any single approach.[84] Well-studied psychosocial/behavioral interventions used in conjunction with pharmacotherapy for OUD include cognitive behavioral therapy (CBT) and contingency management (CM). Cognitive behavioral therapy (CBT) focuses on relapse prevention skills including identification and avoidance of relapse triggers, development of coping skills, understanding cravings, maintaining new lifestyle behaviors, and increasing self-efficacy. Contingency Management

(CM) interventions rely on operant conditioning to shape behavior in accord with specified reinforcers of desired behaviors.[85] Rewards, such as vouchers for providing opioid-negative urine specimens, may escalate in value over time according to a predetermined schedule to facilitate ongoing gains in behavior change, including abstinence from opioid use.

Contingency management has been demonstrated to decrease rates of substance use during methadone and naltrexone treatment over and above rates achieved by routine counseling.[86,87] Studies of behavioral interventions in combination with buprenorphine pharmacotherapy for OUD have largely failed to demonstrate improvement in treatment outcomes associated with behavioral interventions, including CBT and CM, compared to agonist treatment alone.[5,88–90] A secondary analysis of a study of buprenorphine in primary care revealed improved substance use outcomes associated with CBT for primary prescription opioid users but not heroin users.[91]

DISORDERS CO-OCCURRING WITH OUD

To optimize treatment outcomes with pharmacotherapy and ancillary behavioral therapies, other conditions must be addressed in order to improve the overall health of patients and sustain gains from treatment for OUD. Clinicians must be aware of other common co-occurring disorders such as other substance use disorders, psychiatric disorders, and medical disorders.

Other Substance Use Disorders

Individuals with OUD have high rates of other substance use. Problematic use of other substances can undermine stability in treatment and may necessitate additional active interventions. Alcohol use disorder should be treated using one or more behavioral interventions including contingency management, motivational interviewing, or cognitive behavioral therapy for relapse prevention together with approved pharmacotherapy such as naltrexone, disulfiram, or acamprosate. Naltrexone is contraindicated in patients on methadone or buprenorphine because its use will precipitate opioid withdrawal. Additional nonapproved medications with some evidence for the treatment of alcohol use disorder include topiramate and gabapentin.[92] To treat other substance use disorders for which there are no FDA approved medication options, such as cannabis and stimulant use disorders, evidence-based behavioral interventions (e.g., contingency management, cognitive behavioral therapy) remain the mainstay of treatment (e.g., Ref.[93]).

Co-occurring Psychiatric Disorders

Patients with OUD have higher rates of some psychiatric disorders than the general population, including major depression, anxiety disorders, and antisocial personality disorder.[94–96] Careful clinical assessment of co-occurring disorders using a thorough psychiatric interview is warranted. Treatment of psychiatric disorders using medication and behavioral interventions is similar to that delivered to other populations and is ideally integrated with OUD treatment. Primary treatment of OUD is associated with significant reductions in depressive symptoms; however, studies of antidepressant treatment for depressive disorders in individuals with OUD have yielded mixed findings, with some positive but more negative results.[97,98]

Co-occurring Medical Disorders

Opioid use disorder is associated with elevated mortality risk. Certain medical disorders that co-occur with OUD are related to the route of opioid administration. Injection opioid use, for example, is associated with increased risk of infectious diseases including endocarditis, HIV, Hepatitis C, bone and soft tissue infections (e.g.,[99,100]). Chronic pain conditions are also relatively common in individuals with OUD and may be a consequence of co-occurring medical disorders, accidents, or other trauma. When pain occurs, conservative measures such as nonsteroidal anti-inflammatory medications or physical therapy can be attempted. If treatment with opioid pain medications is anticipated or necessary, naltrexone is not a good choice of medication for OUD because it blocks the effects of opioids. Buprenorphine has considerable analgesic activity[101] and may help to stabilize pain in individuals with evidence of opioid misuse.[102] In cases of intractable pain, higher doses of buprenorphine given in divided doses up to 32 mg per day can be attempted, or a switch to methadone maintenance may be considered. However, the analgesic effectiveness of buprenorphine or methadone may be diminished when used for long-term OUD treatment due to opioid-related properties including tolerance, hyperalgesia, and a duration of analgesic activity (4–8 h) that is considerably shorter than suppression of opioid withdrawal (over 24 h[103]).

CONCLUSION

Since opioid use disorder (OUD) and related public health consequences are increasing in prevalence, clinicians need to be aware of potential treatment options for this condition. Individuals with OUD should almost always receive pharmacotherapy because outcomes without medication are often very poor. The three medications approved for treatment of OUD—methadone, buprenorphine, and naltrexone—have unique characteristics and different formulations, which require considerable knowledge and skill for appropriate prescribing and management. Behavioral treatment interventions may be used as an adjunct when combined with pharmacotherapy. When individuals are stabilized on medication for OUD, they also may need interventions for co-occurring substance, psychiatric, and medical disorders to attain optimal treatment outcomes.

REFERENCES

1. American Psychiatric Association. *Diagnostic and Statistical Manual of Mental Disorders*. 5th ed. Washington, DC: Author; 2013.
2. Seth P, Rudd R, Noonan R, Haegerich T. Quantifying the epidemic of prescription opioid overdose deaths. *Am J Public Health*. 2018;108(4):e1–e3.
3. Hedegaard H, Warner M, Miniño AM. *Drug Overdose Deaths in the United States, 1999–2016. NCHS Data Brief, no 294*. Hyattsville, MD: National Center for Health Statistics; 2017.
4. Ball JC, Ross A. *The Effectiveness of Methadone Maintenance Treatment: Clients, Programs, Services, and Outcome*. New York, NY: Springer-Verlag; 1991.
5. Weiss RD, Potter JS, Fiellin DA, et al. Adjunctive counseling during brief and extended buprenorphine-naloxone treatment for prescription opioid dependence: a 2-phase randomized controlled trial. *Arch Gen Psychiatry*. 2011;68(12):1238–1246.
6. Ferrari A, Coccia CPR, Bertolini A, Sternieri E. Methadone—metabolism, pharmacokinetics and interactions. *Pharmacol Res*. 2004;50(6):551–559.
7. Leavitt SB, Shinderman M, Maxwell S, Eap CB, Paris P. When "enough" is not enough: new perspectives on optimal methadone maintenance dose. *Mt Sinai J Med*. 2000;67(5–6):404–411.
8. Inturrisi CE. The role of N-methyl-D-aspartate (NMDA) receptors in pain and morphine tolerance. *Minerva Anestesiol*. 2005;71(7–8):401–403.
9. Eap CB, Buclin T, Baumann P. Interindividual variability of the clinical pharmacokinetics of methadone. *Clin Pharmacokinet*. 2002;41(14):1153–1193.
10. Moody DE, Alburges ME, Parker RJ, Collins JM, Strong JM. The involvement of cytochrome P450 3A4 in the N-demethylation of l-α-acetylmethadol (LAAM), norLAAM, and methadone. *Drug Metabol Dispos*. 1997; 25(12):1347–1353.
11. Eap CB, Broly F, Mino A, et al. Cytochrome P450 2D6 genotype and methadone steady-state concentrations. *J Clin Psychopharmacol*. 2001;21(2):229–234.
12. Kharasch ED, Walker A, Whittington D, Hoffer C, Bedynek PS. Methadone metabolism and clearance are induced by nelfinavir despite inhibition of cytochrome P4503A (CYP3A) activity. *Drug Alcohol Depend*. 2009; 101(3):158–168.
13. Kharasch ED. Current concepts in methadone metabolism and transport. *Clin Pharmacol Drug Develop*. 2017;6(2):125–134.
14. Codd EE, Shank RP, Schupsky JJ, Raffa RB. Serotonin and norepinephrine uptake inhibiting activity of centrally acting analgesics: structural determinants and role in antinociception. *J Pharmacol Exp Ther*. 1995;274(3): 1263–1270.
15. Eap CB, Crettol S, Rougier JS, et al. Stereoselective block of hERG channel by (S)-methadone and QT interval prolongation in CYP2B6 slow metabolizers. *Clin Pharmacol Ther*. 2007;81(5):719–728.
16. Corkery JM, Schifano F, Ghodse AH, Oyefeso A. The effects of methadone and its role in fatalities. *Hum Psychopharmacol Clin Exp*. 2004;19(8):565–576.
17. Chartoff EH, Connery HS. It's MORe exciting than mu: crosstalk between mu opioid receptors and glutamatergic transmission in the mesolimbic dopamine system. *Front Pharmacol*. 2014;5:116.
18. Davis AM, Inturrisi CE. d-Methadone blocks morphine tolerance andN-methyl-D-aspartate-induced hyperalgesia. *J Pharmacol Exp Ther*. 1999;289(2):1048–1053.
19. Strain EC, Bigelow GE, Liebson IA, Stitzer ML. Moderate-vs high-dose methadone in the treatment of opioid dependence: a randomized trial. *JAMA*. 1999;281(11): 1000–1005.
20. McCance-Katz EF, Sullivan LE, Nallani S. Drug interactions of clinical importance among the opioids, methadone and buprenorphine, and other frequently prescribed medications: a review. *Am J Addict*. 2010; 19(1):4–16.
21. Tarumi Y, Pereira J, Watanabe S. Methadone and fluconazole: respiratory depression by drug interaction. *J Pain Symptom Manag*. 2002;23(2):148–153.
22. Armstrong SC, Cozza KL, Oesterheld JR. Med-psych drug-drug interactions update. *Psychosomatics*. 2002;43(1): 77–81.
23. Joy JP, Coulter CV, Duffull SB, Isbister GK. Prediction of torsade de pointes from the QT interval: analysis of a case series of amisulpride overdoses. *Clin Pharmacol Ther*. 2011;90(2):243–245.
24. Thanavaro KL, Thanavaro JL. Methadone-induced torsades de pointes: a twist of fate. *Heart Lung J Acute Crit Care*. 2011;40(5):448–453.
25. Bart G. CSAT's QT interval screening in methadone report: outrageous fortune or sea of troubles? *J Addict Dis*. 2011;30(4):313–317.
26. Perrin-Terrin A, Pathak A, Lapeyre-Mestre M. QT interval prolongation: prevalence, risk factors and pharmacovigilance data among methadone-treated

patients in France. *Fundam Clin Pharmacol.* 2011;25(4): 503–510.

27. Martin JA, Campbell A, Killip T, et al. QT interval screening in methadone maintenance treatment: report of a SAMHSA expert panel. *J Addict Dis.* 2011;30(4): 283–306.

28. Goldenberg I, Zareba W, Moss AJ. Long QT syndrome. *Curr Problems Cardiol.* 2008;33(11):629–694.

29. Schwartz RP, Highfield DA, Jaffe JH, et al. A randomized controlled trial of interim methadone maintenance. *Arch Gen Psychiatry.* 2006;63(1):102–109.

30. Walsh SL, Preston KL, Stitzer ML, Cone EJ, Bigelow GE. Clinical pharmacology of buprenorphine: ceiling effects at high doses. *Clin Pharmacol Ther.* 1994;55(5):569–580.

31. Dahan A, Yassen A, Bijl H, et al. Comparison of the respiratory effects of intravenous buprenorphine and fentanyl in humans and rats. *Br J Anaesth.* 2005;94(6): 825–834.

32. Wedam EF, Bigelow GE, Johnson RE, Nuzzo PA, Haigney MC. QT-interval effects of methadone, levomethadyl, and buprenorphine in a randomized trial. *Arch Intern Med.* 2007;167(22):2469–2475.

33. Comer SD, Sullivan MA, Vosburg SK, et al. Abuse liability of intravenous buprenorphine/naloxone and buprenorphine alone in buprenorphine-maintained intravenous heroin abusers. *Addiction.* 2010;105(4):709–718.

34. Ling W, Casadonte P, Bigelow G, et al. Buprenorphine implants for treatment of opioid dependence: a randomized controlled trial. *JAMA.* 2010;304(14):1576–1583.

35. White J, Bell J, Saunders JB, et al. Open-label dose-finding trial of buprenorphine implants (Probuphine) for treatment of heroin dependence. *Drug Alcohol Depend.* 2009; 103(1–2):37–43.

36. Braeburn Pharmaceuticals. *Titan Pharmaceuticals and Braeburn Pharmaceuticals Announce FDA Advisory Committee Recommends Approval of Probuphine, First 6-Month Implant to Treat Opioid Addiction [online]*; 2015. Available at: https://braeburnpharmaceuticals.com/titan-pharmaceuticals-and-braeburn-pharmaceuticals-announce-fda-advisory-committee-recommends-approval-of-probuphine-first-6-month-implant-to-treat-opioid-addiction/.

37. FDA. *FDA Approves the First Non-opioid Treatment for Management of Opioid Withdrawal Symptoms in Adults;* 2018. https://www.fda.gov/NewsEvents/Newsroom/Press Announcements/ucm607884.htm.

38. *Indivior.* 2017. http://indivior.com/wp-content/uploads/2017/11/SUBLOCADE-Prescribing-Information.pdf.

39. Chiang CN, Hawks RL. Pharmacokinetics of the combination tablet of buprenorphine and naloxone. *Drug Alcohol Depend.* 2003;70(2):S39–S47.

40. Compton P, Ling W, Moody D, Chiang N. Pharmacokinetics, bioavailability and opioid effects of liquid versus tablet buprenorphine. *Drug Alcohol Depend.* 2006;82(1): 25–31.

41. Strain EC, Moody DE, Stoller KB, Walsh SL, Bigelow GE. Relative bioavailability of different buprenorphine formulations under chronic dosing conditions. *Drug Alcohol Depend.* 2004;74(1):37–43.

42. Greenwald MK, Johanson CE, Moody DE, et al. Effects of buprenorphine maintenance dose on μ-opioid receptor availability, plasma concentrations, and antagonist blockade in heroin-dependent volunteers. *Neuropsychopharmacology.* 2003;28(11):2000.

43. Elkader A, Sproule B. Buprenorphine. *Clin Pharmacokinet.* 2005;44(7):661–680.

44. Walsh SL, Eissenberg T. The clinical pharmacology of buprenorphine: extrapolating from the laboratory to the clinic. *Drug Alcohol Depend.* 2003;70(2):S13–S27.

45. Johnson RE, Strain EC, Amass L. Buprenorphine: how to use it right. *Drug Alcohol Depend.* 2003;70(2):S59–S77.

46. Chiou LC, Liao YY, Fan PC, et al. Nociceptin/orphanin FQ peptide receptors: pharmacology and clinical implications. *Curr Drug Targets.* 2007;8(1):117–135.

47. Walsh SL, June HL, Schuh KJ, Preston KL, Bigelow GE, Stitzer ML. Effects of buprenorphine and methadone in methadone-maintained subjects. *Psychopharmacology.* 1995;119(3):268–276.

48. Wesson DR, Ling W. The clinical opiate withdrawal scale (COWS). *J Psychoact Drugs.* 2003;35(2):253–259.

49. Hakkinen M, Launiainen T, Vuori E, Ojanpera I. Benzodiazepines and alcohol are associated with cases of fatal buprenorphine poisoning. *Eur J Clin Pharmacol.* 2012; 68(3):301–309.

50. Mahé I, Chassany O, Grenard AS, Caulin C, Bergmann JF. Methadone and edema: a case-report and literature review. *Eur J Clin Pharmacol.* 2004;59(12):923–924.

51. Langrod J, Lowinson J, Ruiz P. Methadone treatment and physical complaints: a clinical analysis. *Int J Addict.* 1981; 16(5):947–952.

52. Hallinan R, Byrne A, Agho K, McMahon CG, Tynan P, Attia J. Hypogonadism in men receiving methadone and buprenorphine maintenance treatment. *Int J Androl.* 2009;32(2):131–139.

53. Trajanovska AS, Vujovic V, Ignjatova L, Janicevic-Ivanovska D, Cibisev A. Sexual dysfunction as a side effect of hyperprolactinemia in methadone maintenance therapy. *Med Arch.* 2013;67(1):48–50.

54. Kim TW, Alford DP, Malabanan A, Holick MF, Samet JH. Low bone density in patients receiving methadone maintenance treatment. *Drug Alcohol Depend.* 2006;85(3): 258–262.

55. Kim TW, Alford DP, Holick MF, Malabanan AO, Samet JH. Low vitamin d status of patients in methadone maintenance treatment. *J Addict Med.* 2009;3(3):134.

56. Bliesener N, Albrecht S, Schwager A, Weckbecker K, Lichtermann D, Klingmüller D. Plasma testosterone and sexual function in men receiving buprenorphine maintenance for opioid dependence. *J Clin Endocrinol Metab.* 2004;90(1):203–206.

57. Calsyn DA, Malcy JA, Saxon AJ. Slow tapering from methadone maintenance in a program encouraging indefinite maintenance. *J Subst Abuse Treat.* 2006;30(2): 159–163.

58. Ling W, Hillhouse M, Domier C, et al. Buprenorphine tapering schedule and illicit opioid use. *Addiction.* 2009; 104(2):256–265.

59. Nielsen S, Hillhouse M, Thomas C, Hasson A, Ling W. A comparison of buprenorphine taper outcomes between prescription opioid and heroin users. *J Addict Med.* 2013; 7(1):33–38.

60. Gold M, Redmond Jr DE, Kleber H. Clonidine blocks acute opiate-withdrawal symptoms. *Lancet.* 1978; 312(8090):599–602.

61. Yu E, Miotto K, Akerele E, et al. A Phase 3 placebo-controlled, double-blind, multi-site trial of the alpha-2-adrenergic agonist, lofexidine, for opioid withdrawal. *Drug Alcohol Depend.* 2008;97(1):158–168.

62. Ling W, Amass L, Shoptaw S, et al. A multi-center randomized trial of buprenorphine–naloxone versus clonidine for opioid, detoxification: findings from the National Institute on Drug Abuse Clinical Trials Network. *Addiction.* 2005;100(8):1090–1100.

63. Gorodetzky CW, Walsh SL, Martin PR, Saxon AJ, Gullo KL, Biswas K. A phase III, randomized, multi-center, double blind, placebo controlled study of safety and efficacy of lofexidine for relief of symptoms in individuals undergoing inpatient opioid withdrawal. *Drug Alcohol Depend.* 2017;176:79–88.

64. Ndegwa S, Pant S, Pohar S, et al. Injectable extended-release naltrexone to treat opioid use disorder. In: *CADTH Issues in Emerging Health Technologies.* Vol. 2016. Ottawa, ON: Canadian Agency for Drugs and Technologies in Health; 2017:163.

65. Krupitsky E, Nunes EV, Ling W, Illeperuma A, Gastfriend DR, Silverman BL. Injectable extended-release naltrexone for opioid dependence: a double-blind, placebo-controlled, multicentre randomised trial. *Lancet.* 2011;377(9776):1506–1513.

66. Dunbar JL, Turncliff RZ, Dong Q, Silverman BL, Ehrich EW, Lasseter KC. Single-and multiple-dose pharmacokinetics of long-acting injectable naltrexone. *Alcohol Clin Exp Res.* 2006;30(3):480–490.

67. Ciccocioppo R, Martin-Fardon R, Weiss F. Effect of selective blockade of μ 1 or δ opioid receptors on reinstatement of alcohol-seeking behavior by drug-associated stimuli in rats. *Neuropsychopharmacology.* 2002;27(3):391.

68. Lesscher H, Bailey A, Burbach JPH, Van Ree JM, Kitchen I, Gerrits MA. Receptor-selective changes in μ-, δ-and κ-opioid receptors after chronic naltrexone treatment in mice. *Eur J Neurosci.* 2003;17(5): 1006–1012.

69. Meyer MC, Straughn AB, Lo MW, Schary WL, Whitney CC. Bioequivalence, dose-proportionality, and pharmacokinetics of naltrexone after oral administration. *J Clin Psychiatry.* 1984;45(9):15–19.

70. Breyer-Pfaff U, Nill K. Carbonyl reduction of naltrexone and dolasetron by oxidoreductases isolated from human liver cytosol. *J Pharm Pharmacol.* 2004;56(12): 1601–1606.

71. Porter SJ, Somogyi AA, White JM. In vivo and in vitro potency studies of 6ß-naltrexol, the major human metabolite of naltrexone. *Addict Biol.* 2002;7(2):219–225.

72. Miotto K, McCann MJ, Rawson RA, Frosch D, Ling W. Overdose, suicide attempts and death among a cohort of naltrexone-treated opioid addicts. *Drug Alcohol Depend.* 1997;45(1):131–134.

73. Mannelli P, Wu LT, Piendl KS, Swartz MS, Woody GE. Extended-release naltrexone injection is performed in the majority of opioid-dependent patients receiving outpatient induction: a very low dose naltrexone and buprenorphine open-label trial. *Drug Alcohol Depend.* 2014;138:83–88.

74. Sullivan M, Bisaga A, Pavlicova M, et al. Long-acting injectable naltrexone induction: a randomized trial of outpatient opioid detoxification with naltrexone versus buprenorphine. *Am J Psychiatry.* 2017;174(5):459–467.

75. Bisaga A, Mannelli P, Yu M, et al. Outpatient transition to extended-release injectable naltrexone for patients with opioid use disorder. *Drug Alcohol Depend.* 2018;187: 171–178.

76. Minozzi S, Amato L, Vecchi S, Davoli M, Kirchmayer U, Verster A. Oral naltrexone maintenance treatment for opioid dependence. *Cochrane Database Syst Rev.* 2006;1: CD001333.

77. Mattick RP, Kimber J, Breen C, Davoli M. Buprenorphine maintenance versus placebo or methadone maintenance for opioid dependence. *Cochrane Database Syst Rev.* 2014;2.

78. Comer SD, Sullivan MA, Yu E, et al. Injectable, sustained-release naltrexone for the treatment of opioid dependence: a randomized, placebo-controlled trial. *Arch Gen Psychiatry.* 2006;63(2):210–218.

79. Lee JD, Nunes Jr EV, Novo P, et al. Comparative effectiveness of extended-release naltrexone versus buprenorphine-naloxone for opioid relapse prevention (X: BOT): a multicentre, open-label, randomised controlled trial. *Lancet.* 2017;391:309.

80. Tanum L, Solli KK, Benth JŠ, et al. Effectiveness of injectable extended-release naltrexone vs daily buprenorphine-naloxone for opioid dependence: a randomized clinical noninferiority trial. *JAMA Psychiatry.* 2017;74(12): 1197–1205.

81. McAuley A, Aucott L, Matheson C. Exploring the life-saving potential of naloxone: a systematic review and descriptive meta-analysis of take home naloxone (THN) programmes for opioid users. *Int J Drug Policy.* 2015;26: 1183–1188.

82. DHHS. *Surgeon General Advisory*; 2017. https://www.surgeongeneral.gov/priorities/opioid-overdose-prevention/naloxone-advisory.htm.

83. Walley AY, Xuan Z, Hackman HH, et al. Opioid overdose rates and implementation of overdose education and nasal naloxone distribution in Massachusetts: interrupted time series analysis. *BMJ Clin Res.* 2013;346:f174.

84. Dugosh K, Abraham A, Seymour B, McLoyd K, Chalk M, Festinger D. A systematic review on the use of psychosocial interventions in conjunction with medications for the treatment of opioid addiction. *J Addict Med.* 2016; 10(2):91–101.

85. Higgins ST, Alessi SM, Dantona RL. Voucher-based incentives: a substance abuse treatment innovation. *Addict Behav.* 2002;27:887–910.

86. Peirce JM, Petry NM, Stitzer ML, et al. Effects of lower-cost incentives on stimulant abstinence in methadone maintenance treatment: a National Drug Abuse Treatment Clinical Trials Network study. *Arch Gen Psychiatry.* 2006; 63(2):201–208.

87. Carroll KM, Ball SA, Nich C, et al. Targeting behavioral therapies to enhance naltrexone treatment of opioid dependence: efficacy of contingency management and significant other involvement. *Arch Gen Psychiatry.* 2001;58(8):755–761.

88. Fiellin DA, Pantalon MV, Chawarski MC, et al. Counseling plus buprenorphine–naloxone maintenance therapy for opioid dependence. *N Engl J Med.* 2006;355(4): 365–374.

89. Fiellin DA, Barry DT, Sullivan LE, et al. A randomized trial of cognitive behavioral therapy in primary care-based buprenorphine. *Am J Med.* 2013;126(1):74.

90. Ling W, Hillhouse M, Ang A, Jenkins J, Fahey J. Comparison of behavioral treatment conditions in buprenorphine maintenance. *Addiction.* 2013;108(10):1788–1798.

91. Moore BA, Fiellin DA, Cutter CJ, et al. Cognitive behavioral therapy improves treatment outcomes for prescription opioid users in primary care buprenorphine treatment. *J Subst Abuse Treat.* 2016;71:54–57.

92. Winslow BT, Onysko M, Herbert M. Medications for alcohol use disorder. *Am Fam Physician.* 2016;93(6): 457–465.

93. Rawson RA, Huber A, McCann M, et al. A comparison of contingency management and cognitive-behavioral approaches during methadone maintenance treatment for cocaine dependence. *Arch Gen Psychiatry.* 2002;59(9): 817–824.

94. Abbott PJ, Weller SB, Walker SR. Psychiatric disorders of opioid addicts entering treatment: preliminary data. *J Addict Dis.* 1994;13(3):1–11.

95. Brooner RK, King VL, Kidorf M, Schmidt CW, Bigelow GE. Psychiatric and substance use comorbidity among treatment-seeking opioid abusers. *Arch Gen Psychiatry.* 1997;54(1):71–80.

96. Kidorf M, Disney ER, King VL, et al. Prevalence of psychiatric and substance use disorders in opioid abusers in a community syringe exchange program. *Drug Alcohol Depend.* 2004;74(2):115–122.

97. Nunes EV, Sullivan MA, Levin FR. Treatment of depression in patients with opiate dependence. *Biol Psychiatry.* 2004;56(10):793–802.

98. Carpenter KM, Brooks AC, Vosburg SK, Nunes EV. The effect of sertraline and environmental context on treating depression and illicit substance use among methadone maintained opiate dependent patients: a controlled clinical trial. *Drug Alcohol Depend.* 2004;74(2):123–134.

99. Bahorik AL, Satre DD, Kline-Simon AH, et al. Alcohol, cannabis, and opioid use disorders, and disease burden in an integrated health care system. *J Addict Med.* 2017; 11(1):3–9.

100. Backmund M, Reimer J, Meyer K, Gerlach JT, Zachoval R. Hepatitis C virus infection and injection drug users: prevention, risk factors, and treatment. *Clin Infect Dis.* 2005; 40(5):S330–S335.

101. Arendt-Nielsen L, Andresen T, Malver LP, Oksche A, Mansikka H, Drewes AM. A double-blind, placebo-controlled study on the effect of buprenorphine and fentanyl on descending pain modulation: a human experimental study. *Clin J Pain.* 2012;28(7):623–627.

102. Malinoff HL, Barkin RL, Wilson G. Sublingual buprenorphine is effective in the treatment of chronic pain syndrome. *Am J Ther.* 2005;12(5):379–384.

103. Alford DP, Compton P, Samet JH. Acute pain management for patients receiving maintenance methadone or buprenorphine therapy. *Ann Intern Med.* 2006;144(2): 127–134.

FURTHER READING

1. Avants SK, Margolin A, Sindelar JL, et al. Day treatment versus enhanced standard methadone services for opioid-dependent patients: a comparison of clinical efficacy and cost. *Am J Psychiatry.* 1999;156(1):27–33.

2. Berson A, Gervais A, Cazals D, et al. Hepatitis after intravenous buprenorphine misuse in heroin addicts. *J Hepatol.* 2001;34(2):346–350.

3. Calsyn DA, Wells EA, Saxon AJ, et al. Contingency management of urinalysis results and intensity of counseling services have an interactive impact on methadone maintenance treatment outcome. *J Addict Dis.* 1995; 13(3):47–63.

4. Carreno JE, Alvarez CE, Narciso GI, Bascaran MT, Diaz M, Bobes J. Maintenance treatment with depot opioid antagonists in subcutaneous implants: an alternative in the treatment of opioid dependence. *Addict Biol.* 2003;8(4): 429–438.

5. Clausen T, Anchersen K, Waal H. Mortality prior to, during and after opioid maintenance treatment (OMT): a national prospective cross-registry study. *Drug Alcohol Depend.* 2008;94(1):151–157.

6. Collins ED, Kleber HD, Whittington RA, Heitler NE. Anesthesia-assisted vs buprenorphine-or clonidine-assisted heroin detoxification and naltrexone induction: a randomized trial. *JAMA.* 2005;294(8):903–913.

7. Colquhoun R, Tan DY, Hull S. A comparison of oral and implant naltrexone outcomes at 12 months. *J Opioid Manage.* 2005;1(5):249–256.

8. Comer SD, Collins ED, Kleber HD, Nuwayser ES, Kerrigan JH, Fischman MW. Depot naltrexone: long-lasting antagonism of the effects of heroin in humans. *Psychopharmacology.* 2002;159(4):351–360.

9. Cornish JW, Metzger D, Woody GE, et al. Naltrexone pharmacotherapy for opioid dependent federal probationers. *J Subst Abuse Treat.* 1997;14(6):529–534.

10. Digiusto E, Shakeshaft A, Ritter A, O'brien S, Mattick RP. Serious adverse events in the Australian national evaluation of pharmacotherapies for opioid dependence (NEPOD). *Addiction.* 2004;99(4):450–460.

11. Hulse GK, Arnold-Reed DE, O'Neil G, Chan CT, Hansson RC. Achieving long-term continuous blood naltrexone and 6-ß-naltrexol coverage following sequential naltrexone implants. *Addict Biol.* 2004;9(1):67–72.

12. Hulse GK, Tait RJ. Opioid overdose deaths can occur in patients with naltrexone implants. *Med J Aust.* 2007;187(1):54.

13. Fishman M. Precipitated withdrawal during maintenance opioid blockade with extended release naltrexone. *Addiction.* 2008;103(8):1399–1401.

14. Gerra G, Fantoma A, Zaimovic A. Naltrexone and buprenorphine combination in the treatment of opioid dependence. *J Psychopharmacol.* 2006;20(6):806–814.

15. Gowing LR, Farrell M, Bornemann R, Sullivan LE, Ali RL. Brief report: methadone treatment of injecting opioid users for prevention of HIV infection. *J Gen Intern Med.* 2006;21(2):193–195.

16. Hulse GK, Tait RJ, Comer SD, Sullivan MA, Jacobs IG, Arnold-Reed D. Reducing hospital presentations for opioid overdose in patients treated with sustained release naltrexone implants. *Drug Alcohol Depend.* 2005;79(3):351–357.

17. Hulse GK, Morris N, Arnold-Reed D, Tait RJ. Improving clinical outcomes in treating heroin dependence: randomized, controlled trial of oral or implant naltrexone. *Arch Gen Psychiatry.* 2009;66(10):1108–1115.

18. Johansson BA, Berglund M, Lindgren A. Efficacy of maintenance treatment with naltrexone for opioid dependence: a meta-analytical review. *Addiction.* 2006;101(4):491–503.

19. Krupitsky EM, Zvartau EE, Masalov DV, et al. Naltrexone for heroin dependence treatment in St. Petersburg, Russia. *J Subst Abuse Treat.* 2004;26(4):285–294.

20. Krupitsky E, Zvartau E, Woody G. Use of naltrexone to treat opioid addiction in a country in which methadone and buprenorphine are not available. *Curr Psychiatry Rep.* 2010;12(5):448–453.

21. Landabaso MA, Iraurgi I, Jimenez-Lerma JM, et al. A randomized trial of adding fluoxetine to a naltrexone treatment programme for heroin addicts. *Addiction.* 1998;93(5):739–744.

22. Mannelli P, Peindl KS, Wu LT. Pharmacological enhancement of naltrexone treatment for opioid dependence: a review. *Subst Abuse Rehabil.* 2011;2:113.

23. Marsch LA. The efficacy of methadone maintenance interventions in reducing illicit opiate use, HIV risk behavior and criminality: a meta-analysis. *Addiction.* 1998;93(4):515–532.

24. McCann DJ. Potential of buprenorphine/naltrexone in treating polydrug addiction and co-occurring psychiatric disorders. *Clin Pharmacol Ther.* 2008;83(4):627–630.

25. McLellan AT, Arndt IO, Metzger DS, Woody GE, O'brlen CP. The effects of psychosocial services in substance abuse treatment. *Addict Nurs Netw.* 1993;5(2):38–47.

26. Montoya ID, Gorelick DA, Preston KL, et al. Randomized trial of buprenorphine for treatment of concurrent opiate and cocaine dependence. *Clin Pharmacol Ther.* 2004;75(1):34–48.

27. Oviedo-Joekes E, Brissette S, Marsh DC, et al. Diacetylmorphine versus methadone for the treatment of opioid addiction. *N Engl J Med.* 2009;361(8):777–786.

28. Petry NM, Bickel WK, Piasecki D, Marsch LA, Badger GJ. Elevated liver enzyme levels in opioid-dependent patients with hepatitis treated with buprenorphine. *Am J Addict.* 2000;9(3):265–269.

29. Rothenberg JL, Sullivan MA, Church SH, et al. Behavioral naltrexone therapy: an integrated treatment for opiate dependence. *J Subst Abuse Treat.* 2002;23(4):351–360.

30. Saxon AJ, Ling W, Hillhouse M, et al. Buprenorphine/naloxone and methadone effects on laboratory indices of liver health: a randomized trial. *Drug Alcohol Depend.* 2013;128(1):71–76.

31. Sinha R, Kimmerling A, Doebrick C, Kosten TR. Effects of lofexidine on stress-induced and cue-induced opioid craving and opioid abstinence rates: preliminary findings. *Psychopharmacology.* 2007;190(4):569–574.

32. Strain EC, Stitzer ML, Bigelow GE. Early treatment time course of depressive symptoms in opiate addicts. *J Nerv Ment Dis.* 1991;179(4):215–221.

33. Woody GE, McLellan AT, Luborsky L, et al. Severity of psychiatric symptoms as a predictor of benefits from psychotherapy: the Veterans Administration-Penn Study. *Am J Psychiatry.* 1984;141(10):1172–1177.

34. Wu LT, Ling W, Burchett B, et al. Use of item response theory and latent class analysis to link poly-substance use disorders with addiction severity, HIV risk, and quality of life among opioid-dependent patients in the Clinical Trials Network. *Drug Alcohol Depend.* 2011;118(2):186–193.

35. Wu LT, Woody GE, Yang C, Blazer DG. How do prescription opioid users differ from users of heroin or other drugs in psychopathology: results from the National Epidemiologic Survey on Alcohol and Related Conditions. *J Addict Med.* 2011;5(1):28.

CHAPTER 7

The Treatment of Cannabis Use Disorder

ITAI DANOVITCH, MD, MBA, DFASAM, FAPA • DAVID A. GORELICK, MD, PHD, DLFAPA

INTRODUCTION

Cannabis is a flowering plant containing a class of lipophilic hydrocarbons called "cannabinoids." The stem, leaves, and flowers from cannabis have been cultivated throughout history for therapeutic as well as intoxicating purposes. There are dozens of unique cannabinoid substances in cannabis, only several of which have been well characterized.[1] The primary psychoactive component of cannabis is Δ^9-tetrahydrocannabinol (THC). THC produces an intoxication syndrome and promotes release of dopamine in the nucleus accumbens, one of the cornerstone features of reinforcing drugs.[2] Cannabadiol (CBD), which has been associated with some of the therapeutic effects ascribed to cannabis, may influence the effects of THC but does not itself produce intoxication. Cannabis can be bred to contain varying levels of THC, CBD, and other cannabinoids. For this chapter, the term "cannabis" will refer to THC or cannabis species that are bred predominantly for their intoxicating effects.

Cannabis is the most commonly used illicit substance worldwide. In the United States in 2015, 44% of persons over the age of 12 used cannabis at least once in their lifetime[3]; 9.5% used within the past year; in 2013, 2.9% met diagnostic criteria for cannabis use disorder (CUD) within the past year.[4] CUD is characterized by loss of control over cannabis use, harmful consequences from use, and excessive time spent buying, using or recovering from cannabis effects[5] (see DSM-5 Table 7.1). Among individuals who have ever used cannabis, the lifetime risk of developing CUD is estimated at 8%–12%.[3,6] This rate is lower than for many other psychoactive substances (both legal and illegal), but is nonetheless significant considering the high prevalence of cannabis use across the population. Children and young adults have greater susceptibility for developing CUD, a concerning notion

given increased availability of high potency cannabis[7] and reduced perception of risk from cannabis use over the past decade.[8] In 2013, cannabis was reported as the primary substance of misuse by 17% of admissions to publicly funded addiction treatment programs in the US, with one-third of respondents reporting that cannabis use had started prior to age 14.[9]

Epidemiological surveys reveal subtle but significant adverse outcomes associated with CUD. Chronic heavy use is associated with poor educational attainment among youth,[10] an unsurprising association given the fact that chronic cannabis use is associated with cognitive impairment,[11,12,131] with earlier age of onset of cannabis use and greater cumulative cannabis use associated with greater impairment.[14] Prospective longitudinal studies suggest that these impairments start resolving after at least 1 month of abstinence.[15,16] Cannabis use during adolescence carries distinct risk in that, alongside the putative neurobiological consequences of heavy cannabinoid exposure,[17] chronic intoxication may fundamentally alter developmental trajectories.[18,19] Heavy cannabis use has been linked to school failure, early pregnancy, crime, and progression to further drug use,[10,20,21] but some more recent prospective longitudinal studies, which better control for potential confounds, do not demonstrate such associations.[22,23] Even where these associations are demonstrated in prospective, longitudinal studies that control for baseline (i.e., precannabis use) presence of the adverse outcome and known likely confounds (e.g., other substance use, socioeconomic status, psychiatric comorbidity), it remains possible that the observed associations result from convergent risks, reverse causation, or unmeasured or unknown predisposing factors, as much as from direct effects of cannabis use.

One challenge facing treatment of CUD is the high rate of comorbidity with other major psychiatric

The Assessment and Treatment of Addiction. https://doi.org/10.1016/B978-0-323-54856-4.00007-9

TABLE 7.1
DSM5 Cannabis-related Disorders

Cannabis Use Disorder	Cannabis Intoxication	Cannabis Withdrawal

A. A problematic pattern of cannabis use leading to clinically significant impairment or distress, as manifested by at least two of the following, occurring within a 12-month period:
  1. Use in larger amounts or over a longer period than was intended.
  2. Persistent desire or unsuccessful effort to cut back
  3. A great deal of time is spent in activities necessary to obtain, use, or recover effects.
  4. Cravings or persistent desire to use
  5. Failure to fulfill major role obligations at work, school, or home.
  6. Use despite recurrent social or interpersonal problems
  7. Important social, occupational, or recreational activities are given up or reduced
  8. Recurrent use in situations in which it is physically hazardous.
  9. Persistent use despite knowledge of physical or psychological problems caused or exacerbated by using
  10. Tolerance
  11. Withdrawal (refer to Criteria A and B of the criteria set for cannabis withdrawal).
	A. Recent use of cannabis.
	
	B. Clinically significant problematic behavioral or psychological changes (e.g., impaired motor coordination, euphoria, anxiety, sensation of slowed time, impaired judgment, social withdrawal) that developed during, or shortly after, cannabis use.
	
	C. Two (or more) of the following signs or symptoms developing within 2 hours of cannabis use:
	  1. Conjunctival injection.
	  2. Increased appetite
	  3. Dry mouth
	  4. Tachycardia
	
	D. The signs or symptoms are not attributable to another medical condition and are not better explained by another mental disorder, including intoxication with another substance.
		A. Cessation of cannabis use that has been heavy and prolonged
		
		B. Three (or more) of the following signs and symptoms develop within approximately 1 week after Criterion A:
		  1. Irritability, anger, or aggression.
		  2. Nervousness or anxiety
		  3. Sleep difficulty (e.g., insomnia disturbing dreams).
		  4. Decreased appetite or weight loss.
		  5. Restlessness.
		  6. Depressed mood.
		  7. At least one of the following physical symptoms causing significant discomfort: abdominal pain, shakiness/tremors, sweating, fever, chills, or headache.
		
		C. The signs or symptoms in Criterion B cause clinically significant distress or impairment in social, occupational, or other important areas of functioning.
		
		D. The signs or symptoms are not attributable to another medical condition and are not better explained by another mental disorder, including intoxication or withdrawal from another substance.

---

disorders. Large-scale, nationally representative epidemiologic surveys of community-dwelling adults in the US suggest that rates of current major psychiatric disorder among those with current CUD are as follows: any mood disorder—30%—33%, any anxiety disorder—23%—24%, posttraumatic stress disorder (PTSD)—12%, any personality disorder—48%.[24,25] While there are no comparable community-based studies for current schizophrenia (because of low overall-prevalence), large-scale, representative studies in the US and Australia find a 15%—20% prevalence of schizophrenia among hospitalized patients with CUD.[26,27]

CUD poses distinct challenges for treatment providers. The evolving sociocultural context of use for medical (as opposed to intoxication) purposes, public policy liberalization, and societal normalization has contributed to decrease perceived risk and increase acceptability of use.[28–31,320] Simultaneously, the comparatively lower "severity" of cannabis-associated consequences, including the absence of a medically serious withdrawal syndrome (compared with other psychoactive substances),[33] makes it more difficult for some users to recognize adverse consequences from their use and to establish an enduring commitment to change.

These factors, plus the reluctance of many treatment-seekers to accept traditional abstinence-based goals, may account for the low proportion of individuals with CUD who seek treatment. A secondary analysis of data on 7278 adults with current (past-year) moderate-severe CUD (cannabis dependence in DSM-IV terms) in the 2005–13 National Surveys on Drug Use and Health (NSDUH) found that only one out of eight (12.87%, 95% CI 11.62–14.23) received any substance use treatment services that year; only 8.18% (95% CI 7.19–9.29) received cannabis-specific treatment.[34] Notwithstanding these challenges, the high prevalence of CUD, its strong association with comorbid mental health problems, and the difficulty of achieving cannabis cessation ensure that most clinicians will encounter patients with CUD. While no pharmacotherapy has been approved for CUD, several promising approaches are in development. Psychotherapy studies are establishing a number of evidence-based models and techniques and innovative technological platforms promise to increase access to effective treatment. This article reviews established and emerging treatment options for CUD.

PHARMACOTHERAPY
Cannabis Intoxication

Cannabis intoxication is a syndrome recognized in DSM-5 and ICD-10, with both psychological/behavioral (euphoria, relaxation, increased appetite, impaired memory, and concentration) and physical (motor incoordination, tachycardia, orthostatic hypotension, conjunctival reddening) manifestations. These manifestations are mediated by THC activation of the cannabinoid CB1 receptor.[35] Intoxication is usually mild and self-limiting, not requiring pharmacological treatment. The most severe effects (anxiety, panic attack, psychosis) are best treated with a benzodiazepine or second-generation (atypical) antipsychotic medication, as appropriate to acutely control symptoms.[36] No medication is currently approved for the treatment of cannabis intoxication by the US Food and Drug Administration (FDA) or any other national regulatory authority.

Several studies have evaluated the impact of the opioid-antagonist naltrexone on cannabis intoxication. Acute pretreatment with single doses of naltrexone actually increases the reinforcing effects of cannabis,[37] while chronic dosing decreases the subjective effects of cannabis.[38]

Human laboratory studies show that antagonists/inverse agonists of the CB1 receptor block the acute effects of cannabis, so might serve as treatment for acute cannabis intoxication.[39] However, all such compounds were withdrawn from the market and from clinical development a decade ago because of psychiatric side-effects such as suicidality and anxiety.[40]

Cannabis Withdrawal

Cannabis withdrawal is a syndrome that develops upon cessation of prolonged cannabis use and is typically characterized by three or more of the following symptoms: irritability, anger or aggression; nervousness or anxiety; sleep difficulty (i.e., insomnia, disturbing dreams); decreased appetite or weight loss; restlessness; depressed mood.[5] Most symptoms begin during the first week of abstinence and resolve after a few weeks. Up to half of patients in treatment for CUD report symptoms of a withdrawal syndrome.[41–43,44] Although not usually severe, cannabis withdrawal should be a focus of treatment because it may serve as negative reinforcement for relapse to cannabis use in individuals trying to abstain.[41,45]

No medications are approved for the treatment of cannabis withdrawal, but several medications have been evaluated in small clinical studies.[46] One approach is cross-tolerant (cannabinoid CB1 receptor) agonist substitution to suppress the withdrawal syndrome (analogous to using an opioid to suppress heroin withdrawal). This approach can be implemented using synthetic THC (dronabinol), which is legally marketed in many countries, including the US (Marinol), as an oral medication for appetite stimulation and suppression of nausea and vomiting due to chemotherapy. Dronabinol has shown efficacy in several human laboratory studies and open-label case series, at doses up to 30 mg tid, with minimal side effects.[47–49] A controlled clinical trial of dronabinol (20 mg bid), while not showing efficacy for reducing cannabis use (see below), did significantly reduce cannabis withdrawal symptoms.[51] However, a later controlled clinical trial by the same research group found no significant benefit for dronabinol combined with lofexidine (an alpha1-adrenergic receptor agonist found to reduce some cannabis withdrawal symptoms in human laboratory studies).[52]

An alternate cannabinoid agonist approach involves using a combination of THC and CBD (nabiximols) administered as an oromucosal spray. In a two-site controlled trial of nabixomols (maximum daily dose, 86.4 mg THC and 80 mg CBD) for 51 treatment-seeking individuals undergoing inpatient treatment, nabixomols reduced cannabis withdrawal symptoms over 9 days and improved short-term treatment retention, although there was no difference in cannabis use at 28-day follow-up.[53] A smaller (9 subjects) outpatient clinical trial also found that nabiximols reduced cannabis withdrawal symptoms over 5 days, either given as a fixed dose (108 mg THC and 100 mg CBD every hour for 10 hours each day) or self-titrated as needed for withdrawal symptoms.[54]

Lithium, a mood stabilizer used primarily in the treatment of bipolar disorder, has been evaluated in one small open-label clinical study and one randomized controlled trial. In the open-label study, lithium (600−900 mg/day for 6 days) reduced withdrawal symptoms in 4 of the 9 participants, although one of the 4 continued to smoke some cannabis.[55] Abstinence was not verified in the other 8 participants. A placebo-controlled randomized trial of lithium carbonate supplemented with nitrazepam, enrolling 35 treatment-seeking cannabis-dependent adults, showed some improvement on sleep measures but no significant benefit on treatment retention.[56] These results suggest limited therapeutic effect of lithium given during the withdrawal (detoxification) period.

Another approach, which has been evaluated chiefly in human laboratory studies, tries to alleviate symptoms of cannabis withdrawal (e.g., dysphoric mood, disturbed sleep) by influencing the brain circuits that mediate these symptoms, using medications already approved for other psychiatric conditions. In a controlled clinical trial involving 50 treatment-seeking outpatients, the anticonvulsant gabapentin (maximum daily dose 1200 mg/day) significantly reduced cannabis withdrawal symptoms compared with placebo.[57] Human laboratory studies found that the anticonvulsant and mood stabilizer divalproex (1500 mg/day for 29 days) and the antidepressant buproprion (300 mg/day sustained release for 17 days) worsened, rather than improved, some withdrawal symptoms and had no positive effects.[48,58] A single dose of the antidepressant nefazodone (450 mg/day) decreased some, but not the majority, of cannabis withdrawal symptoms.[59]

Cannabis Use Disorder

Several dozen trials have evaluated pharmacological treatment strategies for CUD.[60] No medication has been shown broadly effective in the treatment of CUD, nor is any medication approved for this condition by any national regulatory authority.[61] The medications that have shown the greatest promise, albeit only in single controlled clinical trials, are the anticonvulsant gabapentin (which increases activity of the inhibitory neurotransmitter GABA) and the amino acid derivative N-acetylcysteine (NAC) (which indirectly increases activity of the excitatory neurotransmitter glutamate).

Gabapentin (peak dose of 1200 mg/day) was evaluated in a 12-week, randomized, double-blind, placebo-controlled study enrolling 50 treatment-seeking adult outpatients with cannabis dependence.[57] Gabapentin was associated with improved performance on cognitive tests and short-term reductions in cannabis use relative to placebo. It was well tolerated, with no significant treatment group differences in side-effects.

NAC (1200 mg bid) was evaluated in an 8-week, randomized, double-blind, placebo-controlled study enrolling 116 treatment-seeking youth (15−21 years old) with cannabis dependence.[62] All participants also received contingency management targeted at treatment adherence and abstinence plus weekly brief drug abuse counseling. NAC was associated with significantly better treatment retention and higher proportion of (weekly) urine tests negative for cannabinoids (40.9% vs. 27.2%). NAC was well tolerated, with no significant treatment group differences in adverse events. A subsequent randomized, double-blind, placebo-controlled 12-week study evaluated the same NAC dose (1200 mg bid) in 302 treatment-seeking adults with CUD.[63] As in the prior youth study, all participants also received contingency management targeted at treatment adherence and abstinence plus weekly brief drug abuse counseling. There was no significant treatment effect on cannabis use.

The anticonvulsant topiramate (which both increases GABA activity and blocks glutamate activity) (titrated up to 200 mg/day over 4 weeks to minimize side-effects) was evaluated in a 6-week, randomized, double-blind, placebo-controlled study enrolling 66 treatment-seeking youth (15−24 years old).[64] All participants also received three sessions of motivational enhancement therapy. Topiramate was associated with significantly more cognitive and neurological side-effects and a higher dropout rate due to side-effects (35% vs. 4%). There was no significant treatment effect on cannabis use.

Experimental Pharmacological Targets

Growing knowledge about the endogenous cannabinoid (endocannabinoid) system in the brain and its role in mediating behavior is identifying new targets for the treatment of CUD. The endocannabinoid system includes cannabinoid receptors (CB1 and CB2), endogenous neurotransmitters (anandamide and 2-arachidonoylglyerol), and cannabinoid metabolizing enzymes (fatty acid amide hydrolase and monoacylglycerol lipase). The endocannabinoid system is involved in brain reward signaling to varying degrees, such that pharmacological manipulation may impact the course of CUD, as well as other substance use disorders.[65]

Pharmacological strategies targeting CUD can be generally grouped into three categories: agonist substitution, antagonism at the CB1 receptor, and modulation of other neurotransmitter systems. Though results from studies of these strategies have been mixed, their findings, summarized below, inform an understanding of potential treatment approaches.

One treatment strategy is substitution with a cross-tolerant agonist drug to suppress withdrawal and drug craving, analogous to using nicotine itself to treat tobacco use disorder or methadone for opioid use disorder. For treatment of CUD, this strategy has been evaluated using the legally available agonist dronabinol (synthetic THC). In a controlled clinical trial, dronabinol (20 mg bid for 8 weeks) significantly improved treatment retention and reduced cannabis withdrawal symptoms, but did not improve rates of cannabis abstinence.[51] A subsequent randomized controlled trial of dronabinol combined with the alpha 2 agonist lofexidine (dronabinol 20 mg tid + lofexidine 0.6 mg tid for 11 weeks) did not show clinically significant differences compared to placebo.[52]

An alternative treatment strategy is to use cannabinoid receptor antagonists, or partial or inverse agonists, either to block the reinforcing effects of cannabis or reduce cannabis craving. Studies with the selective CB1 receptor antagonist/inverse agonist rimonabant suggest that CB1 receptors mediate many of the acute effects of cannabis in humans. Human laboratory studies demonstrated that both acute (1 dose) and chronic (2-week) administration of rimonabant attenuated the subjective intoxication and tachycardia caused by an active cannabis cigarette (2.78% THC) smoked double-blind.[39,66] Rimonabant alone did not significantly affect THC pharmacokinetics or produce

significant physiological or psychological effects, suggesting that the observed effects were due to CB1 receptor blockade and not reduced brain THC concentrations. This pattern of findings suggests that CB1 receptor blockade might be beneficial acutely in the treatment of cannabis intoxication or overdose (analogous to the use of the mu-opioid receptor antagonist naloxone in the treatment of opioid overdose) and beneficial as a chronic treatment for CUD (analogous to the use of the long-acting mu-opioid receptor antagonist naltrexone in the treatment of opioid use disorder). However, development of rimonabant and similar CB1 receptor modulators was halted on account of significant psychiatric side-effects (anxiety, depression, suicidality), and there is no medication in this class currently available for human use.[40]

An alternative approach to receptor blockade is modulation of brain concentrations of endocannabinoids. The enzyme fatty acid amide hydrolase (FAAH) catalyzes the breakdown of anandamide. FAAH inhibitors, such as URB597, selectively increase brain anandamide concentrations in rodents and primates. In rodent studies, URB597 produced analgesic, anxiolytic-like, and antidepressant-like effects, but had no effects suggestive of addictive liability, such as self-administration. These findings suggest that enhancing brain endocannabinoid activity with a FAAH inhibitor might offer benefit for the treatment of acute cannabis withdrawal.[67] However, the serious neurotoxicity (including one death) occurring in a recent phase I clinical trial of another FAAH inhibitor suggests the need for caution when pursuing this approach.[68]

Animal studies show that mu-opioid receptor antagonists block acute effects of THC, suggesting that such medications might be useful in the treatment of cannabis intoxication or overdose. Several human laboratory studies have explored this possibility by evaluating whether naltrexone reduces the subjective effects of cannabinoids in humans. Most findings to date have been disappointing. Pretreatment with high doses of naltrexone (50–200 mg) failed to attenuate or enhanced the subjective effects of THC.[69,70,720] A lower, more mu-selective dose of naltrexone (12 mg) decreased the intoxicating effects of 20 mg, but not 40 mg, of THC.[72] A placebo-controlled study in 29 heavy cannabis smokers found that opioid-receptor blockade by naltrexone (12, 25, 50, or 100 mg daily) enhanced the subjective and cardiovascular effects of cannabis.[37] However, a recent human laboratory study administering chronic naltrexone (50 mg daily for 16 days) did find a significant decrease in the acute subjective effects of cannabis and in cannabis self-administration.[38] These findings suggest that chronic (rather than acute) mu-opioid receptor blockade might be a useful therapeutic approach for CUD.

Another strategy is modulation of other neurotransmitter systems to reduce the reinforcing effects of and craving for cannabis. This strategy has been implemented using a variety of medications approved for other psychiatric conditions.

Several small trials did not find enhancement of catecholamine neurotransmitter activity effective in reducing cannabis use. Entacapone inhibits catechol-O-methyl transferase (COMT), an enzyme that metabolizes catecholamine neurotransmitters and regulates dopamine levels in the synapse. In an open-label trial in 36 patients with cannabis dependence (DSM-IV), entacapone (up to 2000 mg/day for 12 weeks) significantly decreased craving for cannabis in 52.7% of the patients (no data on cannabis use was reported).[73] The medication was well tolerated; there were no serious adverse events. Atomoxetine is a selective norepinephrine reuptake inhibitor used in the treatment of attention deficit/hyperactivity disorder (ADHD) and considered to have low addiction potential. In an 11-week open-label study in 13 cannabis-dependent outpatients, atomoxetine (25, 40, or 80 mg/day) showed a trend toward reduction in cannabis use and increase in proportion of abstinent days only in the 8 patients who completed the trial.[74] The majority of patients experienced gastrointestinal adverse events. In a double-blind, placebo-controlled clinical trial in 38 cannabis-dependent outpatients with comorbid ADHD, atomoxetine (25–100 mg/day in escalating doses over 12 weeks) produced no significant change in cannabis use, although there was some improvement in ADHD symptoms.[75]

Buspirone is a 5-HT$_{1A}$ receptor agonist and a D$_2$ receptor antagonist that is used as an anxiolytic. In an open-label trial in 10 cannabis-dependent men, buspirone (up to 60 mg/day for 12 weeks) significantly reduced frequency and duration of cannabis craving and use and reduced irritability and depression.[76] In a placebo-controlled clinical trial in 50 cannabis-dependent outpatients, buspirone (up to 60 mg/day for 12 weeks) in conjunction with motivational interviewing had no significant effect in the intent-to-treat analysis, but significantly increased the proportion of cannabis-negative urine samples by 35% points (95% CI for increase: 7%–63%, $P < .05$) among the 24 patients who completed the entire trial.[77] There was a trend toward faster initiation of abstinence (first cannabis-negative urine) among those receiving buspirone. However, a subsequent randomized trial of

buspirone (up to 60 mg/day for 12 weeks combined with brief motivational enhancement therapy and contingency management) among 175 cannabis-dependent adults did not find any significant benefit.[78]

Divalproex is an anticonvulsant used as a mood stabilizer in the treatment of bipolar disorder. In a 6-week placebo-controlled clinical trial in 25 cannabis-dependent outpatients, divalproex (1500–2000 mg daily for 6 weeks, with target plasma concentration of 50–120 ng/mL) in conjunction with weekly relapse prevention psychotherapy was not significantly more effective than placebo in reducing cannabis use and was poorly tolerated by participants.[79] Lithium (500 mg 2×/day for 7 days) was given to 20 cannabis-dependent inpatients undergoing detoxification.[80] Twelve patients completed the 7-day detoxification program. Over 90 days of follow-up, participants reported being abstinent on 88% of days, with 64% abstinence on Day 10, 65% on Day 24, and 41% on Day 90. Five participants reported continuous abstinence, with cannabis-negative urine tests on day 90.

In a 13-week placebo-controlled clinical trial in 106 cannabis-dependent outpatients, the antidepressants nefazodone (300 mg/day) or bupropion (150 mg sustained release/day) in conjunction with weekly individual coping skills therapy were not significantly better than placebo in reducing cannabis use or symptoms of cannabis withdrawal.[81] Similarly, an 8-week controlled trial of vilazadone (up to 40 mg combined with brief motivational enhancement therapy and contingency management) for 76 cannabis-dependent adults failed to find any advantage over placebo.[82] Finally, in a 9-week controlled trial of escitalopram (10 mg/day combined with cognitive-behavior and motivation-enhancement therapy) for 52 cannabis-dependent adults, escitalopram did not demonstrate any benefit over placebo.[83]

Oxytocin is a hypothalamic neuropeptide that promotes social cognition and prosocial behaviors. A randomized, double-blind, placebo-controlled pilot study enrolling 16 cannabis-dependent adults administered oxytocin (40 IU intranasally) or placebo prior to the first two of three motivational enhancement therapy sessions over a 4-week period.[84] There was no significant treatment group difference in cannabis use.

Cannabis Use Disorder With Psychiatric Comorbidity

Relatively few controlled clinical trials have evaluated pharmacological treatment for adults with diagnosed CUD (rather than just heavy cannabis use) and a comorbid psychiatric disorder. Three studies of antidepressants in outpatients with comorbid depression found mixed results. Two studies evaluated the selective serotonin reuptake inhibitor (SSRI) fluoxetine. A post hoc analysis of 13 adolescents with major depressive disorder and substance dependence who were treated with fluoxetine (20–40 mg daily) showed reduction in both cannabis and alcohol use and depressive symptoms.[85] Five-year follow-up of 10 patients showed that cannabis and alcohol dependence were reduced and academic ability improved, but clinical depression remained problematic. In a placebo-controlled clinical trial in 70 adolescents and young adults with comorbid major depression and CUD, fluoxetine (20 mg daily for 12 weeks) in conjunction with cognitive behavioral/motivational enhancement psychotherapy was no better than placebo in reducing either depressive symptoms or cannabis-related symptoms.[86] A 12-week controlled trial of venlafaxine-extended release (up to 375 mg daily) involving 103 outpatients with cannabis dependence and major depressive disorder or dysthymia found worse outcomes for the active treatment arm.[87] A secondary analysis suggested that subjects may have increased their use of cannabis to self-medicate adverse effects of venlafaxine.[88]

For comorbid bipolar disorder, lithium (targeted to a serum level of 0.9 meq/L) was evaluated in a randomized, double-blind, placebo-controlled study enrolling 25 adolescents with a mood, anxiety, or attention-deficit hyperactivity disorder (70% with bipolar disorder) and a comorbid SUD (56% CUD + alcohol use disorder, 8% CUD only).[89] All participants also received weekly interpersonal therapy. Lithium significantly reduced both mood symptoms and cannabis use (assessed with urine drug tests).

For comorbid schizophrenia spectrum disorders, a few clinical trials suggest that clozapine and quetiapine may be effective in reducing cannabis use, while other second-generation antipsychotic medications are not effective.[90,91] Clozapine (400–560 mg/day) was evaluated in a randomized, double-blind, 12-week study enrolling 31 adults with comorbid CUD and schizophrenia or schizoaffective disorder who continued on their current medication or were switched to clozapine.[92] Clozapine significantly decreased cannabis use (by about 4.5 joints/week) but had no significant effect on schizophrenia symptoms or overall functioning. A second clinical trial openly randomized 30 adults with comorbid CUD and schizophrenia-spectrum disorders to 12 months of clozapine (50–425 mg daily) or ziprasidone (80–400 mg daily).[93] Both treatment groups had significant reductions in cannabis use,

with clozapine producing greater reduction in positive symptoms of schizophrenia and more side effects (primarily hypersalivation). Two open-label within-subject trials that switched 24 and 26 adult patients, respectively, with comorbid SUD (majority CUD) and schizophrenia-spectrum disorders from another antipsychotic medication (not clozapine) to 12 weeks of quetiapine (200–800 mg daily) found significant decreases over time in self-reported cannabis use, as well as improvement in schizophrenia symptoms.[94,95] The quetiapine findings should be interpreted cautiously due to the weak study designs and misuse potential of quetiapine itself.[96]

PSYCHOSOCIAL (NONPHARMACOLOGICAL) TREATMENTS

Psychosocial treatment for CUD has its origins in psychotherapy for substance use disorder in general. The majority of randomized trials of psychosocial treatment for CUD have used manualized treatment methods to study various iterations of motivational enhancement therapy (MET), cognitive behavioral therapy (CBT), or contingency management (CM), as well as community and family interventions. Because the underpinnings of these therapeutic models are complementary, research effort has focused as much on identifying effective combinations than on establishing the superiority of any particular method.

A systematic review and meta-analysis of psychosocial interventions for cannabis use disorder that included 23 randomized controlled trials (involving 4045 participants) found that, based on low-to-moderate-quality evidence overall, psychosocial interventions, compared to treatment as usual or presumably inactive control conditions (e.g., waiting list, single educational session), significantly reduced frequency of cannabis use (mean difference 5.67 [95% CI 3.08–8.26] fewer days per month) and number of cannabis dependence symptoms (standardized mean difference 4.15, 95% CI 1.67–6.63) and increased the likelihood of achieving cannabis abstinence (risk ratio 2.55, 95% CI 1.34–4.83).[97] Participants in the active treatment arms generally did better than inactive controls, and trials delivering greater than four intervention sessions consistently demonstrated improved outcomes. Risk of bias across studies was low to moderate, with frequent limitations related to blinding of subjects or researchers, limited use of bioassays to verify subject self-report, and lack of evaluation of prior treatment or noncannabis substance use during the trial period.

Motivational Enhancement Therapy (MET)

MET is a patient-centered therapy that helps individuals resolve ambivalence in order to generate commitment to change.[98] MET views readiness to change as a dynamic process involving multiple stages: precontemplation, contemplation, preparation, action, and maintenance, and proposes that the role of the therapist is to create the conditions that promote the patient's intrinsic motivation.[99] Five core tenets characterize the motivational "style:" first, maintain empathy and create a respectful, nonjudgmental therapeutic frame through the use of open ended questions and validation; second, develop cognitive discrepancy by identifying goals that are meaningful to the patient and incrementally linking them to contrary behaviors; third, avoid arguments that make patients defensive by letting the patient lead and working from within their perspective; fourth, roll with resistance by using reflective interpretations and reframing rather than confrontations; and fifth, support self-efficacy to engender confidence in the ability to make and sustain change by utilizing support and validation.[98]

MET may be used repeatedly over time as the targets for behavioral change evolve, but in clinical studies MET sessions are typically 60–90 min long, with treatment occurring over one to four sessions. MET has been shown to improve cannabis-related outcomes among treatment-seeking adults,[100] nontreatment seekers,[101] and individuals with psychiatric comorbidity.[102] There have been efforts to computerize motivational interventions,[103–105,1086] simplify them for use in community settings and busy primary care practices, and utilize them in inpatient settings for patients with significant psychiatric comorbidity.[107] Studies of brief motivational interventions show only minimal impact on cannabis use in individuals with severe CUD,[108–110,1131] but show possible benefit for moderating cannabis use in those less severely addicted.[112] It remains to be seen whether brief interventions for nontreatment-seeking cannabis users will increase the possibility of self-directed change by facilitating openness to new information and consideration of future intervention.[108] Most recent studies of MET employ it in combination with other interventions, such as CBT or CM.[97]

Cognitive Behavioral Therapy (CBT)

Cognitive behavioral therapy views drug use as a learned behavior. CBT posits that by identifying the associative links and chain of events precipitating substance use, patients can identify opportunities to alter their behavioral repertoire and use alternative, healthy coping mechanisms.[113] CBT begins by establishing a therapeutic framework and teaching self-monitoring of underlying triggers for substance use. The therapy then moves to the development of relapse prevention skills, such as relaxation techniques, mindfulness, cognitive restructuring, positive self-talk, and assertiveness. The therapist may impart these skills through instruction, modeling, and role playing, but eventually the patient is encouraged to practice those skills outside of therapy (so-called "homework"), such that they develop the skills to adaptively deal with high-risk situations without relapsing.

CBT is typically provided over 6–12 individual or group sessions. The earliest randomized psychotherapy studies for CUD showed small but clinically significant benefits.[114,115] CBT was not superior to MET,[43] but the synergies offered compelling rationale to integrate them.[116] Subsequent studies have demonstrated efficacy for CBT in the context of brief interventions,[114] combination with motivational techniques and contingency management,[117–119] and for individuals with psychiatric comorbidity.[102,107,120,121]

Contingency Management (CM)

Contingency management, based on operant conditioning theory, posits that behaviors will increase or decrease as a function of immediate and directly associated consequences (reward or punishment, respectively). By manipulating the quality and immediacy of external consequences, contingency management attempts to systematically increase the likelihood of desired behaviors, and minimize undesired behaviors. Studies of CM show that rewards (incentives) are generally more effective than punishments and that they do not have to be large or monetary to substantially alter behaviors.[122] For goals that depend on repetitive behavior over time, such as abstinence, escalating values of reward can be very effective (e.g., longer periods of continuous abstinence increase the value of the reinforcer, while relapse resets the reinforcer back to a minimal level).[122,123] Rewards are most effective when they are provided in close temporal proximity to the desired behavior; greater frequency of reinforcement also increases efficacy.[123] CM can link rewards to either treatment outcomes (e.g., abstinence confirmed by toxicological monitoring), treatment adherence (e.g., provision of toxicological samples, attendance at counseling sessions, completion of therapy-related assignments, adherence to medications), or both.

The first randomized study of CM for CUD demonstrated that adding incentives (i.e., vouchers for small payments, gift-certificates, raffle drawings, or products) could improve responses to a motivational behavioral coping skills intervention.[117] CM may nudge the decisional balance in patients who would not otherwise be ready to address their substance use. In clinical studies, CM reliably improves engagement in treatment, thereby facilitating skills acquisition and development of self-efficacy promoted by complementary therapies.[124,125] CM also improves retention among nontreatment seeking adults with CUD, such as those referred by probation,[126] and young adults referred by the criminal justice system.[118] Single studies show promise for utilization of CM among adolescents[127] and for individuals with severe persistent mental illness.[128]

Supportive-Expressive Psychotherapy (SEP)

Supportive-Expressive psychotherapy has characteristics similar to motivational and skills-based treatment. The supportive element of SEP involves establishing a helpful, optimistic, encouraging, and empathic relationship between the patient and therapist. The development of a strong therapeutic alliance enables an expressive component, in which the therapist utilizes reflective listening and interpretation to explore the patient's subjective experience, point out patterns that manifest within the therapeutic relationship, and facilitate development of self-awareness, insight, and adaptive coping.[129] Through self-understanding, SEP aims to help patients achieve greater mastery over problem behavior and improved personal well-being.[130]

In contrast to MET or CBT, SEP is typically delivered over at least 4 months in hour-long sessions once or twice each week and has not been studied in well-controlled, randomized clinical trials. SEP merits mention because it is commonly utilized by community providers of psychotherapy. One study assigned 100 adults with cannabis dependence (using adaptive quasi-randomization with stratification by duration of cannabis use) to 16 weeks of weekly manual-based SEP or to a single session of brief advice and self-help material. At the end of treatment, 58% of participants in the SEP condition reported abstinence, compared with 16% of participants in the control condition (Chi-square = 18.92, $P < .001$). At 12-month follow-up, 28% of those in the SEP condition reported abstinence, compared with 14% of those in the control condition (Chi-square = 2.95, $P = .09$).[131,132]

Family and Systems Interventions

Recognizing the complex interplay of psychosocial factors for many cannabis-dependent youth, system-based interventions have been developed to involve family,

utilize case managers to coordinate care and resources, incorporate community supports to navigate environmental challenges, and collaborate with other stakeholders such as schools. Three manualized "systems" interventions have been studied among cannabis-using adolescents. Family therapy views the family as the patient, taking a systems approach to resolving problems by enhancing intrafamily communication, improving parental limit setting, and facilitating collaborative recovery work.[133] The Adolescent Community Reinforcement Approach (ACRA) is a multisystem behavioral therapy that seeks to integrate cognitive behavioral skills training with collaborative community support and contingency management.[134] Multidimensional family therapy (MDFT) is a comprehensive systems therapy that targets the functioning of the individual within the context of his or her environment by integrating individual therapy, parent coaching, family systems therapy, and engagement of key community stakeholders, such as school, medical supports, juvenile justice, and social services.[135]

In small randomized trials, MDFT has shown greater and more sustainable gains than CBT,[136] group therapy, and MET interventions alone.[137] However, MDFT was not significantly better than other high-quality treatment interventions in the Cannabis Youth Treatment (CYT) study, which randomized 600 adolescents to five different treatment approaches across multiple sites.[138,139] The treatment interventions included ACRA, Family Support Network, MDFT, and five-session and twelve-session versions of combined MET and CBT. The CYT study had good retention rates, acceptability of manual-based interventions to therapists, treatment efficacy, and economic feasibility (costs were comparable to national outpatient program costs). Long-term follow-up data are anticipated, as are initial findings from a large international study of MDFT which is currently under way.[135,140,141,1442]

12-Step Facilitation

Twelve-step programs are often an integral part of the treatment of substance use disorder[143]; manualized protocols for 12-step facilitation have been developed and implemented for alcohol and other substance use disorders.[144] However, twelve-step programs are notably absent from the literature on psychosocial interventions for CUD. In 2009, Marijuana Anonymous World Services published a 12-step workbook.[145] The extent to which 12-step programs are utilized and their long-term efficacy and potential role as an integrated component of psychosocial interventions for CUD have not been examined.

Electronic Technology

Computer and mobile computing platforms may reduce barriers and increase access to psychotherapeutic interventions. New applications, digital platforms, educational tools, and tele-health service delivery models have emerged over the past several years and shown promise in the treatment of substance use disorders. Given the ambivalence toward treatment often shown by users of cannabis, as well as their reluctance to accept traditional abstinence-based goals, digital interventions may generate new entry points to recovery. A recent systematic review and meta-analysis of digital interventions for problematic cannabis users not in formal treatment identified 4 eligible studies involving 1928 participants.[146] These studies employed combinations of MET and/or CBT with interventions ranged from self-guided to clinician-assisted. The largest treatment effects occurred with studies that offered web-based online chat with a trained psychotherapist. Limitations of the studies included reliance on self-report for outcome measures and limited screening for psychiatric comorbidity or other substance use. In recent years, several for-profit companies have sought to develop fee-for-service cannabis interventions employing some of these techniques. To date, there is limited information on the effectiveness of these products and services.

Psychosocial Treatments for CUD With Comorbid Psychiatric Disorders

There are few controlled clinical trials of psychosocial treatments for CUD with comorbid psychiatric disorders; the majority of studies include participants with cannabis and other substance use, but not necessarily CUD.[107,147,148] One clinical trial randomly assigned 97 adults with comorbid major depressive disorder and "problematic" cannabis use (71% of participants) to either one session of motivational interviewing (followed by no further treatment) or to 10 weekly sessions of combined motivational interviewing/CBT, delivered either in person or via computer.[103] The longer treatment was significantly more effective than brief intervention in reducing depressive symptoms and cannabis-related problems over the 12-month follow-up period, with computer-administered therapy showing the largest treatment effect.

A recent systematic review and meta-analysis (including 14 studies involving 1506 participants) of psychosocial treatment for PTSD and comorbid substance use disorder (SUD) found that psychosocial treatments combining trauma-focused and SUD-focused components overall produced significantly more reduction in PTSD symptoms than single-component therapies, but did not significantly reduce substance use.[149] However, none of the included studies involved participants with diagnosed CUD and few involved substantial numbers of cannabis users.

While the large literature on psychosocial treatment of cannabis-using adults with schizophrenia suggests that psychosocial treatment may reduce cannabis use and positive symptoms of schizophrenia,[91,150,151] findings from the small number of controlled clinical trials of psychosocial treatment involving adults with comorbid CUD and schizophrenia-related disorders (i.e., schizophrenia, schizoaffective disorder, or schizophreniform disorder) suggest little or no benefit from CBT and MET. A clinical trial (CapOpus) that enrolled 103 adults with comorbid CUD and psychosis (82% schizophrenia-related) who were randomized to 6 months of treatment as usual (medication and CBT focused on psychosis) without or with weekly CBT/motivational interviewing focused on cannabis use found that psychosocial treatment did not significantly reduce the self-reported frequency of cannabis use at the end of treatment or 4-month follow-up.[121] Participants who received the cannabis-focused treatment had more psychiatric hospital admissions and more psychiatric emergency room contacts over the subsequent 4 years.[152]

A clinical trial that enrolled 88 adults with comorbid cannabis dependence and early onset (within 3 years) psychosis (55% schizophrenia-related) who were randomized to 12 weeks of treatment as usual (multidisciplinary team providing antipsychotic treatment) without or with weekly CBT and motivational interviewing focused on cannabis use found no treatment group difference in cannabis use or psychosis symptoms, although the psychosocial treatment was associated with better subjective quality of life.[153]

A clinical trial that enrolled 130 adults with comorbid current SUD (73% CUD) and psychotic disorder (75% schizophrenia-related) who were randomized to treatment as usual (self-help booklet about substance use) without or with 10 weeks of weekly motivational interviewing/CBT focused on substance use found that the 10-week treatment significantly reduced self-reported frequency of cannabis use at 15 weeks (but not at 6 months or 12 months) and had no significant effect on symptoms of schizophrenia.[120]

A clinical trial that enrolled 31 adults with comorbid schizophrenia and SUD (77% CUD) who were randomized to usual care or 18 months of cognitive enhancement therapy (individual, group, and computer-based sessions focused on goal setting, motivation for treatment, stress and emotion management, and improving social interactions, plus psychoeducation on substance use and schizophrenia) found that the psychosocial treatment had no significant effect on cannabis use, while it did significantly improve social adjustment and emotional function.[154]

For bipolar[155] and anxiety disorders, we are not aware of any clinical trial that focused specifically on comorbid CUD.

CONCLUSIONS

The treatment of CUD can be viewed as a cup half empty or half full. On the one hand, few people who might benefit from treatment actually receive it. Among those who receive treatment in randomized trials, long-term abstinence is achieved by fewer than 20%.[156] Moderate reduction in cannabis use has been associated with decreases in adverse consequences, but the differential impact of such goals on the long-term course of CUD is unknown. Optimal duration of treatment is unclear, and certain populations, particularly patients with psychiatric comorbidity, have not been studied adequately.[107] Twelve-step programs are low-cost, effective for other SUDs, and readily available in most regions of the world. However, their role and efficacy in CUD has not been examined. Finally, no proven effective pharmacological treatments are currently available, although several promising candidates are being investigated.

On the other hand, psychotherapeutic strategies used to treat other substance use disorders can be effective for CUD. A meta-analysis of psychosocial interventions for illicit substance use disorders found that treatments for CUD had a comparable overall effect size ($d = 0.81$, 95% CI = 0.25–1.36) as treatments for cocaine ($d = 0.62$, 95% CI = 0.16–1.08), opioids ($d = 0.39$, 95% CI = 0.18–0.60), and polysubstance use disorders ($d = 0.24$, 95% CI = 0.03–0.44).[157] Combination therapies have proven most effective, particularly those that begin with a motivational intervention, utilize incentives to enhance the commitment to change, and teach behavioral and cognitive copings skills to prevent relapse. Among adolescents, family engagement and collaboration with community stakeholders add substantial value to treatment. Digital interventions show promise to increase accessibility, reduce barriers, and improve fidelity; however, this field is still in the early stages of development.

Although only 8%–12% of regular cannabis users develop CUD, the volume of people who use cannabis ensures that the total number of people in need of help is larger than the current capacity of addiction specialty services. Thus, while efforts to refine and improve the efficacy of treatment interventions continue, innovations that increase the availability and accessibility of treatment are also needed. Computer-based and phone-based interventions, social media, and brief interventions that can be implemented in primary care settings are areas that may hold promise for reaching at-risk populations. Adolescents and persons with psychiatric comorbidity are at particularly high risk of CUD and may suffer disproportionately from cannabis's adverse effects. As in the treatment of other SUDs, there is need for a continuing care model with long-term follow-up that extends past the periods typically evaluated in treatment studies.[158] Additionally, there is a need for further investigation of genetic underpinnings and endophenotypes underlying CUD in order to identify neurobiological mechanisms for targeted intervention.[159] One benefit of the societal focus on cannabis has been a prominent increase in research covering everything from the basic science to the public health impact of cannabis use. Over the next decade, clinicians who provide treatment for individuals with CUD are likely to see their armamentarium of effective interventions expand to the ultimate betterment of patients, their families, and society at large.

DISCLOSURES

Dr. Danovitch has no conflicts of interest to report.
Dr. Gorelick receives royalties from UpToDate for articles about cannabis

REFERENCES

1. Mechoulam R, Hanus LO, Pertwee R, Howlett AC. Early phytocannabinoid chemistry to endocannabinoids and beyond. *Nat Rev Neurosci.* 2014;15(11):757–764.
2. Volkow ND, Hampson AJ, Baler RD. Don't worry, be happy: endocannabinoids and cannabis at the intersection of stress and reward. *Annu Rev Pharmacol Toxicol.* 2017;57:285–308.
3. *National survey on drug Use and health: key substance use and mental health indicators in the United States: results from the 2015 national survey on drug Use and health.* Center for Behavioral Health Statistics and Quality; 2016. SMA 16-4984.
4. Hasin DS, Saha TD, Kerridge BT, et al. Prevalence of marijuana use disorders in the United States between 2001–2002 and 2012–2013. *JAMA Psychiatry.* 2015; 72(12):1235–1242.
5. APA. *Diagnostic and Statistical Manual of Mental Disorders (DSM-5).* American Psychiatric Association; 2013.

6. Swift W, Hall W, Teesson M. Characteristics of DSM-IV and ICD-10 cannabis dependence among Australian adults: results from the national survey of mental health and wellbeing. *Drug Alcohol Depend.* 2001;63(2): 147–153.

7. ElSohly MA, Mehmedic Z, Foster S, Gon C, Chandra S, Church JC. Changes in cannabis potency over the last 2 decades (1995–2014): analysis of current data in the United States. *Biol Psychiatry.* 2016;79(7):613–619.

8. Johnston LD, O'Malley PM, Miech RA, Bachman JG, Schulenberg JE. *Monitoring the Future National Survey Results on Drug Use, 1975–2016: Overview, Key Findings on Adolescent Drug Use.* 2017.

9. SAMHSA. Treatment episode data set (TEDS): 2003–2013. National admissions to substance abuse treatment services. *Subst Abuse Ment Health Serv Adm.* 2015:1–131.

10. Fergusson DM, Horwood LJ, Beautrais AL. Cannabis and educational achievement. *Addiction.* 2003;98(12): 1681–1692.

11. Crane NA, Schuster RM, Fusar-Poli P, Gonzalez R. Effects of cannabis on neurocognitive functioning: recent advances, neurodevelopmental influences, and sex differences. *Neuropsychol Rev.* 2013;23(2):117–137.

12. Curran HV, Freeman TP, Mokrysz C, Lewis DA, Morgan CJ, Parsons LH. Keep off the grass? Cannabis, cognition and addiction. *Nat Rev Neurosci.* 2016;17(5): 293–306.

13. Volkow ND, Swanson JM, Evins AE, et al. Effects of cannabis use on human behavior, including cognition, motivation, and psychosis: a review. *JAMA Psychiatry.* 2016;73(3):292–297.

14. Schulte MH, Cousijn J, den Uyl TE, et al. Recovery of neurocognitive functions following sustained abstinence after substance dependence and implications for treatment. *Clin Psychol Rev.* 2014;34(7):531–550.

15. Schreiner AM, Dunn ME. Residual effects of cannabis use on neurocognitive performance after prolonged abstinence: a meta-analysis. *Exp Clin Psychopharmacol.* 2012; 20(5):420–429.

16. Auer R, Vittinghoff E, Yaffe K, et al. Association between lifetime marijuana use and cognitive function in middle age: the coronary artery risk development in young adults (CARDIA) study. *JAMA Intern Med.* 2016;176(3): 352–361.

17. Medina KL, Hanson KL, Schweinsburg AD, Cohen-Zion M, Nagel BJ, Tapert SF. Neuropsychological functioning in adolescent marijuana users: subtle deficits detectable after a month of abstinence. *J Int Neuropsychol Soc.* 2007;13(5):807–820.

18. Brook JS, Lee JY, Brown EN, Finch SJ, Brook DW. Developmental trajectories of marijuana use from adolescence to adulthood: personality and social role outcomes. *Psychol Rep.* 2011;108(2):339–357.

19. Fontes MA, Bolla KI, Cunha PJ, et al. Cannabis use before age 15 and subsequent executive functioning. *Br J Psychiatry.* 2011;198(6):442–447.

20. Fergusson DM, Boden JM. Cannabis use and later life outcomes. *Addiction.* 2008;103(6):969–976; discussion 977–968.

21. Macleod J, Oakes R, Copello A, et al. Psychological and social sequelae of cannabis and other illicit drug use by young people: a systematic review of longitudinal, general population studies. *Lancet.* 2004;363(9421): 1579–1588.

22. Bechtold J, Simpson T, White HR, Pardini D. Chronic adolescent marijuana use as a risk factor for physical and mental health problems in young adult men. *Psychol Addict Behav J Soc Psychol Addict Behav.* 2015 Sep;29(3): 552–563. https://doi.org/10.1037/adb0000103. Epub 2015 Aug 3. Erratum in: Psychol Addict Behav. 2015 Dec;29(4):ix–x.

23. Meier MH, Hill ML, Small PJ, Luthar SS. Associations of adolescent cannabis use with academic performance and mental health: a longitudinal study of upper middle class youth. *Drug Alcohol Depend.* 2015;156: 207–212.

24. Kerridge BT, Pickering R, Chou P, Saha TD, Hasin DS. DSM-5 cannabis use disorder in the national epidemiologic survey on alcohol and related conditions-III: gender-specific profiles. *Addict Behav.* 2018;76:52–60.

25. Stinson FS, Ruan WJ, Pickering R, Grant BF. Cannabis use disorders in the USA: prevalence, correlates and comorbidity. *Psychol Med.* 2006;36(10):1447–1460.

26. Zhu H, Wu LT. Sex differences in cannabis use disorder diagnosis involved hospitalizations in the United States. *J Addict Med.* 2017;11(5):357–367.

27. Lai HM, Sitharthan T. Exploration of the comorbidity of cannabis use disorders and mental health disorders among inpatients presenting to all hospitals in New South Wales, Australia. *Am J Drug Alcohol Abuse.* 2012; 38(6):567–574.

28. Aggarwal SK, Carter GT, Sullivan MD, ZumBrunnen C, Morrill R, Mayer JD. Medicinal use of cannabis in the United States: historical perspectives, current trends, and future directions. *J Opioid Manag.* 2009;5(3): 153–168.

29. Arbour-Nicitopoulos KP, Kwan MY, Lowe D, Taman S, Faulkner GE. Social norms of alcohol, smoking, and marijuana use within a Canadian university setting. *J Am Coll Health.* 2010;59(3):191–196.

30. Gates P, Copeland J, Swift W, Martin G. Barriers and facilitators to cannabis treatment. *Drug Alcohol Rev.* 2012 May; 31(3):311–319. https://doi.org/10.1111/j.1465-3362.2011. 00313.x. Epub 2011 Apr 26.

31. Hoffmann DE, Weber E. Medical marijuana and the law. *N Engl J Med.* 2010;362(16):1453–1457.

32. Lewis TF, Mobley AK. Substance abuse and dependency risk: the role of peer perceptions, marijuana involvement, and attitudes toward substance use among college students. *J Drug Educ.* 2010;40(3):299–314.

33. Nutt D, King LA, Saulsbury W, Blakemore C. Development of a rational scale to assess the harm of drugs of potential misuse. *Lancet.* 2007;369(9566):1047–1053.

34. Wu LT, Zhu H, Mannelli P, Swartz MS. Prevalence and correlates of treatment utilization among adults with cannabis use disorder in the United States. *Drug Alcohol Depend.* 2017;177:153–162.

35. Cooper ZD, Haney M. Cannabis reinforcement and dependence: role of the cannabinoid CB1 receptor. *Addict Biol.* 2008;13(2):188–195.

36. Wilkins J, Danovitch I, Gorelick D. Management of stimulant, hallucinogen, marijuana, phencyclidine, and club drug intoxication and withdrawal. In: Herron A, Brennan TK, eds. *The ASAM Essentials of Addiction Medicine.* 2nd ed. Torrance, CA: Wolters Kluwer; 2015: 273–282.

37. Cooper ZD, Haney M. Opioid antagonism enhances marijuana's effects in heavy marijuana smokers. *Psychopharmacol Berl.* 2010;211(2):141–148.

38. Haney M, Ramesh D, Glass A, Pavlicova M, Bedi G, Cooper ZD. Naltrexone maintenance decreases cannabis self-administration and subjective effects in daily cannabis smokers. *Neuropsychopharmacology.* 2015; 40(11):2489–2498.

39. Huestis MA, Boyd SJ, Heishman SJ, et al. Single and multiple doses of rimonabant antagonize acute effects of smoked cannabis in male cannabis users. *Psychopharmacol Berl.* 2007;194(4):505–515.

40. Le Foll B, Gorelick DA, Goldberg SR. The future of endocannabinoid-oriented clinical research after CB1 antagonists. *Psychopharmacol Berl.* 2009;205(1): 171–174.

41. Budney AJ, Hughes JR. The cannabis withdrawal syndrome. *Curr Opin Psychiatry.* 2006;19(3):233–238.

42. Budney AJ, Hughes JR, Moore BA, Vandrey R. Review of the validity and significance of cannabis withdrawal syndrome. *Am J Psychiatry.* 2004;161(11):1967–1977.

43. Stephens RS, Roffman RA, Curtin L. Comparison of extended versus brief treatments for marijuana use. *J Consult Clin Psychol.* 2000;68(5):898–908.

44. Budney AJ, Moore BA. Development and consequences of cannabis dependence. *J Clin Pharmacol.* 2002;42(11 suppl):28S–33S.

45. Levin KH, Copersino ML, Heishman SJ, et al. Cannabis withdrawal symptoms in non-treatment-seeking adult cannabis smokers. *Drug Alcohol Depend.* 2010; 111(1–2):120–127.

46. Gorelick DA. Pharmacological treatment of cannabis-related disorders: a narrative review. *Curr Pharm Des.* 2016;22(42):6409–6419.

47. Levin FR, Kleber HD. Use of dronabinol for cannabis dependence: two case reports and review. *Am J Addict.* 2008;17(2):161–164.

48. Haney M, Hart CL, Vosburg SK, et al. Marijuana withdrawal in humans: effects of oral THC or divalproex. *Neuropsychopharmacology.* 2004;29(1):158–170.

49. Budney AJ, Vandrey RG, Hughes JR, Moore BA, Bahrenburg B. Oral delta-9-tetrahydrocannabinol suppresses cannabis withdrawal symptoms. *Drug Alcohol Depend.* 2007;86(1):22–29.

50. Vandrey R, Stitzer ML, Mintzer MZ, Huestis MA, Murray JA, Lee D. The dose effects of short-term dronabinol (oral THC) maintenance in daily cannabis users. *Drug Alcohol Depend.* 2013;128(1–2):64–70.

51. Levin FR, Mariani JJ, Brooks DJ, Pavlicova M, Cheng W, Nunes EV. Dronabinol for the treatment of cannabis dependence: a randomized, double-blind, placebo-controlled trial. *Drug Alcohol Depend.* 2011;116(1–3):142–150.

52. Levin FR, Mariani JJ, Pavlicova M, et al. Dronabinol and lofexidine for cannabis use disorder: a randomized, double-blind, placebo-controlled trial. *Drug Alcohol Depend.* 2016;159:53–60.

53. Allsop DJ, Copeland J, Lintzeris N, et al. Nabiximols as an agonist replacement therapy during cannabis withdrawal: a randomized clinical trial. *JAMA Psychiatry.* 2014;71(3):281–291.

54. Trigo JM, Lagzdins D, Rehm J, et al. Effects of fixed or self-titrated dosages of Sativex on cannabis withdrawal and cravings. *Drug Alcohol Depend.* 2016;161:298–306.

55. Bowen R, McIlwrick J, Baetz M, Zhang X. Lithium and marijuana withdrawal. *Can J Psychiatry.* 2005;50(4): 240–241.

56. Allsop DJ, Bartlett DJ, Johnston J, et al. The effects of lithium carbonate supplemented with nitrazepam on sleep disturbance during cannabis abstinence. *J Clin Sleep Med.* 2015;11(10):1153–1162.

57. Mason BJ, Crean R, Goodell V, et al. A proof-of-concept randomized controlled study of gabapentin: effects on cannabis use, withdrawal and executive function deficits in cannabis-dependent adults. *Neuropsychopharmacology.* 2012;37(7):1689–1698.

58. Haney M, Ward AS, Comer SD, Hart CL, Foltin RW, Fischman MW. Bupropion SR worsens mood during marijuana withdrawal in humans. *Psychopharmacol Berl.* 2001;155(2):171–179.

59. Haney M, Hart CL, Ward AS, Foltin RW. Nefazodone decreases anxiety during marijuana withdrawal in humans. *Psychopharmacol Berl.* 2003;165(2):157–165.

60. Brezing CA, Levin FR. The current state of pharmacological treatments for cannabis use disorder and withdrawal. *Neuropsychopharmacology.* 2018;43(1):173–194.

61. Marshall K, Gowing L, Ali R, Le Foll B. Pharmacotherapies for cannabis dependence. *Cochrane Database Syst Rev.* 2014;(12):CD008940.

62. Gray KM, Carpenter MJ, Baker NL, et al. A double-blind randomized controlled trial of N-acetylcysteine in cannabis-dependent adolescents. *Am Journal Psychiatry.* 2012;169(8):805–812.

63. Gray KM, Sonne SC, McClure EA, et al. A randomized placebo-controlled trial of N-acetylcysteine for cannabis use disorder in adults. *Drug Alcohol Depend.* 2017;177: 249–257.

64. Miranda Jr R, Treloar H, Blanchard A, et al. Topiramate and motivational enhancement therapy for cannabis use among youth: a randomized placebo-controlled pilot study. *Addict Biol.* 2017 May;22(3):779–790. https:// doi.org/10.1111/adb.12350. Epub 2016 Jan 11.

65. Sloan ME, Gowin JL, Ramchandani VA, Hurd YL, Le Foll B. The endocannabinoid system as a target for addiction treatment: trials and tribulations. *Neuropharmacology.* 2017;124:73–83.

66. Huestis MA, Gorelick DA, Heishman SJ, et al. Blockade of effects of smoked marijuana by the CB1-selective cannabinoid receptor antagonist SR141716. *Arch Gen Psychiatry.* 2001;58(4):322–328.

67. Clapper JR, Mangieri RA, Piomelli D. The endocannabinoid system as a target for the treatment of cannabis dependence. *Neuropharmacology.* 2009;56(suppl 1):235–243.

68. Kerbrat A, Ferre JC, Fillatre P, et al. Acute neurologic disorder from an inhibitor of fatty acid amide hydrolase. *N Engl J Med.* 2016;375(18):1717–1725.

69. Greenwald MK, Stitzer ML. Antinociceptive, subjective and behavioral effects of smoked marijuana in humans. *Drug Alcohol Depend.* 2000;59(3):261–275.

70. Wachtel SR, de Wit H. Naltrexone does not block the subjective effects of oral delta(9)-tetrahydrocannabinol in humans. *Drug Alcohol Depend.* 2000;59(3):251–260.

71. Haney M, Bisaga A, Foltin RW. Interaction between naltrexone and oral THC in heavy marijuana smokers. *Psychopharmacol Berl.* 2003;166(1):77–85.

72. Haney M. Opioid antagonism of cannabinoid effects: differences between marijuana smokers and nonmarijuana smokers. *Neuropsychopharmacology.* 2007;32(6):1391–1403.

73. Shafa R. COMT- inhibitors may be a promising tool in treatment of marijuana addiction. *Am J Addict.* 2009;18:322. AAAP 19th Annual Meeting Poster Abstracts.

74. Tirado CF, Goldman M, Lynch K, Kampman KM, Obrien CP. Atomoxetine for treatment of marijuana dependence: a report on the efficacy and high incidence of gastrointestinal adverse events in a pilot study. *Drug Alcohol Depend.* 2008;94(1–3):254–257.

75. McRae-Clark AL, Carter RE, Killeen TK, Carpenter MJ, White KG, Brady KT. A placebo-controlled trial of atomoxetine in marijuana-dependent individuals with attention deficit hyperactivity disorder. *Am J Addict.* 2010;19(6):481–489.

76. McRae AL, Brady KT, Carter RE. Buspirone for treatment of marijuana dependence: a pilot study. *Am J Addict.* 2006;15(5):404.

77. McRae-Clark AL, Carter RE, Killeen TK, et al. A placebo-controlled trial of buspirone for the treatment of marijuana dependence. *Drug Alcohol Depend.* 2009;105(1–2):132–138.

78. McRae-Clark AL, Baker NL, Gray KM, et al. Buspirone treatment of cannabis dependence: a randomized, placebo-controlled trial. *Drug Alcohol Depend.* 2015;156:29–37.

79. Levin FR, McDowell D, Evans SM, et al. Pharmacotherapy for marijuana dependence: a double-blind, placebo-controlled pilot study of divalproex sodium. *Am J Addict.* 2004;13(1):21–32.

80. Winstock AR, Lea T, Copeland J. Lithium carbonate in the management of cannabis withdrawal in humans: an open-label study. *J Psychopharmacol.* 2009;23(1):84–93.

81. Carpenter KM, McDowell D, Brooks DJ, Cheng WY, Levin FR. A preliminary trial: double-blind comparison of nefazodone, bupropion-SR, and placebo in the treatment of cannabis dependence. *Am J Addict.* 2009;18(1):53–64.

82. McRae-Clark AL, Baker NL, Gray KM, Killeen T, Hartwell KJ, Simonian SJ. Vilazodone for cannabis dependence: a randomized, controlled pilot trial. *Am J Addict.* 2016;25(1):69–75.

83. Weinstein AM, Miller H, Bluvstein I, et al. Treatment of cannabis dependence using escitalopram in combination with cognitive-behavior therapy: a double-blind placebo-controlled study. *Am J Drug Alcohol Abuse.* 2014;40(1):16–22.

84. Sherman BJ, Baker NL, McRae-Clark AL. Effect of oxytocin pretreatment on cannabis outcomes in a brief motivational intervention. *Psychiatry Res.* 2017;249:318–320.

85. Cornelius JR, Clark DB, Bukstein OG, Birmaher B, Salloum IM, Brown SA. Acute phase and five-year follow-up study of fluoxetine in adolescents with major depression and a comorbid substance use disorder: a review. *Addict Behav.* 2005;30(9):1824–1833.

86. Cornelius JR, Bukstein OG, Douaihy AB, et al. Double-blind fluoxetine trial in comorbid MDD-CUD youth and young adults. *Drug Alcohol Depend.* 2010;112(1–2):39–45.

87. Levin FR, Mariani J, Brooks DJ, et al. A randomized double-blind, placebo-controlled trial of venlafaxine-extended release for co-occurring cannabis dependence and depressive disorders. *Addiction (Abingdon, Engl).* 2013;108(6):1084–1094.

88. Kelly MA, Pavlicova M, Glass A, et al. Do withdrawal-like symptoms mediate increased marijuana smoking in individuals treated with venlafaxine-XR? *Drug Alcohol Depend.* 2014;144:42–46.

89. Geller B, Cooper TB, Sun K, et al. Double-blind and placebo-controlled study of lithium for adolescent bipolar disorders with secondary substance dependency. *J Am Acad Child Adolesc Psychiatry.* 1998;37(2):171–178.

90. Akerman SC, Brunette MF, Noordsy DL, Green AI. Pharmacotherapy of co-occurring schizophrenia and substance use disorders. *Curr Addict Rep.* 2014;1(4):251–260.

91. Bennett ME, Bradshaw KR, Catalano LT. Treatment of substance use disorders in schizophrenia. *Am J Drug Alcohol Abuse.* 2017;43(4):377–390.

92. Brunette MF, Dawson R, O'Keefe CD, et al. A randomized trial of clozapine vs. other antipsychotics for cannabis use disorder in patients with schizophrenia. *J Dual Diagnosis.* 2011;7(1–2):50–63.

93. Schnell T, Koethe D, Krasnianski A, et al. Ziprasidone versus clozapine in the treatment of dually diagnosed (DD) patients with schizophrenia and cannabis use disorders: a randomized study. *Am J Addict Am Acad Psychiat Alcohol Addict.* 2014;23(3):308–312.

94. Potvin S, Stip E, Lipp O, et al. Quetiapine in patients with comorbid schizophrenia-spectrum and substance use disorders: an open-label trial. *Curr Med Res Opin.* 2006; 22(7):1277−1285.

95. Zhornitsky S, Stip E, Desfosses J, et al. Evolution of substance use, neurological and psychiatric symptoms in schizophrenia and substance use disorder patients: a 12-week, pilot, case-control trial with quetiapine. *Front Psychiatry.* 2011;2:22.

96. Hanley MJ, Kenna GA. Quetiapine: treatment for substance abuse and drug of abuse. *Am J Health-Syst Pharm AJHP.* 2008;65(7):611−618.

97. Gates PJ, Sabioni P, Copeland J, Le Foll B, Gowing L. Psychosocial interventions for cannabis use disorder. *Cochrane Database Syst Rev.* 2016;(5):CD005336.

98. Miller W, Rollnick S. *Motivational Interviewing: Preparing People for Change.* 2nd ed. New York City: The Guilford Press; 2002.

99. Prochaska JO, DiClemente CC, Norcross JC. In search of how people change. Applications to addictive behaviors. *Am Psychol.* 1992;47(9):1102−1114.

100. Babor TF. Brief treatments for cannabis dependence: findings from a randomized multisite trial. *J Consult Clin Psychol.* 2004;72(3):455−466.

101. Stein LA, Lebeau R, Colby SM, Barnett NP, Golembeske C, Monti PM. Motivational interviewing for incarcerated adolescents: effects of depressive symptoms on reducing alcohol and marijuana use after release. *J Stud Alcohol Drugs.* 2011;72(3):497−506.

102. Baker A, Turner A, Kay-Lambkin FJ, Lewin TJ. The long and the short of treatments for alcohol or cannabis misuse among people with severe mental disorders. *Addict Behav.* 2009;34(10):852−858.

103. Kay-Lambkin FJ, Baker AL, Lewin TJ, Carr VJ. Computer-based psychological treatment for comorbid depression and problematic alcohol and/or cannabis use: a randomized controlled trial of clinical efficacy. *Addiction.* 2009; 104(3):378−388.

104. Walker DD, Roffman RA, Picciano JF, Stephens RS. The check-up: in-person, computerized, and telephone adaptations of motivational enhancement treatment to elicit voluntary participation by the contemplator. *Subst Abuse Treat Prev Policy.* 2007;2:2.

105. Christoff Ade O, Boerngen-Lacerda R. Reducing substance involvement in college students: a three-arm parallel-group randomized controlled trial of a computer-based intervention. *Addict Behav.* 2015;45: 164−171.

106. Rooke S, Copeland J, Norberg M, Hine D, McCambridge J. Effectiveness of a self-guided web-based cannabis treatment program: randomized controlled trial. *J Med Internet Res.* 2013;15(2):e26.

107. Baker AL, Hides L, Lubman DI. Treatment of cannabis use among people with psychotic or depressive disorders: a systematic review. *J Clin Psychiatry.* 2010;71(3):247−254.

108. Martin G, Copeland J. The adolescent cannabis check-up: randomized trial of a brief intervention for young cannabis users. *J Subst Abuse Treat.* 2008;34(4):407−414.

109. Walker DD, Roffman RA, Stephens RS, Wakana K, Berghuis J, Kim W. Motivational enhancement therapy for adolescent marijuana users: a preliminary randomized controlled trial. *J Consult Clin Psychol.* 2006;74(3): 628−632.

110. Woolard R, Baird J, Longabaugh R, et al. Project reduce: reducing alcohol and marijuana misuse: effects of a brief intervention in the emergency department. *Addict Behav.* 2013;38(3):1732−1739.

111. Walker DD, Stephens RS, Blevins CE, Banes KE, Matthews L, Roffman RA. Augmenting brief interventions for adolescent marijuana users: the impact of motivational check-ins. *J Consult Clin Psychol.* 2016;84(11): 983−992.

112. Stephens RS, Roffman RA, Fearer SA, Williams C, Burke RS. The Marijuana Check-up: promoting change in ambivalent marijuana users. *Addiction.* 2007;102(6): 947−957.

113. Beck AT, Wright FD, Newman CF, Liese BS. *Cognitive therapy of substance abuse.* New York City: The Guilford Press; 2001.

114. Copeland J, Swift W, Roffman R, Stephens R. A randomized controlled trial of brief cognitive-behavioral interventions for cannabis use disorder. *J Subst Abuse Treat.* 2001;21(2):55−64; discussion 65−66.

115. Stephens RS, Roffman RA, Simpson EE. Treating adult marijuana dependence: a test of the relapse prevention model. *J Consult Clin Psychol.* 1994;62(1):92−99.

116. Stephens R, Roffman R, Copeland J, Swift W. Cognitive-behavioral and motivational enhancement treatments for cannabis dependence. In: Roffman R, Stephens R, eds. *Cannabis Dependence; Its Nature, Consequences and Treatment.* Cambridge: Cambridge University Press; 2006.

117. Budney AJ, Higgins ST, Radonovich KJ, Novy PL. Adding voucher-based incentives to coping skills and motivational enhancement improves outcomes during treatment for marijuana dependence. *J Consult Clin Psychol.* 2000;68(6):1051−1061.

118. Carroll KM, Easton CJ, Nich C, et al. The use of contingency management and motivational/skills-building therapy to treat young adults with marijuana dependence. *J Consult Clin Psychol.* 2006;74(5):955−966.

119. Litt MD, Kadden RM, Petry NM. Behavioral treatment for marijuana dependence: randomized trial of contingency management and self-efficacy enhancement. *Addict Behav.* 2013;38(3):1764−1775.

120. Baker A, Bucci S, Lewin TJ, Kay-Lambkin F, Constable PM, Carr VJ. Cognitive-behavioural therapy for substance use disorders in people with psychotic disorders: randomised controlled trial. *Br J Psychiatry.* 2006;188:439−448.

121. Hjorthoj CR, Fohlmann A, Larsen AM, Gluud C, Arendt M, Nordentoft M. Specialized psychosocial treatment plus treatment as usual (TAU) versus TAU for patients with cannabis use disorder and psychosis: the CapOpus randomized trial. *Psychol Med.* 2013;43(7): 1499−1510.

122. Budney A, Moore B, Sigmon S, Higgins S. Contingency-management interventions for cannabis dependence. In: Roffman R, Stephens R, eds. *Cannabis Dependence; Its Nature, Consequences, and Treatment.* Cambridge: Cambridge University Press; 2007.

123. Petry NM. A comprehensive guide to the application of contingency management procedures in clinical settings. *Drug Alcohol Depend.* 2000;58(1−2):9−25.

124. Budney AJ, Moore BA, Rocha HL, Higgins ST. Clinical trial of abstinence-based vouchers and cognitive-behavioral therapy for cannabis dependence. *J Consult Clin Psychol.* 2006;74(2):307−316.

125. Kadden RM, Litt MD, Kabela-Cormier E, Petry NM. Abstinence rates following behavioral treatments for marijuana dependence. *Addict Behav.* 2007;32(6):1220−1236.

126. Sinha R, Easton C, Renee-Aubin L, Carroll KM. Engaging young probation-referred marijuana-abusing individuals in treatment: a pilot trial. *Am J Addict.* 2003;12(4):314−323.

127. Stanger C, Budney AJ, Kamon JL, Thostensen J. A randomized trial of contingency management for adolescent marijuana abuse and dependence. *Drug Alcohol Depend.* 2009;105(3):240−247.

128. Sigmon SC, Steingard S, Badger GJ, Anthony SL, Higgins ST. Contingent reinforcement of marijuana abstinence among individuals with serious mental illness: a feasibility study. *Exp Clin Psychopharmacol.* 2000;8(4):509−517.

129. Misch DA. Basic strategies of dynamic supportive therapy. *J Psychother Pract Res.* 2000;9(4):173−189.

130. Grenyer B, Luborsky L, Solowij N. *Treatment manual for supportive-expressive dynamic psychotherapy: special adaptation for treatment of cannabis (marijuana) dependence.* Australia: National Drug and Alcohol Research Centre; 1995; 51.

131. Grenyer BSN, Peters R. A comparison of brief versus intensive treatment for cannabis dependence. *Aust Journal Psychology.* 1996;48(suppl 106).

132. Grenyer B, Solowij N. Supportive-expressive psychotherapy for Cannabis dependence. In: Roffman R, Stephens R, eds. *Cannabis Dependence: Its Nature, Consequences and Treatment.* Cambridge: Cambridge University Press; 2006:225−243.

133. Diamond G, Leckrone J, Dennis M, Godley S. *The cannabis youth treatment study: the treatment models and preliminary findings.* Cambridge: Cambridge University Press; 2006.

134. Waldron HB, Kern-Jones S, Turner CW, Peterson TR, Ozechowski TJ. Engaging resistant adolescents in drug abuse treatment. *J Subst Abuse Treat.* 2007;32(2):133−142.

135. Rigter H, Pelc I, Tossmann P, et al. INCANT: a transnational randomized trial of multidimensional family therapy versus treatment as usual for adolescents with cannabis use disorder. *BMC Psychiatry.* 2010;10:28.

136. Liddle HA, Dakof GA, Turner RM, Henderson CE, Greenbaum PE. Treating adolescent drug abuse: a randomized trial comparing multidimensional family therapy and cognitive behavior therapy. *Addiction.* 2008; 103(10):1660−1670.

137. Liddle HA, Dakof GA, Parker K, Diamond GS, Barrett K, Tejeda M. Multidimensional family therapy for adolescent drug abuse: results of a randomized clinical trial. *Am J Drug Alcohol Abuse.* 2001;27(4):651−688.

138. Dennis M, Titus JC, Diamond G, et al. The Cannabis Youth Treatment (CYT) experiment: rationale, study design and analysis plans. *Addiction.* 2002;97(suppl 1):16−34.

139. Diamond G, Godley SH, Liddle HA, et al. Five outpatient treatment models for adolescent marijuana use: a description of the Cannabis youth treatment interventions. *Addiction.* 2002;97(suppl 1):70−83.

140. Schaub MP, Henderson CE, Pelc I, et al. Multidimensional family therapy decreases the rate of externalising behavioural disorder symptoms in cannabis abusing adolescents: outcomes of the INCANT trial. *BMC Psychiatry.* 2014;14:26.

141. Rigter H, Henderson CE, Pelc I, et al. Multidimensional family therapy lowers the rate of cannabis dependence in adolescents: a randomised controlled trial in Western European outpatient settings. *Drug Alcohol Depend.* 2013;130(1−3):85−93.

142. Hendriks V, van der Schee E, Blanken P. Matching adolescents with a cannabis use disorder to multidimensional family therapy or cognitive behavioral therapy: treatment effect moderators in a randomized controlled trial. *Drug Alcohol Depend.* 2012;125(1−2):119−126.

143. Brigham GS. 12-step participation as a pathway to recovery: the Maryhaven experience and implications for treatment and research. *Sci Pract Perspect.* 2003;2(1):43−51.

144. Humphreys K. Professional interventions that facilitate 12-step self-help group involvement. *Alcohol Res Health.* 1999;23(2):93−98.

145. Services MAW, Marijuana Anonymous. *Life with Hope: 12 Step Workbook.* 1st ed. 2009. https://www.marijuana-anonymous.org/12-step-workbook.

146. Hoch E, Preuss UW, Ferri M, Simon R. Digital interventions for problematic cannabis users in non-clinical settings: findings from a systematic review and meta-analysis. *Eur Addict Res.* 2016;22(5):233−242.

147. Kelly TM, Daley DC, Douaihy AB. Treatment of substance abusing patients with comorbid psychiatric disorders. *Addict Behav.* 2012;37(1):11−24.

148. Vujanovic AA, Meyer TD, Heads AM, Stotts AL, Villarreal YR, Schmitz JM. Cognitive-behavioral therapies for depression and substance use disorders: an overview of traditional, third-wave, and transdiagnostic approaches. *Am J Drug Alcohol Abuse.* 2017;43(4):402−415.

149. Roberts NP, Roberts PA, Jones N, Bisson JI. Psychological therapies for post-traumatic stress disorder and comorbid substance use disorder. *Cochrane Database Syst Rev.* 2016; 4:CD010204.

150. Cooper K, Chatters R, Kaltenthaler E, Wong R. Psychological and psychosocial interventions for cannabis cessation in adults: a systematic review short report. *Health Technol Assess Winch Engl.* 2015;19(56):1−130.

151. Hjorthoj CR, Baker A, Fohlmann A, Nordentoft M. Intervention efficacy in trials targeting cannabis use disorders in patients with comorbid psychosis systematic review and meta-analysis. *Curr Pharmaceut Design*. 2014; 20(13):2205–2211.

152. Hjorthoj CR, Orlovska S, Fohlmann A, Nordentoft M. Psychiatric treatment following participation in the CapOpus randomized trial for patients with comorbid cannabis use disorder and psychosis. *Schizophr Res*. 2013;151(1–3):191–196.

153. Madigan K, Brennan D, Lawlor E, et al. A multi-center, randomized controlled trial of a group psychological intervention for psychosis with comorbid cannabis dependence over the early course of illness. *Schizophr Res*. 2013;143(1):138–142.

154. Eack SM, Hogarty SS, Greenwald DP, et al. Cognitive Enhancement Therapy in substance misusing schizophrenia: results of an 18-month feasibility trial. *Schizophr Res*. 2015;161(2–3):478–483.

155. Salloum IM, Brown ES. Management of comorbid bipolar disorder and substance use disorders. *Am J Drug Alcohol Abuse*. 2017;43(4):366–376.

156. Stephens R, Roffman A. The nature, consequences and treatment of cannabis dependence: implications for future research and policy. In: Roffman A, Stephens R, eds. *Cannabis Dependence; Its Nature, Consequences and Treatment*. Cambridge: Cambridge University Press; 2006.

157. Dutra L, Stathopoulou G, Basden SL, Leyro TM, Powers MB, Otto MW. A meta-analytic review of psychosocial interventions for substance use disorders. *Am J Psychiatry*. 2008;165(2):179–187.

158. McLellan AT, Lewis DC, O'Brien CP, Kleber HD. Drug dependence, a chronic medical illness: implications for treatment, insurance, and outcomes evaluation. *JAMA*. 2000;284(13):1689–1695.

159. Solowij N, Michie PT. Cannabis and cognitive dysfunction: parallels with endophenotypes of schizophrenia? *J Psychiatry Neurosci*. 2007;32(1):30–52.

CHAPTER 8

State-of-the-Art Treatment of Alcohol Use Disorder

LARA A. RAY, PHD • EMILY HARTWELL, MA • REJOYCE GREEN, BA • ALEXANDRA VENEGAS, BS

INTRODUCTION

Alcohol use disorder (AUD) is a chronic, relapsing condition, characterized by continued use despite a host of harmful medical, psychological, and social consequences. AUD and its associated consequences remain significant public health problems, as alcohol misuse was deemed the fifth largest risk factor for premature death and disability in 2010. Further, 3.3 million deaths (5.9% of all deaths) and 5.1% of the burden of disease and injury worldwide were attributable to alcohol consumption in 2012. More recently, it has been estimated that alcohol use and misuse contributed to over 200 diseases and injury-related health conditions, including liver cirrhosis, cancers, and injuries.[1]

Recent findings from a major epidemiological study, the National Epidemiological Survey on Alcohol and Related Conditions III (NESARC-III) conducted between 2012 and 2013 by the National Institute on Alcohol Abuse and Alcoholism,[2] indicated that the prevalence of *DSM-5* 12-month and lifetime AUD in the general population of adults in the United States was 13.9% and 29.1%, respectively. Stratifying by severity, 12-month prevalence of AUD was estimated to be 7.3% for mild AUD, 3.2% for moderate AUD, and 3.4% for severe AUD. Lifetime diagnosis rates broken down by severity revealed a similar pattern, with a prevalence of mild AUD of 8.6%, 6.6% for moderate AUD, and 13.9% for severe AUD. Mean age of AUD onset, of any severity, was found to be 26.2 years. Age of onset seems to decrease with increasing severity, with the age of onset approximating 30.1 years for mild AUD and 23.9 years for severe AUD.[2]

In terms of sociodemographic differences, the incidence of both a 12-month and lifetime AUD, of any severity, were greater among men (17.6% and 36.0%) than women (10.4% and 22.7%). Conversely, rates of lifetime AUD were found to be lower among black

(14.4%), Asian or Pacific Islander (15.6%), and Hispanic (22.9%) respondents than Caucasians (32.6%).[2] The prevalence of AUDs also varied by age, such that individuals between the ages of 18 and 29 had the highest rates of *DSM-5* AUD with a prevalence estimate of 26.7% for 12-month and 37.0% for lifetime compared to 16.2% 12-month and 34.4% lifetime for individuals between the ages of 30 and 44.[2]

Results from NESARC-III compared to previous epidemiological studies of alcohol use disorders show a marked increase in prevalence of AUD since 2002. Previous NESARC data[3] compared to the latest NESARC results[2] suggest that both the 12-month and lifetime prevalence of *DSM-IV* AUD substantially increased over the past decade, from 8.5% to 12.7% and from 30.3% to 43.6%, respectively. These observed significant increases may be attributable to significant increases in high-risk drinking from 2002 to 2013.[2] It is important to note that a striking cohort effect has been documented in that the gender gap between the prevalence of AUD between men and women appears to be narrowing.[4,5] Possible explanations for this effect include the notion that drinking norms may have become more liberal among women, coupled with increased educational and occupational opportunities for women as compared to previous decades, perhaps leading to increased alcohol use in general among women. These factors may explain the marked increase in high-risk drinking among women in more recent cohorts, yet further studies of this recently identified effect are warranted.

Overall, results from the most recent epidemiological study of alcohol use disorder and related conditions [NESARC] show that 13.9% of the adult population in the United States suffer from an alcohol use disorder in a given year, and 29.1% will suffer from an alcohol use disorder in their lifetime, with affected individuals

The Assessment and Treatment of Addiction. https://doi.org/10.1016/B978-0-323-54856-4.00008-0

totaling roughly 44.6 million and 93.4 million, respectively.[2] Further, it is estimated that the economic burden of alcohol use disorder treatment is $250 billion nationally.[6] These figures overtly highlight the gravity of alcohol use disorder as an important public health and economic concern and call for an effort for the development and implementation of effective treatments to address alcohol-related problems in the US. The remainder of this chapter addresses the issue of best practices in the treatment of AUD, including both psychosocial and pharmacological interventions with a focus on identifying those receiving the most empirical support.

TREATMENT

Although the recent increases in high-risk drinking and alcohol use disorder prevalence convey a significant public health concern, treatment rates for AUD remain extremely low. Among those with 12-month and lifetime diagnoses of AUD, only 7.7% and 19.8%, respectively, sought treatment from 2012 to 2013. Of those who did seek treatment, the most commonly accessed treatment modalities included 12-step groups, healthcare practitioners, and outpatient and inpatient rehabilitation facilities.[2] It was previously estimated that there is an average lag of approximately 8 years between the age of onset and the age at first treatment episode,[7] but more recent estimates suggest that this gap between onset and treatment-seeking is approximately 14 years, which is much longer than formerly determined.[8]

Those who eventually seek AUD treatment differ from those who do not on a host of sociodemographic, personality, psychological, and alcohol use pattern measures, and these inherent inconsistencies also predict differential clinical outcomes. Specifically, those who seek treatment for AUD tend to be older, report more AUD symptoms, have a longer duration of AUD symptoms, have a family history of AUD, and consume more alcohol, on average, than nontreatment seekers with a current AUD diagnosis. Treatment seekers also tend to be female, less ethnically diverse,[8,9] have higher numbers of negative social consequences and have higher rates of drug and psychiatric severity.[10]

There is also a robust body of literature on natural recovery from AUD, which is successful recovery without formal treatment. These data show that natural recovery is not only the most commonly reported method to mitigating negative consequences of continued use, but also that it is feasible for a large subset of those suffering from AUD. Two Canadian surveys showed that more than 75% of those who recovered from an alcohol problem for a year or more did so without

formal treatment, and even maintained recovery for over 5 years.[11] Additional findings uphold the notion that social support is fundamental in recovery; while those with low social support manage to reach unassisted recovery, as long as their alcohol-related issues are mild in nature, and conversely, those with severe alcohol problems require greater amounts of social support in order to reach their recovery goals.[12] It is important for clinicians to recognize that natural recovery is part of the landscape of AUD, particularly for individuals in the mild range of the disorder. As documented by brief intervention studies for AUD,[13] there is ample support to the notion that a brief intervention may promote natural recovery, particularly among individuals in the mild range of AUD, whereas those in the moderate-to-severe range are more likely to require specialized interventions as discussed in details below.

Psychosocial Treatments

Numerous psychosocial treatments for alcohol use disorders (AUD) exist, though they vary in the degree to which they have received empirical support. In other words, various treatments have not been sufficiently tested scientifically or have failed to show superiority in randomized controlled trials. Next, we provide a brief overview of psychosocial treatments for AUD that are considered evidence-based, or in other words, that have been empirically supported through controlled trials.

1. *Brief interventions* (BI) entail a succinct screening for alcohol use, negotiation of a behavioral change, and encouragement of follow-up or engagement with other resources. BI is typically delivered in a single session by a healthcare professional, with no apparent benefit from extended interventions.[14] Research samples have typically been opportunistic, yet meta-analyses have consistently shown a benefit in the reduction of alcohol use.[15–17] In nontreatment-seeking heavy users, BI can be a powerful tool to reduce use; however, BI should not replace long-term, specialist-delivered treatment for treatment seekers or severely dependent individuals.[13,17] Notably, the evidence for BI is weak as levels of AUD and heavy drinking increase.[13]

2. *Motivational interviewing* or *motivational enhancement therapy* (MET) seeks to enhance the motivation and commitment to change in the individual. The therapist helps the patient develop discrepancies between the factors maintain substance use and the problems that they are also experiencing. Typically delivered in 1–4 sessions, or in conjunction with other therapies,[18] MET is designed to meet patients where they are at along the continuum of change in

a collaborative, empathetic, and nonconfrontational manner.[19] Several meta-analyses have supported the efficacy of this modality, particularly in emergency departments[20] and primary care[21] settings. More recently, the consensus in the field is that MET is best used when in combination with skills-based approaches, particularly CBT. The reason being that motivation alone may not be sufficient to promote recovery, particularly among more severe cases of AUD.

3. *Cognitive behavioral therapies* (CBT) typically begin with a functional analysis of alcohol use which serves to elucidate the individual's cycles of thoughts, feelings, and behaviors underlying excessive drinking. Subsequently, the therapist provides psychoeducation, teaches skills to cope with cravings and fluctuations in mood, identifies and plans for triggers, and works to develop a plan to prevent relapse.[22] A host of studies and reviews have empirically supported CBT for the treatment of AUD.[23-25] Despite CBT demonstrating consistently significant effect sizes in meta-analyses, it has been posited that CBT may be less effective for AUD compared to other substances of abuse, such as cannabis, and may be more effective for women than men.[24,26] While those findings warrant replication, the take-home message is that CBT is one of the most widely studied and empirically supported treatments for AUD developed to date.

4. *Behavioral couple therapy* (BCT) presupposes a reciprocal relationship between substance use and relationship distress such that the two feed the other. Thus, BCT treats substance use within the dyad of the substance user and their partner. Interventions typically include psychoeducation, communication skills, behavioral activation to increase positive shared activities, negotiation of sobriety contracts, and relapse prevention with the goals of improving relationship functioning, teaching coping, and decreasing use.[27] This treatment has been shown to be superior to individual treatment in reducing frequency and consequences of use, increasing relationship satisfaction, and improving treatment retention for married and cohabitating individuals with AUD.[27,28] Of particular note, BCT has been associated with reduced risk of domestic violence.[27] As reviewed recently by McCrady and colleagues (2016),[29] new directions in couples therapy for alcohol problems include adaptions to nontraditional couples as well as the development of flexible models to enhance dissemination (e.g., technology-based delivery systems).

5. *Behavioral treatments* are typically based in operant conditioning theory and assume that alcohol use in itself is inherently rewarding. Therefore, for a treatment to be effective, the reinforcing value of alcohol must be decreased and the value of reinforcement in other activities must increase. The community reinforcement approach (CRA) aims to help individuals reorganize their lives to increase healthy, pleasurable, drug-free behaviors and teaches the skills to sustain this lifestyle.[30] Evidence for CRA is generally favorable for AUD and can be paired with contingency management (CM) and pharmacology treatment.[31] CM programs provide incentives based upon the demonstration of an agreed to behavior (e.g., negative breathalyzer, clean urine drug screen), which have typically shown good efficacy.[32] These approaches have shown utility in a number of settings, across diverse populations, and with different substances in addition to increasing engagement and attendance.[32,33] However, limitations of behavioral treatments include the relatively high cost, intensive labor to set up and continue, and the concern that treatment gains weaken over time,[32] and may in fact degrade quickly once reinforcements are no longer in place.

6. *Cue-exposure therapy* (CET), based in classical conditioning theory, involves repeated exposure to alcohol-related stimuli, without the reinforcement of alcohol consumption, to produce a decrease in alcohol craving and an increase in self-efficacy for coping with urges and high-risk situations.[34] CET has received some empirical support from a number of studies, including a comparison to CBT,[35,36] in conjunction with pharmacotherapies,[37] and in fMRI work.[38] However, despite the theory driven approach of CET, data have not been unanimously supportive. One study did not show that CET have additional benefits beyond CBT alone.[39] Two meta-analyses have shown the overall effect size of CET to be small ($d < 0.10$[34]) and to have little to no impact on drinking outcomes,[40] thus suggesting that CET does not significantly improve abstinence rates for AUD. Nevertheless, novel approaches to the delivery of CET are currently under investigation, specifically via smartphone applications.[41]

7. *Twelve-step therapies* (TST) include Alcoholics Anonymous (AA) and 12-step facilitation (TSF) which are rooted in the AA tradition. TST represent a widely available, free resource for individuals with alcohol problems, which espouses the goal of long-term, complete abstinence. Thus, according to the TST program psychological wellbeing, ability to cope,

and adaptation to a sober lifestyle are foundational elements of recovery. Experimental research into AA has historically been difficult, with no studies demonstrating unequivocal efficacy for TST.[42] However, strengths of TST include the length of treatment, cost, ease, social support, and self-regulated exposure to common therapeutic components.[43] Given the accessibility of TST as well as the evidence for its efficacy, we encourage clinicians to support their patients in seeking a TST group that is a good fit for them.

8. *Mindfulness-based therapies* are based in Buddhist traditions regarding mediation and mindfulness techniques. Promoted concepts include awareness of the "here and now" and nonjudgmental stances toward one's current state, emotional and otherwise. In AUD treatment, mindfulness is used to cope with urges, such as cravings, and to prevent relapse. Specifically, Mindfulness-Based Relapse Prevention (MBRP)[44] aims to increase cognizance of triggers, habitual behavioral patterns, and reactions, and the automatic responses to these discomforts in order to modify response.[45] Though newer and not as widely tested, MBRP has shown initial efficacy at reducing substance use and craving.[46,47] A meta-analysis of 42 studies published in 2017 found that MBRP had significant effects on the reduction of craving, reducing substance misuse, and lessening stress levels.[48] Based on the literature thus far, we encourage clinicians to consider mindfulness-based interventions in their practice with individuals with AUD.

In summary, the psychosocial treatment modalities described above show at least some level of empirical support for the treatment of AUD. However, no single treatment has surpassed all others at treating this complex, relapsing disorder.[49] Psychosocial treatments may be at their best when combined with another psychosocial modality and/or with pharmacotherapy. Over the years, some research has begged the question of how to best match patients with the optimal modality. For example, Project MATCH[50,51] compared the efficacy of CBT, TSF, and motivational enhancement therapy (MET). Two groups were enrolled in the study, outpatients and aftercare patients who were recently discharged from inpatient alcohol treatment. Patients' alcohol use was measured at one and 3 years after treatment. At 1-year follow-up, TSF appeared to slightly outperform the other two modalities; however, this difference had dissipated at 3-year follow-up. The overall abstinence rate across conditions was approximately 30% at 3-year follow-up, although there was an effect

of condition such that the patients in aftercare had higher rates of abstinence compared to the outpatients, 35% versus 20% respectively.[51] Moreover, few of the proposed moderator variables impacted treatment outcome, with the notable exception of pretreatment anger level and severity of alcohol dependence which responded better to MET and TSF, respectively.[50] Subsequent work has also proposed the importance of additional clinical variables in treatment matching, such as impulsivity[52] and drinking goal.[53,54] The role of drinking goal was analyzed in the COMBINE Study and found that individuals whose goal was complete abstinence had the best abstinence rates, whereas individuals whose goal was controlled drinking had the least drinks per drinking day.[53] Further, for those individuals who did not have a goal of complete abstinence, combined behavioral intervention was the best treatment condition compared to medication management alone.[53] Ultimately, further research is needed into the specific clinical characteristics and moderators that will make treatments more efficacious for subgroups of individuals with AUD.

Another consideration in the current landscape of AUD treatment is the role and implementation of technology-based interventions. A recent NIAAA study compared a computer-based delivery platform, *Take Control*, to traditional therapist-delivered interventions.[55] *Take Control* is a seven module intervention rooted in principles of psychoeducation, skill building, goal setting, and AUD treatment education. In the study by Devine and colleagues (2016), Take Control was comparable to traditionally administered interventions on participant retention, medication adherence, and placebo response rate, indicating that this type of intervention may be a viable alternative and cost-saving tool to traditional face-to-face individual interventions. Other platforms include internet-based education and skill-building platforms, screening tools, smart phone applications, and online support groups.[56-58] However, efficacy testing for these novel approaches has been variable and many available studies pertain only to college-age populations.[56,58,59] Such technology-based interventions have a host of potential benefits, including reduction of therapist bias in randomized control trials, increased ability to detect medication effects, and decreased cost.[55] Furthermore, these computer-based interventions may have the unique ability to reach groups that have historically been underserved including women, younger individuals, and other at-risk populations. As the landscape of mental health continues to adapt to the era of social media and mobile technology, so does the arena of AUD interventions. Thus, we recommend that clinicians become familiar with the latest developments in evidence-based applications of psychological principles to AUD treatment through mobile technology and computerized interventions. These resources, much like TSF, represent highly accessible options to patients with AUD and as such deserve our consideration in order to broaden the scope of care.

Pharmacological Treatment

Pharmacotherapy for alcoholism is used less often than psychosocial interventions. Aside from withdrawal management, when pharmacological agents are often used to manage alcohol withdrawal symptoms, few community programs combine pharmacotherapy and psychosocial interventions to treat AUD. The limited use of pharmacotherapy for AUD is due, in part, to the relative lack of effective pharmacological options to treat alcohol use disorders.

Food and Drug Administration (FDA) approved medications

The only pharmacotherapies currently approved by the FDA for the treatment of AUD are disulfram (Antabuse - average maintenance dose 250mg/day), naltrexon (50 mg daily), acamprosate (2g daily), and Vivitrol—an injectable longer acting form of naltrexone.[60–62]

Naltrexone is the most studied of these medications. Naltrexone is a highly selective opioid antagonist, with the highest affinity for the mu-opioid receptor. The neurobiological basis for the use of naltrexone stems from the route through which alcohol exerts its effects.[63,64] Alcohol increases release of endogenous opioids in the mesolimbic dopamine system contributing to the pleasurable effects of alcohol[63,64]; thus, an opioid antagonist is proposed to block these reinforcing effects. Naltrexone was approved by the FDA in 1994 after initial trials suggested that naltrexone resulted in significantly fewer drinking days and lower rates of relapse (23% relapse rate for naltrexone vs. 54% relapse rate for placebo) following 3 months of treatment.[65,66] These initial results have been largely supported by more recent trials of naltrexone that have generally demonstrated naltrexone to reduce the subjective pleasurable effects of alcohol,[67,68] craving for alcohol,[69,70] drinks per drinking day,[71] rates of relapse,[72,73] and time to first relapse.[74,75] However, the support for naltrexone is not uniform. A few trials, including a recent large multisite trial, have reported no significant outcome differences between naltrexone- and placebo-treated patients.[76–78] Moreover, the effect sizes of previous findings are often modest even when they reach statistical significance. In sum, studies of naltrexone to date suggest only a modest effect on the reduction of alcohol use.

Acamprosate was approved by the FDA in 2004. While the specific mechanisms of action for acamprosate are still under investigation, recent studies suggest that acamprosate acts as an N-Methyl-D-aspartic acid (NMDA) receptor modulator.[79] It is proposed to be more effective in achieving and maintaining abstinence as opposed to preventing relapse if drinking occurs.[80] This effect was supported in a recent review demonstrating reduced risk of returning to any drinking, as well as fewer drinking days, while taking acamprosate in comparison with placebo.[81] Acamprosate has also been suggested to have neuroprotective factors,[82,83] which may be particularly important in AUD treatment considering neuronal changes that may occur following frequent alcohol consumption.[84,85]

Disulfiram was the first medication approved for the treatment of AUD in 1951. Disulfiram is an aldehyde dehydrogenase inhibitor that exerts its clinical effect by blocking the metabolism of alcohol, thus producing an aversive unpleasant response after alcohol intake that results in severe nausea and vomiting.[86] Disulfiram has demonstrated mixed clinical efficacy.[87,88] In the context of more recent medications, disulfiram has been suggested to still have a role in AUD treatment if an individual is having difficulty attaining sobriety[89]; however, compliance and medical management issues significantly limit the widespread utilization of disulfiram in clinical practice for AUD.

Seeking to improve the clinical efficacy of two approved AUD pharmacotherapies, naltrexone and acamprosate, through combination with psychosocial treatments, NIAAA conducted an ambitious multisite trial of naltrexone, acamprosate, or placebo in combination with a behavioral intervention (combine behavioral intervention; CBI) or medication management using a multifactorial research design.[90,91] In this project, CBI was designed to combine several elements of empirically supported psychosocial treatments previously tested in Project MATCH, such as motivation enhancement therapy, cognitive-behavioral therapy, and facilitation of involvement in mutual-help groups.[92]

Results from the COMBINE Study found that patients receiving medical management (MM) with naltrexone, CBI, or both fared better on drinking outcomes, whereas acamprosate showed no evidence of efficacy, with or without CBI. No combination of medications produced better efficacy than naltrexone or CBI alone in the presence of medical management.[93] The authors concluded that naltrexone with medical management could be delivered in healthcare settings, thus serving alcohol-dependent patients who might otherwise not receive treatment. In brief, the COMBINE Project supported the efficacy of naltrexone for AUD and its results were used to disseminate this knowledge to physicians who can prescribe naltrexone in conjunction with medication management practices.

In addition to the main effects of the COMBINE Project, a strong pharmacogenetic, or personalized medicine, angle was explored. Specifically, the COMBINE Project examined whether a single-nucleotide polymorphism (SNP) in the mu-opioid receptor (OPRM1) gene, the Asn40Asp SNP predicts clinical response to naltrexone, an opioid antagonist. Results of the COMBINE project indicated that if treated with MM alone and naltrexone, 87.1% of Asp40 carriers had a good clinical outcome, compared with only 54.8% of individuals with the Asn40/Asn40 genotype (odds ratio, 5.75; confidence interval, 1.88–17.54), while, if treated with placebo, 48.6% of Asp40 carriers and 54.0% of individuals with the Asn40/Asn40 genotype had a good clinical outcome.[94] These findings are consistent with controlled laboratory studies suggesting that individuals with this polymorphism of the OPRM1 gene had a stronger hedonic response to alcohol in the laboratory,[95,96] in the natural environment,[97] and in the context of molecular imaging whereby dopamine release was measured during alcohol administration.[98] Further, controlled studies suggest that naltrexone attenuates the rewarding effects of alcohol more strongly among Asp40 carriers.[67,96,99] As reviewed in detail elsewhere,[100] the naltrexone × OPRM1 gene interaction is a prime example of pharmacogenetics in the field of alcoholism. Nevertheless, a recent using prospective genotyping did not support this pharmacogenetics effect,[101] in casts doubt onto whether this finding may be replicable and clinically meaningful.

Promising off-label medications

Numerous promising pharmacotherapies have been examined as possible treatments for AUD. In fact, in 2007 the National Institute on Alcohol Abuse and Alcoholism (NIAAA) established the Clinical Investigations Group (NCIG) as a formalized effort to support Phase II clinical trials that may further examine additional medications. To date, NCIG has completed 4 Phase II multisite, placebo-controlled, randomized trials. Next, we review several pharmacotherapies recently tested off-label for the treatment of AUD.

Nalmafene and varenicline are two recent pharmacotherapies currently under study that show promise for the treatment of Alcohol Dependence. Nalmafene is an opioid antagonist that is approved for the treatment of alcohol dependence in Europe. Initial results have supported the efficacy for nalmafene to prevent relapse to heavy drinking in comparison to placebo,[102,103] although some studies have found no superiority of nalmafene compared to placebo.[104] Varenicline is a partial α4β2 nicotinic agonist and full α7 agonist that is currently FDA approved for the treatment of nicotine dependence. Varenicline was examined as part of the NCIG initiative,[105] and found to significantly reduce weekly percentage of heavy drinking days, drinks per day, drinks per drinking day, as well as alcohol craving. Varenicline was also well tolerated suggesting that it may serve as a promising option for AUD treatment. The FDA did issue a black box warning for varenicline in 2009 due to possible adverse neuropsychiatric events. Recent reports suggest while there is an increased risk of nausea with varenicline, there is not an increased risk of depression or suicidality.[106] Recent studies have supported these effects in heavy-drinking smokers as well.[107,108]

Another class of medications that have been examined are anticonvulsants, which target GABA-ergic activity. Gabapentin is proposed to modulate GABA activity by indirectly interacting with voltage-gated calcium channels.[109] A recent 12-week clinical trial revealed that gabapentin significantly improved rates of heavy drinking and abstinence, and was well tolerated with no serious adverse events.[110] Additional single-site RCTs have demonstrated initial efficacy for gabapentin to reduce drinking outcomes[111,112] and in combination with naltrexone produce superior effects than naltrexone alone.[113] A Cochrane Review found gabapentin to significantly reduce rates of heavy drinking, but reported no effects on attenuating alcohol craving or maintaining abstinence.[114]

Another promising anticonvulsant medication is topiramate. While the precise mechanisms of action remain unclear, topiramate is thought to reduce neuronal excitability through inhibition at glutamate AMPA/kainate receptors and L-type calcium channels. This could conceivably decrease the distress associated with protracted withdrawal from alcohol. Topiramate also facilitates brain GABA function and may even increase GABA levels. Both of these effects (i.e., glutamate blockade, GABA facilitation) can in turn reduce or inhibit mesolimbic DA activity. It has been suggested that topiramate may indirectly influence midbrain dopaminergic activity, thereby reducing craving.[115] A trial found that topiramate reduced drinking and alcohol craving over a 12-week treatment period.[115] A more recent trial found topiramate to reduce drinks per day, percentage of days drinking, and percentage of days heavy drinking.[116] Side effects of topiramate include some cognitive impairment, such as slight reductions in verbal fluency and working memory.[116] A recent review concluded that topiramate demonstrates clinical efficacy in various drinking outcomes; however, longer-term trials of topiramate are warranted to further establish the optimal treatment dose, duration, and tolerability.[117] Lastly, zonisamide, an FDA approved adjunct treatment for partial seizures, has shown initial efficacy in reducing number of heavy drinking day and drinks per week,[118] as well as reduce urge to drink.[119] Additional trials of zonisamide are currently underway.

Two additional medications that have shown initial efficacy but are currently awaiting ongoing trials are baclofen and ondansetron. Baclofen is a GABA$_B$ agonist that is currently FDA approved for muscle spasticity. While preclinical trials have shown reduced alcohol intake,[120] clinical trials have shown mixed results.[121–123] Ondansetron is a 5-HT3 antagonist that has demonstrated effectiveness, relative to placebo, in the reduction of drinking among early onset alcoholics.[124] Although the mechanism of action is unclear, it has been speculated that ondansetron might address the serotonergic dysfunction thought to characterize early onset AUD[124,125] and that it might reduce craving for alcohol through the influence of 5-HT3 projections to mesolimbic dopaminergic connections in the midbrain.[124,125]

In addition to the promising medications reviewed above, a series of pharmacotherapies have been tested and results suggested poor efficacy despite initial promising findings. Quetiapine is often used in treating psychiatric disorders as it is an atypical antipsychotic; however, it showed initial efficacy in heavy drinkers.[126–128] The proposed mechanism of action for quetiapine is to reduce craving by targeting mesocorticolimbic dopamine function. However, an examination of quetiapine as part of the NCIG trials found no significant differences were found between placebo and quetiapine on percentage of heavy drinking days.[129] Quetiapine did improve sleep and decrease the number of depressive symptoms in comparison with placebo. Levetiracetam is another medication that has shown poor efficacy as a treatment for AUD despite early promising results. Levetiracetam is an anticonvulsant that initially showed promise in limiting harmful drinking in both animal models[130] and reducing alcohol withdrawal symptoms in clinical sample.[131] When examined in NCIG, levetiracetam was no different than placebo on primary and secondary outcome measures.[132]

Other medications showing poor efficacy are selective serotonin reuptake inhibitors (SSRIs). The efficacy of SSRIs in reducing drinking has been largely modest,[120,133] although it has been suggested that they may work better in certain genetic subgroups.[134] Another medication showing poor efficacy is a novel arginine vasopressin V1B receptor antagonist ABT-436. This medication was examined as part of the NCIG trials.[135] The basis for this was vasopressin receptors have a regulatory role during alcohol consumption, as well in stress and anxiety.[136] Results from this NCIG trial revealed no significant differences in percentage of heavy drinking days between ABT-436 and placebo.[135] There was a significant difference in percentage of abstinent days, such that participants receiving ABT-436 had a greater percentage of abstinent days. This medication appears to exert some selective effects on specific drinking outcomes that may serve as a target in AUD treatment.

In summary, randomized clinical trials have provided sufficient evidence of the efficacy, albeit modest efficacy, for acamprosate, naltrexone, and Vivitrol for AUD treatment.[76,137–139] Of the NCIG trials conducted to date, Varenicline appears to be the most promising off-label medication.[105] In addition, there are a number of opportunities for research in the field of pharmacotherapies for alcohol-use disorders, including the need to identify psychosocial predictors of medication compliance and efficacy,[76] expand our knowledge of dosing issues,[140] improve the dissemination of research findings to clinicians in the field,[141] examine the combined effects of psychosocial and pharmacotherapy treatments,[142] and study the role of genetic factors in predicting treatment response to pharmacotherapies. Perhaps most importantly, there is a strong recommendation that novel targets and novel compounds be screened for efficacy for AUD treatment,[143,144] given the recognition that repurposing psychiatric medications for AUD treatment has been met with limited success. Thus, we anticipate that future AUD clinical trials will branch toward novel compounds and targets that can more effectively mitigate the neurotoxic effects of alcohol and ameliorate alcohol-induced neuroadaptations.

SUMMARY AND FUTURE DIRECTIONS

Alcohol use disorder has multifaceted etiology, maintenance, and relapse processes. Research reviewed in this chapter underscores the complex nature of AUD and its treatment. Some of the broad assertions from the work reviewed herein are that while AUD is highly prevalent, treatment-seeking for AUD is not. There is substantial naturalistic recovery and brief intervention may be able to catalyze recovery in mild cases, yet the vast majority of individuals with moderate-to-severe AUD will require specialized treatment to overcome this disorder. To that end, identifying treatments that are evidence-based is a challenging task, to the extent that NIAAA has launched a new initiative called NIAAA Alcohol Treatment Navigator (https://alcoholtreatment.niaaa.nih.gov/). The goal of the Alcohol Treatment Navigator is to help patients and families identify evidence-based care. We encourage providers to become familiar with the resources in the NIAAA Alcohol Treatment Navigator and to consider using it in their practice. This chapter sought to characterize the literature on evidence-based care for AUD at the level of psychosocial and pharmacological interventions. As reviewed here, there are a host of behavioral and pharmacological treatments that have shown compelling evidence of efficacy for the treatment of AUD. While none of those treatments is the so-called "silver bullet" for alcoholism, they each have the potential to significantly improve the odds of recovery for individuals with AUD. Personalized treatment, or identification of best treatment matches for individual patients, looms as an important promise to improve care, yet specific matches are not reliable in their research evidence to warrant clinical dissemination. Nonetheless, there is a strong recognition among providers and patients alike that "more is better" and that giving patients access to multiple evidence-based resources for behavioral and pharmacological management of AUD is likely to improve each individual's chances of sustained recovery from AUD. As the field of AUD treatment moves toward the development of novel pharmacotherapies and the adaptation of behavioral therapies to the high-technology environment we live in, we are reminded that decades of research have produce the currently available treatments that are evidence-based and that each individual patient is entitled to receive those treatments as they embark on their recovery from alcoholism.

ACKNOWLEDGMENTS

Supported by NIH grants DA041226, AA026006, and AA023669 (LR) and T32 DA007272 (AV).

REFERENCES

1. World Health Organization & WHO. Management of substance unit. *Glob Status Rep Alcohol Heal*. 2014;2014 (World Health Organization).
2. Grant BF, Goldstein RB, Saha TD, et al. Epidemiology of DSM-5 alcohol use disorder results from the national epidemiologic survey on alcohol and related conditions III. *JAMA Psychiatry*. 2015;72(8):757−766. https://doi.org/10.1001/jamapsychiatry.2015.0584.
3. Grant BF, Dawson DA, Stinson FS, Chou SP, Dufour MC, Pickering RP. The 12-month prevalence and trends in DSM-IV alcohol abuse and dependence: United States, 1991−1992 and 2001−2002. *Drug Alcohol Depend*. 2004;74(3):223−234. https://doi.org/10.1016/j.drugalcdep.2004.02.004.
4. Grant BF, Chou SP, Saha TD, et al. Prevalence of 12-month alcohol use, high-risk drinking, and DSM-IV alcohol use disorder in the United States, 2001−2002 to 2012−2013: results from the national epidemiologic survey on alcohol and related conditions. *JAMA Psychiatry*. 2017;74(9):911−923. https://doi.org/10.1001/jamapsychiatry.2017.2161.
5. Keyes KM, Grant BF, Hasin DS. Evidence for a closing gender gap in alcohol use, abuse, and dependence in the United States population. *Drug Alcohol Depend*. 2008;93(1):21−29.
6. Sacks JJ, Gonzales KR, Bouchery EE, Tomedi LE, Brewer RD. 2010 national and state costs of excessive alcohol consumption. *Am J Prev Med*. 2015; 49(5):e73−e79. https://doi.org/10.1016/j.amepre.2015.05.031.
7. Hasin DS, Stinson FS, Ogburn E, Grant BF. Prevalence, correlates, disability, and comorbidity of DSM-IV alcohol abuse and dependence in the United States: results from the national epidemiologic survey on alcohol and related conditions. *Arch Gen Psychiatry*. 2007;64(7):830−842. https://doi.org/10.1001/archpsyc.64.7.830.
8. Ray LA, Bujarski S, Yardley MM, Roche DJO, Hartwell EE. Differences between treatment-seeking and non-treatment-seeking participants in medication studies for alcoholism: do they matter? *Am J Drug Alcohol Abuse*. 2017:1−8. https://doi.org/10.1080/00952990.2017.1312423.
9. Rohn MCH, Lee MR, Kleuter SB, Schwandt ML, Falk DE, Leggio L. Differences between treatment-seeking and nontreatment-seeking alcohol-dependent research participants: an exploratory analysis. *Alcohol Clin Exp Res*. 2017;41(2):414−420. https://doi.org/10.1111/acer.13304.
10. Weisner C, Matzger H. A prospective study of the factors influencing entry to alcohol and drug treatment. *J Behav Health Serv Res*. 2002;29(2):126−137. https://doi.org/10.1007/BF02287699.
11. Sobell LC, Cunningham JA, Sobell MB. Recovery from alcohol problems with and without treatment: prevalence in two population surveys. *Am J Public Health*. 1996;86(7):966−972. https://doi.org/10.2105/AJPH.86.-7.966.
12. Bischof G, Rumpf HJ, Hapke U, Meyer C, John U. Types of natural recovery from alcohol dependence: a cluster analytic approach. *Addiction*. 2003;98(12):1737−1746. https://doi.org/10.1111/j.1360-0443.2003.00571.x.
13. Saitz R. Alcohol screening and brief intervention in primary care: absence of evidence for efficacy in people with dependence or very heavy drinking. *Drug Alcohol Rev*. 2010;29(6):631−640.

14. Kaner E, Dickinson H, Beyer F, et al. Effectiveness of brief alcohol interventions in primary care populations (Review). *Cochrane Database Syst Rev.* 2007. https://doi.org/10.1002/14651858.CD004148.pub3.

15. Bertholet N, Daeppen J, Wietlisback V, Fleming M, Burnand B. Reduction of alcohol consumption by brief alcohol intervention in primary care. *Arch Intern Med.* 2005;165(9):986–995. https://doi.org/10.1001/archinte.165.9.986.

16. D'Onofrio G, Degutis LC. Preventive care in the emergency department: screening and brief intervention for alcohol problems in the emergency department: a systematic review. *Acad Emerg Med.* 2002;9(6):627–638. https://doi.org/10.1197/aemj.9.6.627.

17. Moyer A, Finney J, Swearingen C, Vergun P. Brief interventions for alcohol problems: a meta-analytic review of controlled investigations in treatment seeking and non treatment seeking populations. *Addiction.* 2002;97:279–292. https://doi.org/10.1046/j.1360-0443.2002.00018.x.

18. Riper H, Andersson G, Hunter SB, de Wit J, Berking M, Cuijpers P. Treatment of comorbid alcohol use disorders and depression with cognitive-behavioural therapy and motivational interviewing: a meta-analysis. *Addiction.* 2014;109(3):394–406. https://doi.org/10.1111/add.12441.

19. Miller WR, Rollnick S. *Motivational Interviewing: Helping People Change.* Guilford Press; 2012.

20. Schmidt CS, Schulte B, Seo H-N, et al. Meta-analysis on the effectiveness of alcohol screening with brief interventions for patients in emergency care settings. *Addiction.* 2016;111(5):783–794. https://doi.org/10.1111/add.13263.

21. Jonas D, Grbutt J, Amick H, et al. Annals of internal medicine review behavioral counseling after screening for alcohol misuse in primary. *Ann Intern Med.* 2012;157(9):645–654.

22. Monti PM. *Treating Alcohol Dependence: A Coping Skills Training Guide.* Guilford Press; 2002.

23. Carroll KM, Kiluk BD. Cognitive behavioral interventions for alcohol and drug use disorders: through the stage model and back again. *Psychol Addict Behav.* 2017;31(8):847–861. https://doi.org/10.1037/adb0000311.

24. Magill M, Ray LA. Cognitive-behavioral treatment with adult alcohol and illicit drug users: a meta-analysis of randomized controlled trials. *J Stud Alcohol Drugs.* 2009;70(4):516–527. https://doi.org/10.15288/jsad.2009.70.516.

25. McHugh KR, Hearon BA, Otto MW. Cognitive-behavioral therapy for substance use disorders. *Psychiatr Clin North Am.* 2010;33(3):511–525. https://doi.org/10.1016/j.psc.2010.04.012.

26. Hofmann SG, Asnaani A, Vonk IJJ, Sawyer AT, Fang A. The efficacy of cognitive behavioral therapy: a review of meta-analyses. *Cogn Ther Res.* 2012;36(5):427–440. https://doi.org/10.1007/s10608-012-9476-1.

27. O'Farrell TJ, Fals-Stewart W. Behavioral couples therapy for alcoholism and drug abuse. *J Subst Abuse Treat.* 2000;18(1):51–54.

28. Powers MB, Vedel E, Emmelkamp PMG. Behavioral couples therapy (BCT) for alcohol and drug use disorders: a meta-analysis. *Clin Psychol Rev.* 2008;28(6):952–962. https://doi.org/10.1016/j.cpr.2008.02.002.

29. McCrady BS, Wilson AD, Muñoz RE, Fink BC, Fokas K, Borders A. Alcohol-focused behavioral couple therapy. *Fam Process.* 2016;55(3):443–459. https://doi.org/10.1111/famp.12231.

30. Meyers RJ, Roozen HG, Smith JE. The community reinforcement approach: an update of the evidence. *Alcohol Res Heal.* 2011;33(4):380–388.

31. Roozen HG, Boulogne JJ, Van Tulder MW, Van Den Brink W, De Jong CAJ, Kerkhof AJFM. A systematic review of the effectiveness of the community reinforcement approach in alcohol, cocaine and opioid addiction. *Drug Alcohol Depend.* 2004;74(1):1–13. https://doi.org/10.1016/j.drugalcdep.2003.12.006.

32. Davis DR, Kurti AN, Skelly JM, Redner R, White TJ, Higgins ST. A review of the literature on contingency management in the treatment of substance use disorders, 2009–2014. *Prev Med.* 2016;92:36–46.

33. Fitzsimons H, Tuten M, Borsuk C, Lookatch S, Hanks L. Clinician-delivered contingency management increases engagement and attendance in drug and alcohol treatment. *Drug Alcohol Depend.* 2015;152:62–67. https://doi.org/10.1016/j.drugalcdep.2015.04.021.

34. Conklin CA, Tiffany ST. Applying extinction research and theory to cue-exposure addiction treatments. *Addiction.* 2002;97(2):155–167. https://doi.org/10.1046/j.1360-0443.2002.00014.x.

35. Loeber S, Croissant B, Heinz A, Mann K, Flor H. Cue exposure in the treatment of alcohol dependence: effects on drinking outcome, craving and self-efficacy. *Br J Clin Psychol.* 2006;45(4):515–529. https://doi.org/10.1348/014466505X82586.

36. Rohsenow DJ, Monti PM, Rubonis AV, et al. Cue exposure with coping skills training and communication skills training for alcohol dependence: 6- and 12-month outcomes. *Addiction.* 2001;96(8):1161–1174.

37. Monti PM, Rohsenow DJ, Swift RM, et al. Naltrexone and cue exposure with coping and communication skills training for alcoholics: treatment process and 1-year outcomes. *Alcohol Clin Exp Res.* 2001;25(11):1634–1647. https://doi.org/10.1111/j.1530-0277.2001.tb02170.x.

38. Vollstädt-Klein S, Loeber S, Kirsch M, et al. Effects of cue-exposure treatment on neural cue reactivity in alcohol dependence: a randomized trial. *Biol Psychiatry.* 2011;69(11):1060–1066. https://doi.org/10.1016/j.biopsych.2010.12.016.

39. Kavanagh DJ, Sitharthan G, Young RM, et al. Addition of cue exposure to cognitive-behaviour therapy for alcohol misuse: a randomized trial with dysphoric drinkers. *Addiction.* 2006;101(8):1106–1116. https://doi.org/10.1111/j.1360-0443.2006.01488.x.

40. Mellentin AI, Skøt L, Nielsen B, et al. Cue exposure therapy for the treatment of alcohol use disorders: a meta-analytic review. *Clin Psychol Rev.* 2017;57:195–207. https://doi.org/10.1016/j.cpr.2017.07.006.

41. Mellentin AI, Stenager E, Nielsen B, Nielsen AS, Yu FA. Smarter pathway for delivering cue exposure therapy? The design and development of a smartphone app targeting alcohol use disorder. *JMIR mHealth uHealth.* 2017;5(1).

42. Ferri M, Amato L, Davoli M. Alcoholics Anonymous and other 12-step programmes for alcohol dependence. *Cochrane Collab.* 2006;(3).

43. Kelly JF, Magill M, Stout RL. How do people recover from alcohol dependence? A systematic review of the research on mechanisms of behavior change in Alcoholics Anonymous. *Addict Res Theory.* 2009;17(3):236–259. https://doi.org/10.1080/16066350902770458.

44. Witkiewitz K, Marlatt GA, Walker D. Mindfulness-based relapse prevention for alcohol and substance use disorders. *J Cogn Psychother.* 2005;19(3):211–228.

45. Bowen S, Chawla N, Marlatt GA. *Mindfulness-based Relapse Prevention for Addictive Behaviors.* New York: The Guilford Press; 2011.

46. Bowen S, Witkiewitz K, Clifasefi SL, et al. Relative efficacy of mindfulness-based relapse prevention, standard relapse prevention, and treatment as usual for substance use disorders. *JAMA Psychiatry.* 2014;71(5):547–556. https://doi.org/10.1001/jamapsychiatry.2013.4546.

47. Witkiewitz K, Bowen S, Douglas H, Hsu SH. Mindfulness-based relapse prevention for substance craving. *Addict Behav.* 2013;38(2):1563–1571. https://doi.org/10.1016/j.addbeh.2012.04.001.

48. Li W, Howard MO, Garland EL, McGovern P, Lazar M. Mindfulness treatment for substance misuse: a systematic review and meta-analysis. *J Subst Abuse Treat.* 2017;75:62–96. https://doi.org/10.1016/j.jsat.2017.01.008.

49. Litten RZ, Ryan ML, Falk DE, Reilly M, Fertig JB, Koob GF. Heterogeneity of alcohol use disorder: understanding mechanisms to advance personalized treatment. *Alcohol Clin Exp Res.* 2015;39(4):579–584. https://doi.org/10.1111/acer.12669.

50. Allen J, Anton RF, Babor TF, Carbonari J. Project MATCH secondary a priori hypotheses. *Addiction.* 1997;92(12):1671.

51. Group PMR. Matching patients with alcohol disorders to treatments: clinical implications from Project MATCH. *J Ment Heal.* 1998;7(6):589–602.

52. Tomko RL, Bountress KE, Gray KM. Personalizing substance use treatment based on pre-treatment impulsivity and sensation seeking: a review. *Drug Alcohol Depend.* 2016;167(supplement C):1–7.

53. Bujarski S, O'Malley SS, Lunny K, Ray LA. The effects of drinking goal on treatment outcome for alcoholism. *J Consult Clin Psychol.* 2013;81(1):13. https://doi.org/10.1037/a0030886.

54. Gueorguieva R, Wu R, O'Connor PG, et al. Predictors of abstinence from heavy drinking during treatment in COMBINE and external validation in PREDICT. *Alcohol Clin Exp Res.* 2014;38(10):2647–2656. https://doi.org/10.1111/acer.12541.

55. Devine EG, Ryan ML, Falk DE, Fertig JB, Litten RZ. An exploratory evaluation of take control: a novel computer-delivered behavioral platform for placebo-controlled pharmacotherapy trials for alcohol use disorder. *Contemp Clin Trials.* 2016;50:178–185.

56. Donoghue K, Patton R, Phillips T, Deluca P, Drummond C. The effectiveness of electronic screening and brief intervention for reducing levels of alcohol consumption: a systematic review and meta-analysis. *J Med Internet Res.* 2014;16(6):e142.

57. Hester RK, Lenberg KL, Campbell W, Delaney HD. Overcoming addictions, a web-based application, and SMART recovery, an online and in-person mutual help group for problem drinkers, Part 1: three-month outcomes of a randomized controlled trial. *J Med Internet Res.* 2003;15(7):e134.

58. White A, Kavanagh D, Stallman H, et al. Online alcohol interventions: a systematic review. *J Med Inter Res.* 2010;12(5):e62.

59. Scott-Sheldon LAJ, Carey KB, Elliott JC, Garey L, Carey MP. Efficacy of alcohol interventions for first-year college students: a meta-analytic review of randomized controlled trials. *J Consult Clin Psychol.* 2014;82(2):177–188. https://doi.org/10.1037/a0035192.

60. Petrakis IL. A rational approach to the pharmacotherapy of alcohol dependence. *J Clin Psychopharmacol.* 2006;26:S3–S12.

60a. Center for Substance Abuse Treatment. Incorporating Alcohol Pharmacotherapies Into Medical Practice. Rockville (MD): Substance Abuse and Mental Health Services Administration (US); 2009. (Treatment Improvement Protocol (TIP) Series, No. 49.) Chapter 3—Disulfiram. Available from: https://www.ncbi.nlm.nih.gov/books/NBK64036/.

61. Pettinati HM, Rabinowitz AR. Choosing the right medication for the treatment of alcoholism. *Curr Psychiatry Rep.* 2006;8(5):383–388. https://doi.org/10.1007/s11920-006-0040-0.

62. Zindel LR, Kranzler HR. Pharmacotherapy of alcohol use disorders: seventy-five years of progress. *J Stud Alcohol Drugs Suppl.* 2014;75(suppl 17):79–88. https://doi.org/10.15288/JSADS.2014.S17.79.

63. Mitchell JM, O'Neil JP, Janabi M, Marks SM, Jagust WJ, Fields HL. Alcohol consumption induces endogenous opioid release in the human orbitofrontal cortex and nucleus accumbens. *Sci Transl Med.* 2012;4(116):116ra6-116ra6. https://doi.org/10.1126/scitranslmed.3002902.

64. Nestler EJ. Is there a common molecular pathway for addiction? *Nat Neurosci.* 2005;8(11):1445–1449. https://doi.org/10.1038/nn1578.

65. O'Malley S, Jaffe A, Chang G, Schottenfeld RS, Meyer RE, RB. Naltrexone and coping skills therapy for alcohol dependency. A controlled study. *Arch Gen Psychiatry*. 1992; 49(3):881–887.

66. Volpicelli JR, Alterman AI, Hayashida M, OCP. Naltrexone in the treatment of alcohol dependence. *Subst Abus*. 1992;49(11):876–880.

67. Ray LA, Hutchison KE. Effects of naltrexone on alcohol sensitivity and genetic moderators of medication response: a double-blind placebo-controlled study. *Arch Gen Psychiatry*. 2007;64(9):1069–1077. https://doi.org/ 10.1001/archpsyc.64.9.1069.

68. Drobes DJ, Anton RF, Thomas SE, Voronin K. Effects of naltrexone and nalmefene on subjective response to alcohol among non-treatment-seeking alcoholics and social drinkers. *Alcohol Clin Exp Res*. 2004;28(9):1362–1370. https://doi.org/10.1097/ 01.ALC.0000139704.88862.01.

69. O'Malley SS, Krishnan-Sarin S, Farren C, Sinha R, Kreek M. Naltrexone decreases craving and alcohol self-administration in alcohol-dependent subjects and activates the hypothalamo-pituitary-adrenocortical axis. *Psychopharmacol Berl*. 2002;160(1):19–29. https:// doi.org/10.1007/s002130100919.

70. Richardson K, Baillie A, Reid S, et al. Do acamprosate or naltrexone have an effect on daily drinking by reducing craving for alcohol? *Addiction*. 2008;103(6):953–959. https://doi.org/10.1111/j.1360-0443.2008.02215.x.

71. O'Malley SS, Corbin WR, Leeman RF, et al. Reduction of alcohol drinking in young adults by naltrexone: a double-blind, placebo-controlled, randomized clinical trial of efficacy and safety. *J Clin Psychiatry*. 2015;76(2): e207–e213. https://doi.org/10.4088/JCP.13m08934.

72. Morris PL, Hopwood M, Whelan G, Gardiner J, Drummond E. Naltrexone for alcohol dependence: a randomized controlled trial. *Addiction*. 2001;96(11): 1565–1573. https://doi.org/10.1080/ 09652140120080705.

73. Carmen B, Angeles M, Ana M, María AJ. Efficacy and safety of naltrexone and acamprosate in the treatment of alcohol dependence: a systematic review. *Addiction*. 2004;99(7):811–828. https://doi.org/10.1111/j.1360- 0443.2004.00763.x.

74. Kiefer F. Comparing and combining naltrexone and acamprosate in relapse prevention of alcoholism: a double-blind, placebo-controlled study. *Arch Gen Psychiatry*. 2003;60(1):92. https://doi.org/10.1001/archpsyc.60.1.92.

75. Guardia J, Caso C, Arias F, et al. A double-blind, placebo-controlled study of naltrexone in the treatment of alcohol-dependence disorder: results from a multicenter clinical trial. *Alcohol Clin Exp Res*. 2002;26(9):1381–1387. https://doi.org/10.1097/01.ALC.0000030561.15921.A9.

76. Kranzler HR, Modesto-Lowe V, Van Kirk J. Naltrexone vs. nefazodone for treatment of alcohol dependence: a placebo-controlled trial. *Neuropsychopharmacology*. 2000; 22(5):493–503. https://doi.org/10.1016/S0893- 133X(99)00135-9.

77. Krystal JH, Cramer JA, Krol WF, Kirk GF, Rosenheck RA. *Naltrexone Treat Alcohol Depend*. 2001;345(24): 1734–1739.

78. Streeton C, Whelan G. Naltrexone, a relapse prevention maintenance treatment of alcohol dependence: a meta-analysis of randomized controlled trials. *Alcohol Alcohol*. 2001;36(6):544–552. https://doi.org/10.1093/alcalc/ 36.6.544.

79. Mason BJ, Heyser CJ. Acamprosate: a prototypic neuromodulator in the treatment of alcohol dependence. *CNS Neurol Disord Drug Targets*. 2010;9(1):23–32. https://doi.org/10.2174/187152710790966641.

80. Rösner S, Leucht S, Lehert P, Soyka M. Acamprosate supports abstinence, Naltrexone prevents excessive drinking: evidence from a meta-analysis with unreported outcomes. *J Psychopharmacol*. 2008;22(1):11–23. https://doi.org/10.1177/0269881107078308.

81. Jonas DE, Amick HR, Feltner C, et al. Pharmacotherapy for adults with alcohol use disorders in outpatient settings: a systematic review and meta-analysis. *JAMA J Am Med Assoc*. 2014;311(18):1889–1900. https://doi.org/ 10.1001/jama.2014.3628.

82. Koob GF, Mason BJ, De Witte P, Littleton J, Siggins GR. Potential neuroprotective effects of acamprosate. *Alcohol Clin Exp Res*. 2002;26(4):586–592.

83. Littleton JM. Acamprosate in alcohol dependence: implications of a unique mechanism of action. *J Addict Med*. 2007;1(3):115–125.

84. Grant KA, Valverius P, Hudspith M, Tabakoff B. Ethanol withdrawal seizures and the NMDA receptor complex. *Eur J Pharmacol*. 1990;176(3):289–296.

85. Davidson M, Shanley B, Wilce P. Increased NMDA-induced excitability during ethanol withdrawal – a behavioral and histological study. *Brain Res*. 1995; 674(1):91–96. https://doi.org/10.1016/0006-8993(94) 01440-S.

86. Vallari RC, Pietruszko R. Human aldehyde dehydrogenase: mechanism of inhibition of disulfiram. *Sci (80-)*. 1982;216(4546):637–639.

87. Fuller RK, Branchey L, Brightwell DR, et al. Disulfiram treatment of alcoholism: a veterans administration cooperative study. *JAMA*. 1986;256(11):1449. https://doi.org/ 10.1001/jama.1986.03380110055026.

88. Garbutt JC, West SL, Carey TS, Lohr KN, Crews FT. Pharmacological treatment of alcohol dependence: a review of the evidence. *JAMA*. 1999;281(14):1318–1325.

89. Fuller RK, Gordis E. Does disulfiram have a role in alcoholism treatment today? *Addiction*. 2004;99(1):21–24. https://doi.org/10.1111/j.1360-0443.2004.00597.x.

90. COMBINE Study Research Group. Testing combined pharmacotherapies and behavioral interventions for alcohol dependence (the COMBINE study): a pilot feasibility study. *Alcohol Clin Exp Res*. 2003;27(7):1123–1131.

91. COMBINE Study Research Group. Testing combined pharmacotherapies and behavioral interventions in alcohol dependence: rationale and methods. *Alcohol Clin Exp Res*. 2003;27(7):1107–1122.

92. Combined behavioral intervention manual: a clinical research guide for therapists treating people with alcohol dependence. In: Miller WR, ed. *COMBINE Monograph Series, 1*. 1st ed. Bethesda, MD: National Institute on Alcohol Abuse and Alcoholism; 2004 (NIH 04-5288).

93. Anton RF, O'Malley SS, Ciraulo DA, et al. Combined pharmacotherapies and behavioral interventions for alcohol dependence. *JAMA*. 2006;295(17):2003. https://doi.org/10.1001/jama.295.17.2003.

94. Anton RF, Orozszi G, O'Malley S, et al. An evaluation of μ-opioid receptor (OPRM1) as a predictor of naltrexone response in the treatment of alcohol dependence: results from the combined pharmacotherapies and behavioral interventions for alcohol dependence (COMBINE) study. *Arch Gen Psychiatry*. 2008;65(2):135–144. https://doi.org/10.1001/archpsyc.65.2.135.

95. Ray LA, Hutchison KE. A polymorphism of the μ,-opioid receptor gene (OPRM1) and sensitivity to the effects of alcohol in humans. *Alcohol Clin Exp Res*. 2004; 28(12):1789–1795. https://doi.org/10.1097/01.ALC.-0000148114.34000.B9.

96. Ray LA, Bujarski S, Chin PF, Miotto K. Pharmacogenetics of naltrexone in Asian Americans: a randomized placebo-controlled laboratory study. *Neuropsychopharmacology*. 2012;37(2):445–455. https://doi.org/10.1038/npp.2011.192.

97. Ray LA, Miranda Jr R, Tidey JW, et al. Polymorphisms of the μ-opioid receptor and dopamine D₄ receptor genes and subjective responses to alcohol in the natural environment. *J Abnorm Psychol*. 2010;119(1):115.

98. Ramchandani VA, Umhau J, Pavon FJ, et al. A genetic determinant of the striatal dopamine response to alcohol in men. *Mol Psychiatry*. 2011;16(8):809–817. https://doi.org/10.1038/mp.2010.56.

99. Setiawan E, Pihl RO, Cox SML, et al. Influence of the OPRM1 A118G polymorphism on alcohol-induced euphoria, risk for alcoholism and the clinical efficacy of naltrexone. *Alcohol Clin Exp Res*. 2011;35(6):1134–1141.

100. Ray LA, Barr CS, Blendy JA, Oslin D, Goldman D, Anton RF. The role of the Asn40Asp polymorphism of the mu opioid receptor gene (OPRM1) on alcoholism etiology and treatment: a critical review. *Alcohol Clin Exp Res*. 2012;36(3):385–394. https://doi.org/10.1111/j.1530-0277.2011.01633.x.

101. Oslin DW, Leong SH, Lynch KG, et al. Naltrexone vs placebo for the treatment of alcohol dependence: a randomized clinical trial. *JAMA Psychiatry*. 2015;72(5):430–437. https://doi.org/10.1001/jamapsychiatry.2014.3053.

102. Mason BJ, Salvato FR, Williams LD, Ritvo EC, Cutler RB. A double-blind, placebo-controlled study of oral nalmefene for alcohol dependence. *Arch Gen Psychiatry*. 1999; 56(8):719–724.

103. Mann K, Bladström A, Torup L, Gual A, Van Den Brink W. Extending the treatment options in alcohol dependence: a randomized controlled study of As-needed nalmefene. *Biol Psychiatry*. 2013;73(8):706–713. https://doi.org/10.1016/j.biopsych.2012.10.020.

104. Anton RF, Pettinati H, Zweben A, et al. A multi-site dose ranging study of nalmefene in the treatment of alcohol dependence. *J Clin Psychopharmacol*. 2004; 24(4):421–428. https://doi.org/10.1097/01.jcp.0000130555.63254.73.

105. Litten RZ, Ryan ML, Fertig JB, et al. A double-blind, placebo-controlled trial assessing the efficacy of varenicline tartrate for alcohol dependence. *J Addict Med*. 2013;7(4):277–286. https://doi.org/10.1097/ADM.0b013e31829623f4.

106. Gibbons RD, Mann JJ. Varenicline, smoking cessation, and neuropsychiatric adverse events. *Am J Psychiatry*. 2013;170(12):1460–1467. https://doi.org/10.1176/appi.ajp.2013.12121599.

107. Mckee SA, Harrison ELR, Malley SSO, et al. Varenicline reduces alcohol self-administration in heavy- drinking smokers. *Biol Psychiatry*. 2009;66(2):185–190. https://doi.org/10.1016/j.biopsych.2009.01.029.

108. Mitchell JM, Teague CH, Kayser AS, Bartlett SE, Fields HL. Varenicline decreases alcohol consumption in heavy-drinking smokers. *Psychopharmacol Berl*. 2012;223(3):299–306. https://doi.org/10.1007/s00213-012-2717-x.

109. Sills GJ. The mechanisms of action of gabapentin and pregabalin. *Curr Opin Pharmacol*. 2006;6(1):108–113. https://doi.org/10.1016/j.coph.2005.11.003.

110. Mason BJ, Quello S, Goodell V, Shadan F, Kyle M, Begovic A. Gabapentin treatment for alcohol dependence a randomized clinical trial. *JAMA Intern Med*. 2014;174(1):70–77. https://doi.org/10.1001/jamainternmed.2013.11950.

111. Brower KJ, Myra Kim H, Strobbe S, Karam-Hage MA, Consens F, Zucker RA. Randomized double-blind pilot trial of gabapentin versus placebo to treat alcohol dependence and comorbid insomnia. *Alcohol Clin Exp Res*. 2008;32(8):1429–1438.

112. Furieri FA, Nakamura-Palacios EM. Gabapentin reduces alcohol consumption and craving: a randomized, double-blind, placebo-controlled trial. *J Clin Psychiatry*. 2007;68(11):1691–1700.

113. Anton RF, Myrick H, Wright TM, et al. Gabapentin combined with naltrexone for the treatment of alcohol dependence. *Am J Psychiatry*. 2011;168(7):709–717. https://doi.org/10.1176/appi.ajp.2011.10101436.

114. Pani PP, Trogu E, Pacini M, Maremmani I. Anticonvulsants for alcohol dependence. *Cochrane Database Syst Rev*. 2010:2.

115. Johnson BA, Ait-Daoud N, Bowden CL, et al. Oral topiramate for treatment of alcohol dependence: a randomised controlled trial. *Lancet*. 2003;361(9370): 1677–1685. https://doi.org/10.1016/S0140-6736(03)13370-3.

116. Knapp CM, Ciraulo DA, Sarid-Segal O, et al. Zonisamide, topiramate, and levetiracetam efficacy and neuropsychological effects in alcohol use disorders. *J Clin Psychopharmacol*. 2015;35(1):34–42. https://doi.org/10.1097/JCP.0000000000000246.

117. Olmsted CL, Kockler DR. Topiramate for alcohol dependence. *Ann Pharmacother.* 2008;42:1475−1480. https://doi.org/10.1345/aph.1L157.

118. Arias AJ, Feinn R, Oncken C, Covault J, Kranzler HR. Placebo-controlled trial of zonisamide for the treatment of alcohol dependence. *J Clin Psychopharmacol.* 2010;30(3):318−322. https://doi.org/10.1097/JCP.0b013e3181db38bb.

119. Sarid-Segal O, Knapp CM, Burch W, et al. The anticonvulsant zonisamide reduces ethanol self-administration by risky drinkers. *Am J Drug Alcohol Abuse.* 2009;35(5):316−319. https://doi.org/10.1080/00952990903060150.

120. Litten RZ, Fertig J, Mattson M, Egli M. Development of medications for alcohol use disorders: recent advances and ongoing challenges. *Expert Opin Emerg Drugs.* 2005; 10(2):323−343.

121. Addolorato G, Caputo F, Capristo E, et al. Baclofen efficacy in reducing alcohol craving and intake: a preliminary double-blind randomized controlled study. *Alcohol Alcohol.* 2002;37(5):504−508. https://doi.org/10.1093/alcalc/37.5.504.

122. Garbutt JC, Kampov-polevoy AB, Ph D, Gallop R, Flannery BA. Efficacy and safety of baclofen for alcohol dependence: a randomized, double-blind,. *Placebo-controlled Trial.* 2010;34(11):1849−1857. https://doi.org/10.1111/j.1530-0277.2010.01273.x.

123. Morley KC, Baillie A, Leung S, Addolorato G, Leggio L, Haber PS. Baclofen for the treatment of alcohol dependence and possible role of comorbid anxiety. *Alcohol Alcohol.* 2014;49(6):654−660. https://doi.org/10.1093/alcalc/agu062.

124. Johnson B, Ait-Daoud N, Prihoda TJ. Combining ondansetron and naltrexone effectively treats biologically predisposed alcoholics: from hypotheses to preliminary clinical evidence. *Alcohol Clin Exp Res.* 2000; 24(5):737−742. https://doi.org/10.1111/j.1530-0277.2000.tb02048.x.

125. Johnson BA, Ait-Daoud N. Neuropharmacological treatments for alcoholism: scientific basis and clinical findings. *Psychopharmacol Berl.* 2000;149(4):327−344.

126. Martinotti G, Andreoli S, Di Nicola M, Di Giannantonio M, Sarchiapone M, Janiri L. Quetiapine decreases alcohol consumption, craving, and psychiatric symptoms in dually diagnosed alcoholics. *Hum Psychopharmacol Clin Exp.* 2008;23(5):417−424.

127. Monnelly EP, Ciraulo DA, Knapp C, LoCastro J, Sepulveda I. Quetiapine for treatment of alcohol dependence. *J Clin Psychopharmacol.* 2004;24(5):532−535. https://doi.org/10.1097/01.jcp.0000138763.23482.2a.

128. Sattar SP, Bhatia SC, Petty F. Potential benefits of quetiapine in the treatment of substance dependence disorders. *J Psychiatry Neurosci.* 2004;29(6):452−457.

129. Litten RZ, Fertig JB, Falk DE, et al. A double-blind, placebo-controlled trial to assess the efficacy of quetiapine fumarate XR in very heavy-drinking alcohol-dependent patients. *Alcohol Clin Exp Res.* 2012;36(3):406−416. https://doi.org/10.1111/j.1530-0277.2011.01649.x.

130. Zalewska-Kaszubska J, Bajer B, Gorska D, Andrzejczak D, Dyr W, Bieńkowski P. Voluntary alcohol consumption and plasma beta-endorphin levels in alcohol preferring rats chronically treated with lamotrigine. *Physiol Behav.* 2015; 139:7−12. https://doi.org/10.1016/j.physbeh.2014.11.026.

131. Muller CA, Schafer M, Schneider S, et al. Efficacy and safety of levetiracetam for outpatient alcohol detoxification. *Pharmacopsychiatry.* 2010;43(5):184−189.

132. Fertig JB, Ryan ML, Falk DE, et al. A double-blind, placebo-controlled trial assessing the efficacy of levetiracetam extended-release in very heavy drinking alcohol-dependent patients. *Alcohol Clin Exp Res.* 2012; 36(8):1421−1430. https://doi.org/10.1111/j.1530-0277.2011.01716.x.

133. Johnson BA. Update on neuropharmacological treatments for alcoholism: scientific basis and clinical findings. *Biochem Pharmacol.* 2008;75(1):34−56. https://doi.org/10.1016/j.bcp.2007.08.005.

134. Kranzler HR, Armeli S, Tennen H, et al. A double-blind, randomized trial of sertraline for alcohol dependence: moderation by age of onset and 5-hydroxytryptamine transporter-linked promoter region genotype. *J Clin Psychopharmacol.* 2011;31(1):22−30. https://doi.org/10.1097/JCP.0b013e31820465fa.

135. Ryan ML, Falk DE, Fertig JB, et al. A Phase 2, double-blind, placebo-controlled randomized trial assessing the efficacy of ABT-436, a novel V1b receptor antagonist, for alcohol dependence. *Neuropsychopharmacology.* 2017;42(5): 1012−1023. https://doi.org/10.1038/npp.2016.214.

136. Caldwell HK, Wersinger SRYWS. The role of the vasopressin 1b receptor in aggression and other social behaviours. *Prog Brain Res.* 2008;170:65−72.

137. Mann K. Pharmacotherapy of alcohol dependence. *CNS Drugs.* 2004;18(8):485−504.

138. Myrick H, Brady KT, Malcolm R. New developments in the pharmacotherapy of alcohol dependence. *Am J Addict.* 2001; 10(s1). https://doi.org/10.1080/10550490150504092.

139. Schaffer A, Naranjo CA. Recommended drug treatment strategies for the alcoholic patient. *Drugs.* 1998;56(4): 571−585. https://doi.org/10.2165/00003495-199856040-00005.

140. Mason BJ. Dosing issues in the pharmacotherapy of alcoholism. *Alcohol Clin Exp Res.* 1996;20(s7).

141. Meza E, Kranzler H. Closing the gap between alcoholism research and practice: the case for pharmacotherapy. *Psychiatr Serv.* 1996;47(9):917−920.

142. McCaul ME, Petry NM. The role of psychosocial treatments in pharmacotherapy for alcoholism. *Am J Addict.* 2003;12(s1).

143. Litten RZ, Falk DE, Ryan ML, Fertig JB. Discovery, development, and adoption of medications to treat alcohol use disorder: goals for the phases of medications development. *Alcohol Clin Exp Res.* 2016;40(7): 1368−1379. https://doi.org/10.1111/acer.13093.

144. Litten RZ, Egli M, Heilig M, et al. Medications development to treat alcohol dependence: a vision for the next decade. *Addict Biol.* 2012;17(3):513−527. https://doi.org/10.1111/j.1369-1600.2012.00454.x.

CHAPTER 9

Applying Best Practice Guidelines on Chronic Pain in Clinical Practice— Treating Patients Who Suffer From Pain and Addiction

KEITH G. HEINZERLING, MD, MPH

Pain is defined as "an unpleasant sensory and emotional experience associated with actual or potential tissue damage, or described in terms of such damage" and chronic pain is defined as "pain that persists beyond normal tissue healing time, which is assumed to be 3 months."[1] An estimated 126.1 million United States (US) adults report some pain in the previous 3 months while 25.2 million (11.2%) report chronic pain.[2] Costs to US society in medical expenditures and lost productivity from chronic pain are estimated to be $560–$635 billion, more than the yearly costs of heart disease ($309 billion), cancer ($243 billion), and diabetes ($188 billion).[3]

Opioid prescribing in the US increased dramatically since 1999 largely due to increased prescribing of opioids to treat chronic pain. Opioid prescriptions in the US peaked in 2010 at 782 morphine milligram equivalents (MME) per capita and then decreased to 640 MME per capita in 2015, although the 2015 US prescribing rate was still three times as high as 1999 and four times higher than the prescribing rate for Europe in 2015.[4] The United States consumes 80% of all the opioids manufactured globally each year.[5] The large increase in prescribing has occurred with little data to support the effectiveness of chronic opioid therapy for non-cancer pain and an explosion of data regarding serious adverse effects of opioid therapy including fatal overdoses. Clinical trials of opioids for chronic low back pain have found short-term reductions in pain relative to placebo but have not assessed complications of chronic opioid therapy including opioid misuse, overdose, or addiction.[6] Prevalence of prescription and illicit opioid use disorder have also increased, with 2 million Americans reporting misuse of prescription opioids and nearly 600,000 reporting heroin use disorder in 2015.[7,8] Furthermore, paralleling the increase in opioid prescribing has been an equally dramatic increase in deaths due to opioid overdose. Drug overdose rates in the US tripled from 1999 to 2015, with 52,404 Americans dead from a drug overdose in 2015, of which 63% involved an opioid, compared to 16,849 overdose deaths in the US in 1999.[9]

Pain, substance use disorders, and psychological conditions are commonly comorbid. Prevalence of pain among people receiving substance use disorder treatment ranges from 40% to 60%.[10–12] Estimates of substance use disorders among chronic pain patients are highly variable ranging from 0.05% to 26% for opioid use disorder, from 3% to 48% for substance use disorders not restricted to opioids, and from 8% to 29% for opioid misuse.[10] Anxiety and depression are also common among patients with chronic pain and are risk factors for prescription opioid misuse and overdose.[13] Patients with chronic pain are four times as likely to have anxiety or depression than those without chronic pain[14] and in a sample of patients on opioids for chronic pain, 37% had an anxiety disorder and 34% depression.[15] Pain catastrophizing, a negative cognitive–affective response to anticipated or actual pain, is associated with increased risk of chronic pain, higher levels of pain intensity and interference, greater disability, and worse treatment outcomes.[16] Higher levels of pain catastrophizing and pain-related anxiety are associated with lower heat pain threshold and tolerance in patients with chronic pain[17] while pain catastrophizing, distress intolerance, depression, and

The Assessment and Treatment of Addiction. https://doi.org/10.1016/B978-0-323-54856-4.00009-2

anxiety are associated with prescription opioid misuse.[18-20] Negative affect, a cluster of negative emotions and thoughts manifesting as high levels of depression, anxiety, and catastrophizing is common in chronic pain. Negative affect is associated with lower opioid analgesia, higher opioid doses, increased rates of opioid misuse, and increased risk for the development of opioid-induced hyperalgesia (OIH) among patients treated with opioids for chronic low back pain.[21,22]

Recent research into the neurobiology of chronic pain has emphasized the affective and motivational dimensions of the chronic pain syndrome, the role of brain reward systems in pain chronification, and overlap between the brain areas involved in chronic pain and addiction.[23] Pain is a multimodal subjective experience with both sensory and affective dimensions[24] with different brain systems processing each of these dimensions.[25] In particular, deficits in dopaminergic functioning similar to those found in addictive disorders have been found in chronic pain[26] and the mesolimbic reward system plays a critical role in mediating the affective and motivational aspects of chronic pain and analgesia.[27] In a series of neuroimaging studies, baseline structural and functional connectivity within the mesocorticolimbic system, not areas related to pain sensation, predicted the development of chronic low back pain among patients undergoing imaging at the onset of acute back pain.[28] Of note, the same brain areas involved in affect and motivation that predict onset of chronic pain are also critically involved in addiction.[29] Opioids relieve the affective aspect of pain, and the boost in mood some patients receive from opioids is rewarding.[30,31] In light of the shared neurobiology underlying chronic pain and substance use disorders, it is not surprising that the dramatic increase in opioid prescribing for chronic pain has been accompanied by increases in opioid use disorder and overdose.

Clinicians and patients face multiple challenges and barriers to successfully treating pain in the context of substance use disorders. Many medications used for pain have an abuse liability and carry a risk of overdose especially when combined, including opioids, benzodiazepines, skeletal muscle relaxants, and gabapentinoids. Patients with active substance use problems prescribed pain medications may misuse the prescribed medications and/or combine them in a dangerous fashion with illicit drugs or alcohol. Patients with past substance use disorders in remission and their clinicians may have concerns that exposure to potentially addictive medications may trigger a relapse. While these are legitimate clinical concerns, patients also fear that addiction-related issues may result in their pain being undertreated leading to loss of trust, conflict, and breakdown of the doctor–patient relationship thereby further complicating treatment.[32,33] Navigating these potential conflicts requires clinicians to strike a balance between acknowledging the patient's perspective and avoiding iatrogenic harm by emphasizing a collaborative and shared approach to decision-making.[34]

In response to the US epidemic of opioid abuse and overdose, the Centers for Disease Control and Prevention issued guidelines for prescribing opioids for chronic pain.[35] The guidelines strongly recommend against opioids for chronic noncancer pain, instead recommending nonpharmacologic and nonopioid pharmacologic therapy. If opioids are started for chronic pain the guidelines recommend avoiding dose escalation and keeping the dose to less than 50 morphine milligram equivalents (MME)/day. Doses $\geq$90 mg MME/day are high risk for overdose and should be avoided. Opioids and benzodiazepines should not be prescribed concomitantly due to synergistic overdose risk. If opioids are used for acute pain, the guidelines recommend limiting opioids to a short course of the lowest dose of an immediate-release opioid for 3 days or rarely as long as 7 days. Offering or providing medication-assisted treatment with approved medications, e.g., methadone, buprenorphine, and long-acting injectable naltrexone, along with behavioral treatment, for patients with opioid use disorder is also recommended.

While avoiding prescribing opioids in patients with substance use disorders may be the safest option, this is not possible or even clinically appropriate in all situations such as severe acute pain, surgical/procedural pain, cancer pain, end of life/palliative care, and even some cases of chronic noncancer pain. Tailoring treatment to each patient's needs to maximize potential benefits and mitigate risks is most likely to produce good clinical outcomes such as a reduction in pain and suffering while minimizing iatrogenic harms. Below, we review the evidence for a variety of pharmacologic and nonpharmacologic pain management treatments in patients with opioid use disorder as well as nonopioid substance use disorders. We aim to provide clinicians and patients with evidence with which to pursue a shared decision-making process aimed at identifying treatment plans to alleviate pain and suffering while mitigating risk of developing or worsening addiction.

METHADONE

Methadone is a synthetic mu-opioid agonist with a long half-life (range 5–55 h) used as an analgesic and an approved treatment for opioid use disorder.[36] In the US, physicians can prescribe methadone to treat pain but methadone maintenance treatment for opioid use disorder must be dispensed within the context of highly structured and regulated opioid treatment programs[37] with once-daily supervised dosing aimed at minimizing the risk of methadone misuse or diversion.[38] Evidence from multiple randomized clinical trials shows that methadone maintenance treatment for opioid use disorder reduces illicit opioid use and increases treatment retention relative to placebo[39] and methadone retains patients in opioid use disorder treatment longer than buprenorphine.[40] Although years of clinical experience support methadone's analgesic effects, the few studies of methadone for cancer and chronic pain have been small and of short duration finding methadone to be similar to morphine but with a greater risk of sedation.[41] Methadone is an NMDA-receptor antagonist resulting in methadone's purported efficacy for chronic neuropathic pain although results of the small, low quality clinical studies of methadone for neuropathic pain are mixed.[42]

There are several potential serious adverse effects with methadone. There is a risk of serious cardiac events with higher doses of methadone including QT prolongation, torsade de pointes, ventricular arrhythmias, and cardiac arrest[43,44] and patients on doses ≥120 mg a day should be monitored with electrocardiograms and assessed for other pro-arrhythmic factors such as electrolyte abnormalities and concomitant prescription of HIV antiretrovirals.[45,46] In the US, methadone prescribed for pain outside of methadone maintenance programs has been responsible for a disproportionate number of prescription overdose deaths, with methadone accounting for 2% of US opioid prescriptions in 2009 but approximately 30% of prescription opioid overdose deaths.[47] Prescribing of methadone to patients with substance use disorders for pain outside of methadone maintenance programs should be approached with great caution due to the risk of accidental overdose especially if methadone is combined with other sedatives such as benzodiazepines or alcohol. The long and variable half-life of methadone combined with multiple possible drug-drug interactions contribute to the high risk of overdose with methadone and require that methadone be initiated at a low dose and titrated very slowly with clinical monitoring.[46]

Chronic pain is common among methadone maintenance patients with prevalence from 50% to 60% compared to approximately 30% among adults in the US general population.[11] Opioid-induced hyperalgesia (OIH) is clinically characterized by increasing pain intensity over time, pain spreading to other locations beyond the initial site of pain, and increased pain sensation in response to external stimuli, in the context of exposure to opioids.[48] OIH has been demonstrated in animal models[49] and following short-term, intraoperative use of opioids[50] but whether chronic opioid use, such as with illicit opioid use, methadone maintenance, or chronic pain treatment, results in clinically meaningful hyperalgesia is less clear.

Studies have consistently found that methadone maintenance patients are hyperalgesic to experimental pain induced by the cold pressor test[51–54] but studies have less consistently demonstrated hyperalgesia via electrical, thermal, or pressure pain stimulation.[51,55–57] A few small studies found that history of chronic pain, but not methadone dose, was a significant predictor of pain threshold in methadone maintenance patients[52,55] and additional studies examining the influence of methadone dose and chronic pain status on hyperalgesia in methadone patients are warranted. Heroin users were also hyperalgesic via cold pressor prior to starting methadone/buprenorphine treatment[56] while abstinent heroin users are less hyperalgesic than those receiving methadone treatment[58–62] suggesting that hyperalgesia results from ongoing opioid exposure and is not unique to methadone. In fact, hyperalgesia was similar among methadone maintenance patients and chronic pain patients treated with methadone or morphine.[57]

OIH is thought to be mediated in part by activation of excitatory NMDA glutamate receptors.[63] Methadone is an NMDA antagonist[64] and how to rectify this with findings of OIH in methadone maintenance patients is not clear. Ketamine is an NMDA antagonist and reduces postoperative hyperalgesia but whether ketamine may be useful as an adjuvant to prevent or reduce hyperalgesia with methadone treatment has not been established.[65] Dextromethorphan, also an NMDA-receptor antagonist, did not reduce hyperalgesia more than placebo in a randomized trial among methadone maintenance patients.[66] Gabapentin significantly increased pain threshold and tolerance more than placebo in a small randomized clinical trial in a methadone maintenance treatment program, although nonadherent and nonopioid abstinent participants were excluded from the analysis and chronic pain status of the participants is not described.[67]

Studies of hyperalgesia among methadone maintenance patients are limited by small sample size, observational designs, and inconsistent results using pain measures other than the cold pressor test.[48,68] Prospective studies of hyperalgesia among chronic pain patients have conflicting results with some studies finding that prescription opioid use predicted the onset of hyperalgesia[69] and others failing to find an effect.[70] In a randomized, double-blind, placebo controlled trial, patients with chronic low back pain did not develop hyperalgesia after 1 month of morphine treatment[71] although longer treatment and/or higher doses may be necessary for the development of OIH. Larger, prospective, well-controlled studies assessing the effect of methadone maintenance on hyperalgesia and the impact, if any, of hyperalgesia to experimental pain on important clinical outcomes, such as opioid relapse and quality of life, are needed.

Pain management in methadone maintained patients is complicated by cross-tolerance between methadone and other opioid analgesics such that high opioid doses may be needed to achieve analgesia.[52,72] Also methadone's analgesic effects last 4−6 h and methadone for pain should be dosed two to three times daily[36,73] as compared to once-daily methadone maintenance dosing. Strategies to address this include adding an additional short-acting opioid to the methadone or splitting the daily methadone dose into twice or thrice daily dosing and slowly titrating methadone to achieve analgesia. The addition of another opioid to methadone maintenance treatment must be done cautiously and in coordination with methadone maintenance dosing to reduce the risk of accidental overdose. There are no randomized trials addressing questions related to pain management during methadone maintenance treatment and the available studies are limited to small observational studies and case reports.[74] A retrospective study found that providing additional analgesic methadone on top of the methadone maintenance dosing resulted in a reduction in pain scores among 53 patients with HIV and chronic pain undergoing methadone maintenance treatment.[75] Additional methadone was titrated to approximately 200% of the initial methadone maintenance dose and was well tolerated and rates of heroin use were relatively low (13% opioid positive urine drug screens at 12 months). Cognitive behavioral therapy is effective for pain management, but many methadone program counselors are not trained or equipped to address pain and studies to integrate behavioral approaches to pain management within substance use counseling programs are needed.[76,77]

BUPRENORPHINE

Buprenorphine is a mu-opioid partial agonist that is approved by the US Food and Drug Administration (FDA) for treatment of opioid use disorder and pain. Buprenorphine is available in sublingual and buccal formulations of buprenorphine/naloxone and newly approved long-acting buprenorphine depot formulations for opioid use disorder as well as transdermal, buccal, and intravenous buprenorphine formulations approved for treating pain. The addition of naloxone to buprenorphine is to deter intravenous buprenorphine use as naloxone is poorly absorbed when administered sublingually but precipitates opioid withdrawal if buprenorphine/naloxone is injected. As a partial opioid agonist, buprenorphine has a ceiling effect for respiratory depression making it safer than methadone, although there is still a risk of overdose when buprenorphine is combined with sedatives such as benzodiazepines or alcohol. Risk of cardiac arrhythmias and QT prolongation with buprenorphine is much lower than with methadone.[43,78,79] The improved safety profile and lower risk of misuse and overdose with buprenorphine relative to methadone led to the approval in the US of buprenorphine for the treatment of opioid use disorder in office-based settings by certified physicians as opposed to highly regulated and controlled methadone clinic settings. Buprenorphine reduces heroin use compared to placebo but may be less effective than high-dose methadone in cases of severe opioid use disorder.[40]

Buprenorphine is more effective for treating chronic pain than placebo and similar in analgesic effect to full opioid agonists in multiple clinical trials for cancer pain and noncancer pain including low back pain, joint pain, and neuropathic pain.[80] The majority of these studies evaluated transdermal and buccal buprenorphine formulations approved for pain as opposed to the sublingual buprenorphine/naloxone formulation approved for treating opioid use disorder, and few studies included patients with opioid addiction. In a large, multisite clinical trial (N = 653) of buprenorphine/naloxone treatment for prescription opioid use disorder in which 42% of participants reported chronic pain at baseline, prevalence of chronic pain as well as scores for pain intensity and interference decreased significantly with buprenorphine/naloxone.[81,82] A past history of heroin use, but not baseline chronic pain, among participants with prescription opioid use disorder was associated with increased opioid use during buprenorphine/naloxone treatment,[82] although higher pain severity at baseline did predict higher buprenorphine/naloxone dose during initial stabilization.[83] The majority of participants with prescription opioid use disorder and chronic pain at study baseline reported that their first source of prescription opioids was a legitimate prescription taken for physical pain.[84] Higher pain severity scores in a given week during buprenorphine/naloxone treatment was significantly associated with opioid use in the subsequent week, with an increase from one pain severity category to the next (e.g., from mild to moderate pain) associated with a 32%–52% increase in the odds of opioid use in the following week.[84] Together these findings suggest that buprenorphine is an effective analgesic with an improved safety profile compared to full opioid agonists in patients with and without opioid use disorder and that worsening pain during buprenorphine/naloxone treatment for opioid use disorder is a risk factor for opioid relapse.

Similar to methadone, patients with opioid use disorder and pain may require different dosing of buprenorphine for treatment of pain versus opioid use disorder. While once-daily buprenorphine dosing is recommended for treating opioid use disorder, improved analgesia may result from splitting the daily dose to three or four times daily.[85] There has been controversy concerning whether buprenorphine's partial agonist "ceiling effect" may limit the analgesia obtained from buprenorphine. Early rodent studies suggested a ceiling effect on analgesia hypothesized to be due to buprenorphine effects at the antinociceptive ORL1 receptor, but clinical studies have failed to demonstrate an analgesic ceiling for buprenorphine in humans.[86] Buprenorphine has a very high affinity for the mu-opioid receptor and a long half-life and as a result doses sufficient to saturate available mu receptors (>16 mg sublingual buprenorphine) will block the euphoric and analgesic effects of other opioids.[87] Of note, patients sometimes misattribute this opioid antagonizing effect of buprenorphine to naloxone in the buprenorphine/naloxone formulation but when taken sublingually naloxone is poorly absorbed. While blocking of opioid agonist effects is an advantage of buprenorphine when treating opioid use disorder, high doses of buprenorphine may also antagonize the analgesic effects of other opioids thereby complicating management of pain in patients maintained on high-dose buprenorphine. Transdermal and buccal buprenorphine formulations approved for treating pain can be used with short-acting opioid full agonists for management of "breakthrough pain" although use of these formulations in patients with opioid use disorder should be done with caution as analgesic doses of buprenorphine may

not antagonize euphorigenic opioid effects or deter concomitant use of opioids including heroin.[88]

Management of surgical or procedural analgesia in patients maintained on opioid blocking doses of buprenorphine is complicated. Randomized trials to determine the optimal management strategy are lacking but current consensus is that for minor surgical or diagnostic procedures buprenorphine can be continued and nonopioid analgesics added but there is controversy regarding the best plan for major surgery or procedures expected to result in significant pain. Some experts recommend buprenorphine be discontinued at least 72 h prior to a major surgery/procedure to avoid buprenorphine antagonizing other opioid analgesics followed by close monitoring for potential opioid relapse off buprenorphine and pain management with high affinity full opioid agonists (e.g., fentanyl) and nonopioid modalities.[89] Others recommend continuing buprenorphine and supplementing with high affinity full opioid agonists able to compete with buprenorphine thereby providing additional analgesia while reducing opioid withdrawal and relapse risk related to discontinuing buprenorphine.[90,91] Although potential antagonism of opioid analgesic effects was not examined, buprenorphine blockade of other opioid agonist effects (subjective, reinforcing, and physiologic effects) is dose dependent and high doses (>24–32 mg sublingually) are required to significantly antagonize other opioids.[88] Controlled clinical trials to identify the optimal strategy for managing surgical/procedural pain in buprenorphine maintained patients are needed, especially in light of newly approved buprenorphine depot formulations which will make discontinuing buprenorphine prior to surgery/procedure impossible in some cases.

Buprenorphine may be less likely to induce opioid-induced hyperalgesia than full opioid agonists including methadone. There was no difference in hyperalgesia between buprenorphine maintained (N = 18) and methadone maintained (N = 18) patients with opioid use disorder, but in the subgroup of patients abstinent from illicit opioids, hyperalgesia was less with buprenorphine than with methadone treatment suggesting that illicit opioid use may have counteracted antihyperalgesic effects of buprenorphine.[53] A small study found reductions in pain severity and interference and improvements in mood among chronic pain patients on more than 100 mg morphine equivalent following transition to buprenorphine although changes in pain tolerance and threshold assessed via Quantitative Sensory Testing were not statistically significant and many of the improvements in pain and mood had regressed by 6 months.[92] A similar small study found significant reductions in pain intensity scores and improvement in quality of life measures among chronic pain patients transferred from high-dose opioids (mean daily morphine equivalent 550 mg) to buprenorphine.[93] In a randomized, double-blind clinical trial, perioperative buprenorphine had lower rates of postoperative hyperalgesia measured by quantitative sensory testing and lower postoperative pain scores compared to morphine in patients receiving remifentanil infusion during general anesthesia for major lung surgery.[94] Buprenorphine is a kappa opioid receptor antagonist and may reduce hyperalgesia by blocking spinal dynorphin, an endogenous nociceptive kappa opioid agonist.[95]

Pain, especially the chronic pain syndrome, involves strong affective and motivational components and depression and anxiety disorders commonly accompany pain conditions.[24] Buprenorphine has antidepressant effects thought to be mediated by kappa opioid antagonism that may be useful in treating the affective and motivational aspects of pain. Low doses of buprenorphine (0.2−2 mg per day sublingual) have shown promise in improving mood and reducing suicidality among opioid naïve patients with treatment-resistant depression although additional randomized, placebo-controlled trials are needed to determine efficacy of buprenorphine for depression.[96] Buprenorphine increased evoked functional MRI responses to noxious heat in limbic/mesolimbic circuits, brain regions important in the affective component of pain processing, among healthy volunteers.[97] High levels of negative affect are associated with lower analgesic effect and increased hyperalgesia during opioid treatment for chronic low back pain.[21,22] In addition to treating opioid use disorder and providing analgesia in patients with pain and opioid use disorder, buprenorphine may also reduce the affective aspects of pain and depressive symptoms.

Induction of buprenorphine from high doses of prescription opioids and/or long-acting opioids can be challenging. As a partial opioid agonist with a high affinity for the mu-opioid receptor, buprenorphine will displace other mu-opioid agonists thereby precipitating opioid withdrawal. To avoid precipitating withdrawal, other opioids must be discontinued for 12−72 h and at least moderate physical opioid withdrawal symptoms should be present prior to administering the first dose of buprenorphine. Failure to complete buprenorphine induction may occur when inducting from high opioid doses, due to severe opioid withdrawal symptoms, or when inducting from long-acting opioids due to the need to wait 48−72 h or more prior to starting buprenorphine in order to avoid precipitating withdrawal. Several investigators have demonstrated that very low doses of sublingual or transdermal buprenorphine can be started immediately after stopping full agonist opioids without precipitating withdrawal thereby facilitating buprenorphine induction.[98,99] Additional studies assessing this method as well as other novel buprenorphine induction strategies would be of great clinical utility especially for patients with pain and opioid use disorder.

NALTREXONE

Naltrexone is an opioid antagonist FDA approved in the US for the treatment of opioid and/or alcohol use disorder. Oral formulations for once daily administration as well as monthly long-acting injectable depot formulations aimed at reducing nonadherence with oral naltrexone are available. As compared to methadone and buprenorphine, which have analgesic effects and therefore may treat opioid use disorder and pain simultaneously, naltrexone is a mu-opioid receptor antagonist that does not produce analgesia and antagonizes opioid analgesic effects. As a result, naltrexone is not suitable for patients with significant analgesic requirements such as in the context of acute, surgical, or cancer-related pain. But in opioid and/or alcohol use disorder with chronic noncancer pain, where guidelines recommend avoiding opioids in favor of nonopioid analgesics, naltrexone may be an underutilized option.

Low-dose naltrexone (1−4.5 mg orally daily) has antiinflammatory effects thought to be mediated by blockade of Toll-like Receptor 4. Low-dose naltrexone has been shown to be safe and well tolerated and to reduce pain and improve quality of life in a small number of preliminary clinical studies in multiple sclerosis and fibromyalgia but additional randomized, placebo-controlled trials are needed to determine whether low-dose naltrexone is effective for these conditions.[100] Of note, low doses of naltrexone may not be appropriate in patients with pain and opioid use disorder as higher doses (50 mg daily for oral naltrexone and 380 mg monthly for long-acting depot formulations) are needed to provide opioid blockade and reduce risk of opioid relapse.

ABUSE-DETERRENT OPIOID FORMULATIONS

Use of opioid analgesics in patients with substance use disorders carries a risk of misuse, diversion, and complications of interactions between opioids and other substances of abuse including overdose in combination with alcohol and sedatives. Avoiding opioid analgesics in patients with substance use disorders is optimal but may be unavoidable especially in cases of severe acute pain and in the perioperative and postoperative periods. While merely taking more of an opioid analgesic than prescribed is the most common form of prescription opioid misuse or abuse, crushing or chewing opioid tablets to allow intranasal, inhalation, or intravenous administration are also common. Abuse-deterrent opioid formulations incorporate strategies such as the formation of a viscous gel when the tablet is crushed and exposed to liquid (e.g., Reformulated OxyContin tablets) or the inclusion of a core of naltrexone that remains sequestered when the tablet is taken orally but is released and precipitates opioid withdrawal when the tablet is crushed for nonoral administration (e.g., Embeda or morphine sulfate and naltrexone hydrochloride extended-release capsules). In human laboratory studies, nondependent "recreational" opioid users report lower scores for drug liking and less interest in taking the drug again for abuse-deterrent formulations and postmarketing studies suggest a greater reduction in OxyContin diversion, misuse, overdose, and doctor shopping since introduction of Reformulated OxyContin in 2010 than was observed with other standard opioid formulations over the same time period.[101] However, reductions in OxyContin abuse were accompanied by increases in abuse of other standard opioid analgesic formulations and heroin suggesting that abuse-deterrent formulations are helpful but not sufficient to reduce overall rates of opioid misuse.[102] Of note, rates of misuse and overdose for transdermal buprenorphine are much lower than that for other long-acting opioids in postmarketing studies.[103]

Tapentadol (Nucynta) is a schedule II controlled substance in the US that is a mu-opioid receptor agonist with additional norepinephrine reuptake activity that is approved to treat moderate to severe acute or chronic pain. Tapentadol is available in a crush-resistant extended release formulation and an immediate release formulation. Volunteers with experience abusing nontamper-resistant oxycodone extended-release tablets reported being less likely to tamper with and snort tamper-resistant extended-release tapentadol tablets than nontamper-resistant oxycodone tablets.[104] Postmarketing surveillance data suggest that overall rates of abuse and diversion of tapentadol is low; although after adjusting for drug availability, tapentadol abuse rates were similar to hydrocodone and tramadol.[105]

Initial data suggest that abuse-deterrent opioid formulations are misused and diverted less than standard opioid formulations. For patients with substance use disorders needing analgesia with full opioid agonists, use of an abuse-deterrent formulation is advisable although there is still risk of overdose if full agonists are combined with sedatives even when taken orally. None of the abuse-deterrent formulations are approved to treat opioid use disorder and in patients with cooccurring opioid use disorder and pain, buprenorphine has the advantage of treating both conditions and having a lower risk of overdose and misuse.

NONPHARMACOLOGIC/BEHAVIORAL PAIN TREATMENTS

Psychosocial and behavioral therapies are a mainstay of treatment for substance use disorders[106–108] and have also been evaluated for chronic pain. A large number of randomized trials have found small to moderate effect sizes for cognitive behavioral therapy (CBT) for reducing pain and disability and improving mood in chronic noncancer pain although many of the studies are small with methodological issues.[109] Depression and anxiety symptoms and sleep problems are frequently comorbid with chronic pain and substance use disorders and CBT is effective for mood and sleep disorders.[110] CBT can reduce pain catastrophizing and improve pain-related outcomes when targeted to patients with high levels of catastrophizing.[111] Although fewer studies have been done, initial results also suggest that CBT can reduce postsurgical pain intensity and disability.[112] Other behavioral therapies with evidence for treating chronic pain include mindfulness practices[113] and Acceptance and Commitment Therapy[114] although additional randomized trials assessing these interventions for pain are needed.

A large number of clinical trials have found physical activity and exercise have small to moderate effects on reducing pain intensity and improving physical functioning but not psychological function or quality of life although conclusions are limited as the majority of trials had small size and short-term follow-up.[115] Motor control exercises which aim to develop the core muscles that support the spine were slightly more effective than general exercise in reducing pain and improving functioning in chronic low back pain.[116] Exercise reduces pain and improves quality of life in fibromyalgia.[117,118] Exercise-reduced methamphetamine use compared to an educational control intervention among participants with lower severity methamphetamine use disorder[119] possibly mediated by exercise-induced increases in striatal dopaminergic functioning[120] and further investigation of exercise for comorbid chronic pain and opioid use disorder would be of interest. Yoga reduces pain intensity and improves functioning compared to general exercise for a variety of chronic pain conditions in some but not all trials although the difference is small.[116,121] Tai chi reduces pain in a few small trials with neck pain, knee arthritis, and fibromyalgia.[121] Patients receiving acupuncture had lower postoperative pain and opioid requirements compared to no-acupuncture control[121] and acupuncture reduces pain more than sham as well as no acupuncture control in nonspecific musculoskeletal pain, osteoarthritis, chronic headache, and shoulder pain.[122] Chiropractic spinal manipulation and mobilization reduces pain and disability in chronic low back pain although optimal techniques, dosing, and duration of treatment have not been established.[123]

Several randomized trials have investigated behavioral therapies targeted to patients receiving chronic opioid therapy for chronic pain. In a randomized trial, patients on chronic opioid therapy for low back pain at high risk of prescription opioid misuse randomized to a brief behavioral therapy consisting of monthly urine screens, compliance checklists, and individual and group motivational counseling were significantly less likely to have signs of opioid misuse compared to patients randomized to standard care.[124] In a pilot randomized clinical trial, a mindfulness-based intervention decreased opioid misuse, desire for opioids, pain severity, and overall pain-related functional interference compared to a standard support group among patients on chronic opioid therapy for noncancer pain.[125] In a small study of patients with chronic musculoskeletal pain, an automated telephone-based behavioral support intervention reduced opioid use, pain intensity, and increased coping behaviors compared to standard care control group (which increased opioid use) following 11 weeks of pain-CBT.[126,127] In a randomized trial, a behavioral intervention for facilitating opioid tapering that included psychiatric consultation, opioid dose tapering, and 18 weekly meetings with a physician assistant to explore motivation for tapering and learn pain self-management skills significantly reduced self-reported pain interference, and prescription opioid problems, and improved pain self-efficacy compared to standard physician tapering.[128] Both intervention and control group patients reduced daily opioid dose but the difference between groups was not significant.

Combining behavioral therapies, especially cognitive behavioral therapy, for substance use disorders and pain management may result in the best outcomes for patients with comorbid substance use disorders and pain. Unfortunately, barriers to integrating pain and substance use behavioral therapies exist and pain often goes unaddressed by addiction therapists while pain specialists may struggle to address and manage substance use issues.[32,76,129] Additional studies to determine the best models for integrating behavioral therapies for pain and substance use disorders are needed.

NONOPIOID PHARMACOLOGIC TREATMENTS

For chronic noncancer pain, guidelines recommend prioritizing nonopioid medications over opioid analgesics in all patients but particularly in patients with substance use disorders.[35] The choice of pharmacotherapy in this case typically is made on the basis of the type of pain syndrome(s) present along with consideration of any comorbid conditions such as depression or anxiety.

Nonsteroidal anti-inflammatories (NSAIDs), but not acetaminophen, have been shown to be more effective than placebo in reducing pain in a variety of acute and chronic pain conditions including acute pain, arthritis, headache, and back pain.[6,130,131] Serious adverse events with NSAIDs in back pain trials were rare and cyclooxygenase-2-selective NSAIDs had a lower risk of adverse events than nonselective NSAIDs.[6] Although frequently recommended, there is little quality clinical trial evidence to support the efficacy of acetaminophen for a variety of acute and chronic pain conditions.[130]

Comorbid depression is common in pain conditions and with chronic opioid use and substance use disorders[132–134] and chronic pain is a risk factor for suicide.[135] Opioids relieve the unpleasantness and affective aspects of pain[30] and patients who start opioids for pain relief may continue opioid use as a means of managing unpleasant affective symptoms including depression and anxiety.[136] Buprenorphine has antidepressant effects, potentially due to its kappa opioid antagonist effects, and has been considered for clinical development as an antidepressant.[137,138] Treating cooccurring depression may reduce pain and improve mood and thereby facilitate tapering or cessation of opioid use.[139] Antidepressants with noradrenergic activity such as serotonin norepinephrine reuptake inhibitors (SNRIs) and tricyclic antidepressants (TCAs) reduce pain by facilitating antinociceptive descending inhibitory systems.[140] Duloxetine, an SNRI, but not TCAs or selective serotonin reuptake inhibitors (SSRIs), produced greater reductions in low back pain intensity and interference than placebo although the effects were small to moderate.[6] SNRIs and TCAs are effective for neuropathic pain[141] while SSRIs and TCAs are effective in reducing abdominal pain in Irritable Bowel Syndrome and other functional gastrointestinal disorders.[142] Duloxetine and low doses of amitriptyline are modestly effective, but SSRIs are not effective for treating fibromyalgia.[143-145]

Gabapentinoids, including gabapentin and pregabalin, are antiseizure medications that modulate pain-related neurotransmission by acting on the alpha-2 delta-2 subunit of voltage-dependent calcium channels. Gabapentin and pregabalin are effective for neuropathic pain with the best evidence in postherpetic neuralgia and peripheral diabetic neuropathy.[141,146] Pregabalin is more effective in reducing pain intensity in fibromyalgia than placebo[147] while data to assess gabapentin for fibromyalgia is limited due to a lack of high-quality placebo-controlled trials.[148] There is no reliable evidence from clinical trials that gabapentin or pregabalin is effective for low back pain.[6,149] Common adverse effects with gabapentin or pregabalin include dizziness, fatigue, sedation, edema, and weight gain[150] and these CNS depressant effects are a concern when used in patients with substance use disorders. Data suggest that misuse and diversion of gabapentinoids is increasing in particular among people with opioid use disorder.[151] There are reports of opioid users combining gabapentin with buprenorphine or methadone in order to obtain an enhanced opioid high[152-154] and opioid users prefer pregabalin over gabapentin.[155] While gabapentin and pregabalin alone have a relatively low risk of fatal overdose, risk of overdose increases when gabapentinoids are combined with other substances especially opioids.[156,157]

Nonbenzodiazepine skeletal muscle relaxants are more effective than placebo for short-term (<1 week) pain relief in acute low back pain but quality trials of muscle relaxants in chronic back pain are lacking.[6] Examples include baclofen, a $GABA_B$ agonist, tizanidine, a centrally acting alpha-2 agonist related to clonidine, carisoprodol, which is metabolized to meprobamate an anxiolytic similar to barbiturates, and cyclobenzaprine, similar to tricyclic antidepressants, and methocarbamol which likely work primarily via producing sedation.[158] Muscle relaxants may produce excess sedation and carry a risk of misuse and overdose especially when combined with other central nervous system sedatives such as opioids, benzodiazepines, or alcohol.[159,160]

Ketamine is an NMDA receptor antagonist that is used for perioperative anesthesia and analgesia. Multiple studies have demonstrated that intravenous ketamine is effective in reducing postoperative opioid use.[161] Several randomized clinical trials have found that intraoperative intravenous ketamine significantly reduced postoperative opioid use and pain intensity compared to placebo among opioid-dependent patients undergoing back surgery.[162,163] There were no serious psychiatric adverse events, such as hallucinations or serious perceptual disturbances, with ketamine at the relatively low doses and short course used in these trials. Initial studies also suggest that intravenous ketamine at "subanesthetic doses" can produce a rapid but short-lived antidepressant effect in patients with treatment-resistant depression[164] and ketamine may be an option for patients with treatment-resistant depression and chronic pain/substance use disorders although additional clinical trials in these populations are needed. Low doses of ketamine for acute pain management in the emergency department produce a similar analgesic effect to opioids with lower risk of respiratory depression and evidence of opioid sparing[165,166] and this may be of particular utility in managing acute pain in patients who should avoid opioids including those with substance use disorders. Initial small preliminary trials suggest that ketamine may reduce pain intensity more than the placebo in chronic pain but studies were short with small sample size, and higher doses seem necessary for analgesia than antidepressant effects and as a result psychiatric adverse events are more common.[167] Side effects with long-term use of ketamine in chronic pain have not been adequately evaluated. Ketamine has been reported to facilitate opioid tapering in chronic pain patients on high opioid doses and future placebo-controlled trials to assess this would be of great interest.[168-170] Recreational use of ketamine for its hallucinogenic effects and perceptual disturbances does occur,[171] and abuse potential could be a concern with use of ketamine in patients with existing substance use disorders. At the same time, ketamine has shown some promise as a treatment for substance use disorders, including alcohol, heroin, and cocaine, potentially by promoting a mystical experience in the user.[172,173] In light of the potential antidepressant, analgesic, antihyperalgesic, and antiaddictive effects of ketamine, adequately powered and well-controlled clinical trials in patients with chronic pain and substance use disorders are needed.

MEDICAL CANNABIS

Prevalence of cannabis use in the US has risen significantly from 6.7% of US adults in 2005%−12.9% in

2015.[174] Twenty-eight US states and the District of Columbia have made medicinal use of cannabis legal with over 90% of patients reporting they use medical cannabis to treat severe pain.[175] The major psychoactive compound found in cannabis is Δ9-tetrahydrocannabinol (THC), which binds to cannabinoid receptors (CB1 and CB2) and is thought to be responsible for many of the potential negative consequences of cannabis use including addiction, psychosis, cognitive impairment, weight gain, anhedonia, and rebound anxiety and insomnia. In contrast, cannabidiol (CBD) is a negative allosteric modulator of CB1, interacts with multiple other receptors including partial agonism at the 5-HT_{1A} receptor, and has anti-inflammatory and antianxiety effects.[176] The medical marijuana landscape is complex due to the existence of thousands of different cannabis chemovars, each containing different concentrations of THC, CBD, and multiple other chemical constituents of cannabis that may have pharmacologic activity, as well as cannabis extracts with high concentrations of THC and/or CBD which can be administered via smoking, vaporization, orally, sublingually, or topically.[176]

Marijuana is not FDA approved in the US for any indication and remains a schedule I controlled substance although dronabinol, a synthetic form of THC, is approved for weight loss with Acquired Immune Deficiency Syndrome (AIDS) and dronabinol and nabilone, a synthetic cannabinoid similar to THC, are approved for refractory chemotherapy-induced nausea and vomiting.[177] Nabiximols is an oromucosal spray containing 2.7 mg of THC and 2.5 mg of CBD that is approved in the European Union and Canada for spasticity due to multiple sclerosis but is not approved in the US. As of 2018, CBD is under review for approval in the US and Europe for the treatment of seizures associated with two rare forms of childhood-onset epilepsy, Lennox-Gastaut syndrome (LGS), and Dravet syndrome.[178]

Multiple randomized controlled trials and meta-analyses have found marijuana and cannabinoids reduce pain intensity more than placebo in chronic noncancer pain, especially when delivered via inhalation, although not all studies demonstrated a clinically significant analgesic effect such as a reduction of two or more points on a 0–10 numeric pain scale.[175,179,180] There is strong evidence that access to medical marijuana in the US reduces prescription opioid overdose rates most likely due switching from opioids to cannabis for pain control.[181,182] Medical marijuana laws are associated with increased pediatric exposures to cannabis, mostly by unintentional ingestion,[183] and increased cannabis use, but not increased rates of cannabis use disorder, among adults[184] but there is no evidence that medical marijuana laws increase adolescent cannabis use[185] or traffic accidents[186] and in fact reduction in opioid-related traffic fatalities occurs with access to medical marijuana.[187] Smoked cannabis increased the analgesic effect of a subanalgesic dose of oxycodone in a human laboratory study but also slightly increased measures of oxycodone abuse liability.[188] Together these studies suggest that cannabis and cannabinoids reduce pain in chronic noncancer pain and may have opioid sparing effects in some patients, thereby reducing reliance on prescription opioids and risk of opioid-related complications including overdose. Additional randomized controlled trials to determine the safety and effectiveness of smoked or inhaled cannabis as well as other novel cannabinoid formulations for chronic pain and opioid sparing are needed.

CLINICAL MONITORING DURING OPIOID PRESCRIBING

Drug testing is commonly used for assessing and monitoring patients for illicit drug use during treatment for substance use disorders and can also be used to monitor adherence and detect diversion among patients prescribed medications for pain. Urine drug testing is most common but blood, hair, sweat, or saliva can also be tested with large variation in the window of drug detection across specimen type with detection within hours of use for blood or saliva, days for urine, and weeks to months for hair.[189] Immunoassay tests are inexpensive and can be done point-of-care in the office but provide qualitative (above or below a concentration cutoff) not quantitative results and are indirect screening tests subject to false-positive and false-negative results especially with synthetic/semisynthetic opioids and benzodiazepines.[190] Confirmatory tests using gas chromatography-mass spectrometry or liquid chromatography-mass spectrometry provide quantitative levels of the specific drugs and metabolites present avoiding false-positive and false-negative results but are expensive and require laboratory testing with a delay in results compared to point-of-care drug screen results.[189] A thorough understanding of the metabolism of the drugs tested for as well as the performance of the assays used is essential for proper interpretation of drug test results and application of results to clinical decision-making with patients. The most cost-effective strategy for drug testing, including the frequency of testing and when to use screening versus confirmatory testing depends on the prevalence of different substances in the population being tested but routine urine drug screen testing with confirmatory tests reserved for unexpected or clinically ambiguous screen results is an algorithm commonly used.[191] Guidelines recommend at least yearly urine drug screening in patients on chronic opioid therapy for pain[192] and although studies to determine the optimal frequency of urine drug screening in patients treated for pain are lacking, drug testing of patients with substance use disorders is typically more frequent (e.g., weekly early in treatment and monthly in more stable patients) and more frequent testing in patients with risk factors for medication misuse is likely warranted.

Prescription drug monitoring programs (PDMP) give clinicians access to data on controlled substances dispensed to a patient with the aim of reducing misuse and diversion of opioids due to overprescribing and "doctor shopping." PDMPs in the US are managed by state governments and implementation and utilization vary considerably state to state. While opioid prescribing has been decreasing in the US in response to an epidemic of opioid overdoses, the precise role that PDMPs have played in reduced prescribing versus overall trends in attitudes and awareness regarding the dangers of opioid prescribing is not clear.[193,194] Also, studies have found both reductions and increases in opioid overdose rates following implementation of PDMPs potentially due to prescription users switching to illicit opioids especially heroin and fentanyl.[195–198] Despite these outstanding questions, checking the PDMP prior to prescribing controlled substances to patients with a substance use disorder is warranted to avoid "doctor shopping" and coordinate prescribing in patients who may be under the care of multiple clinicians including addiction medicine, pain management, and psychiatry. Clinicians should be aware that methadone treatment programs for opioid use disorder do not report to PDMPs.[199]

A variety of questionnaires are available to assess risk of prescription opioid misuse among chronic pain patients including the Current Opioid Misuse Measure (COMM), Opioid Risk Tool (ORT), and Screener and Opioid Assessment for Patients with Pain—Revised (SOAPP-R). Unfortunately, the clinical utility of these measures is limited by a lack of quality prospective studies demonstrating changes in clinically meaningful outcomes such as patient or clinician behavior or overdose rates and the time required to administer the measures, which has resulted in limited use of these measures outside of research studies and specialty pain clinics.[10] The Pain average, interference with Enjoyment of life, and interference with General activity (PEG) Assessment Scale is an easy to administer 3-item scale used to assess pain intensity and interference derived from the longer Brief Pain Inventory.[200] The PEG can be easily administered to track response to opioid analgesic treatment with a 30% reduction in PEG score suggesting a clinically meaningful improvement in pain and/or functioning.[201]

Treatment agreements that outline provider and patient expectations regarding opioid prescribing and pain management, such as requirements for urine drug testing, what happens if there is diversion of medication or requests for early refills, and stipulations that prescriptions be obtained from one clinician only, also have not been shown to reduce prescription opioid misuse or abuse and implementation in real-world settings has been limited.[10]

NALOXONE FOR OPIOID OVERDOSE

Naloxone is an opioid antagonist that is FDA approved for reversing sedation and respiratory depression due to opioid overdose. Intravenous, intramuscular, intranasal, subcutaneous, or nebulized administration of naloxone is all effective for opioid overdose reversal with less evidence supporting endotracheal administration.[202] Initially, naloxone was approved only for use in hospitals or by emergency medical services (EMS) but reluctance of drug users to call EMS due to fear of arrest lead to activists and clinicians developing programs to distribute naloxone to intravenous drug users for administration without medical supervision. Currently, a naloxone nasal spray and an autoinjector have been approved in the US for administration by laypersons. Studies of community programs providing drug users and other laypersons with take home naloxone kits for intramuscular or intranasal administration and training on overdose prevention and naloxone administration have found take home naloxone to be safe, acceptable, and successfully administered by laypersons although most of these studies have been observational and lacking a control group.[203] A recent randomized trial of emergency department-delivered overdose prevention training and an off-label naloxone intranasal take home kit versus usual care for persons at increased risk of opioid overdose failed to find a significant difference in subsequent opioid overdose or emergency room/hospital utilization between intervention and control groups suggesting that additional studies are needed to clarify in what populations take home naloxone is effective.[204] Of note, overdose rates due to illicit fentanyl often found as a contaminant in heroin have increased dramatically in the US and due to fentanyl's very high potency successful reversal of a fentanyl overdose may require immediate naloxone administration as well as multiple administrations of higher than standard naloxone doses.[205-207]

The majority of studies and experience with take-home naloxone has been with users of heroin or illicit opioid analgesics but pilot studies of coprescribing take home naloxone to chronic pain patients on opioid therapy have found it to be acceptable and safe although randomized clinical trials to determine the effectiveness of naloxone in this population are warranted.[208-211] Clinicians treating pain in patients with substance use disorders should consider providing take home naloxone to reduce the risk of fatal opioid overdose. Among patients prescribed opioids for chronic pain, higher opioid doses, concomitant use of opioids and other central nervous system sedatives especially benzodiazepines and muscle relaxants, and use of long-acting as opposed to short-acting opioids are associated with increased risk of overdose and avoiding these prescribing practices in patients with pain and substance use disorders is an additional intervention that may reduce overdose risk.[212,213]

CONCLUSIONS

Managing pain in patients with substance use disorders is a clinical challenge and frequent source of frustration for clinicians and patients. Major increases in opioid prescribing for chronic noncancer pain in the US has resulted in an epidemic of opioid use disorder and overdose and consensus now favors avoiding opioids in chronic pain and limiting opioid duration and dose when used for other indications in all populations but particularly in patients with substance use disorders. Optimally, treatment of pain and substance use disorders would be integrated and coordinated and combine effective pharmacologic and nonpharmacologic treatments for both pain and addiction but such comprehensive treatment is rarely available under one roof. Additional training of clinicians in the comanagement of pain and substance use disorders is needed as well as studies to identify and develop safer and more effective approaches to managing pain than currently available opioids. While avoiding opioids is advisable, evidence suggests that as opioid prescribing has decreased patients have increasingly turned to illicit opioids including heroin and reducing opioid prescribing without a coordinated increase in the availability of nonopioid pain management as well as treatment for opioid use disorder, including buprenorphine and methadone, will likely only worsen the current epidemic of opioid overdose and abuse.[214] Use of

buprenorphine is likely to continue to increase both for the comanagement of pain and opioid use disorder and as a safer alternative to full opioid agonists for pain in patients at high risk of opioid complications or with nonopioid substance use disorders. Increased availability and accessibility of behavioral treatments for pain including better training of substance use counselors to address pain and its connection to substance use is also needed. Novel treatments such as ketamine and cannabinoids show promise but require additional randomized, placebo-controlled trials to clarify their potential role in reducing the impact of opioid misuse and opioid use disorder and improving outcomes in comorbid pain and substance use disorders.

While waiting for novel treatments to reach the clinic, clinicians can act now to improve outcomes in patients with pain and substance use disorders by avoiding problems with conflict and erosion of trust between clinician and patient during discussions and decision making regarding opioids and pain management. As is the case with many conditions, positive pretreatment patient expectations predict good clinical outcomes in the treatment of chronic pain.[215] Developing rapport and a strong therapeutic alliance with patients and communicating empathy and understanding regarding the patient's suffering and priorities can assist clinicians in avoiding distrust and counteracting negative patient expectations even when treatment options may be limited due to severe pain and/or serious substance use disorders.[216] By acknowledging and legitimizing each patient's unique perspective and concerns, clinicians may help their patients to find relief from suffering even if pain endures.[217]

DISCLOSURE STATEMENT

Dr. Heinzerling has received research support and study medication, but no salary, from Alkermes, Medicinova, and Denovo pharmaceuticals.

REFERENCES

1. Task Force on Taxonomy of the International Association for the Study of Pain. *Classification of Chronic Pain. Descriptions of Chronic Pain Syndromes and Definitions of Pain Terms. Prepared by the International Association for the Study of Pain, Subcommittee on Taxonomy*. 1986. 0167-6482 (Print) 0167-6482.
2. Nahin RL. Estimates of pain prevalence and severity in adults: United States, 2012. *J Pain*. 2015;16(8):769-780.
3. Gaskin DJ, Richard P. The economic costs of pain in the United States. *J Pain*. 2012;13(8):715-724.
4. Guy Jr GP, Zhang K, Bohm MK, et al. Vital signs: changes in opioid prescribing in the United States, 2006-2015. *MMWR Morb Mortal Wkly Rep*. 2017;66(26):697-704.

5. Brown Jr RE, Sloan PA. The opioid crisis in the United States: chronic pain physicians are the answer, not the cause. *Anesth Analg.* 2017;125(5):1432–1434.

6. Chou R, Deyo R, Friedly J, et al. Systemic pharmacologic therapies for low back pain: a systematic review for an American College of Physicians Clinical Practice Guideline. *Ann Intern Med.* 2017;166(7):480–492.

7. Han B, Compton WM, Jones CM, Cai R. Nonmedical prescription opioid use and use disorders among adults aged 18 through 64 years in the United States, 2003-2013. *JAMA.* 2015;314(14):1468–1478.

8. O'Donnell JK, Gladden RM, Seth P. Trends in deaths involving heroin and synthetic opioids excluding methadone, and law enforcement drug product reports, by census region - United States, 2006-2015. *MMWR Morb Mortal Wkly Rep.* 2017;66(34):897–903.

9. Rudd RA, Seth P, David F, Scholl L. Increases in drug and opioid-involved overdose deaths - United States, 2010-2015. *MMWR Morb Mortal Wkly Rep.* 2016;65(5051):1445–1452.

10. Voon P, Karamouzian M, Kerr T. Chronic pain and opioid misuse: a review of reviews. *Subst Abuse Treat Prev Policy.* 2017;12(1):36.

11. Voon P, Hayashi K, Milloy MJ, et al. Pain among high-risk patients on methadone maintenance treatment. *J Pain.* 2015;16(9):887–894.

12. Eyler EC. Chronic and acute pain and pain management for patients in methadone maintenance treatment. *Am J Addict.* 2013;22(1):75–83.

13. Velly AM, Mohit S. Epidemiology of pain and relation to psychiatric disorders. *Prog Neuropsychopharmacol Biol Psychiatry.* 2017. https://doi.org/10.1016/j.pnpbp.2017.05.012.

14. Gureje O, Von Korff M, Simon GE, Gater R. Persistent pain and well-being: a World Health Organization study in primary care. *JAMA.* 1998;280(2):147–151.

15. Saffier K, Colombo C, Brown D, Mundt MP, Fleming MF. Addiction severity index in a chronic pain sample receiving opioid therapy. *J Subst Abuse Treat.* 2007;33(3):303–311.

16. Wertli MM, Eugster R, Held U, Steurer J, Kofmehl R, Weiser S. Catastrophizing-a prognostic factor for outcome in patients with low back pain: a systematic review. *Spine J.* 2014;14(11):2639–2657.

17. Terry MJ, Moeschler SM, Hoelzer BC, Hooten WM. Pain catastrophizing and anxiety are associated with heat pain perception in a community sample of adults with chronic pain. *Clin J Pain.* 2016;32(10):875–881.

18. McHugh RK, Weiss RD, Cornelius M, Martel MO, Jamison RN, Edwards RR. Distress intolerance and prescription opioid misuse among patients with chronic pain. *J Pain.* 2016;17(7):806–814.

19. Martel MO, Wasan AD, Jamison RN, Edwards RR. Catastrophic thinking and increased risk for prescription opioid misuse in patients with chronic pain. *Drug Alcohol Depend.* 2013;132(1–2):335–341.

20. Arteta J, Cobos B, Hu Y, Jordan K, Howard K. Evaluation of how depression and anxiety mediate the relationship between pain catastrophizing and prescription opioid misuse in a chronic pain population. *Pain Med.* 2016;17(2):295–303.

21. Wasan AD, Michna E, Edwards RR, et al. Psychiatric comorbidity is associated prospectively with diminished opioid analgesia and increased opioid misuse in patients with chronic low back pain. *Anesthesiology.* 2015;123(4):861–872.

22. Edwards RR, Dolman AJ, Michna E, et al. Changes in pain sensitivity and pain modulation during oral opioid treatment: the impact of negative affect. *Pain Med.* 2016;17(10):1882–1891.

23. Porreca F, Navratilova E. Reward, motivation, and emotion of pain and its relief. *Pain.* 2017;158(suppl 1):S43–S49.

24. Fields HL. Pain: an unpleasant topic. *Pain.* 1999;(suppl 6):S61–S69.

25. Coghill RC. Individual differences in the subjective experience of pain: new insights into mechanisms and models. *Headache.* 2010;50(9):1531–1535.

26. Taylor AM, Becker S, Schweinhardt P, Cahill C. Mesolimbic dopamine signaling in acute and chronic pain: implications for motivation, analgesia, and addiction. *Pain.* 2016;157(6):1194–1198.

27. Finan PH, Remeniuk B, Dunn KE. The risk for problematic opioid use in chronic pain: what can we learn from studies of pain and reward? *Prog Neuropsychopharmacol Biol Psychiatry.* 2017. https://doi.org/10.1016/j.pnpbp.2017.07.029.

28. Vachon-Presseau E, Tetreault P, Petre B, et al. Corticolimbic anatomical characteristics predetermine risk for chronic pain. *Brain.* 2016;139(Pt 7):1958–1970.

29. Volkow ND, Koob GF, McLellan AT. Neurobiologic advances from the brain disease model of addiction. *N Engl J Med.* 2016;374(4):363–371.

30. Price DD, Von der Gruen A, Miller J, Rafii A, Price C. A psychophysical analysis of morphine analgesia. *Pain.* 1985;22(3):261–269.

31. Oertel BG, Preibisch C, Wallenhorst T, et al. Differential opioid action on sensory and affective cerebral pain processing. *Clin Pharmacol Ther.* 2008;83(4):577–588.

32. Buchman DZ, Ho A, Illes J. You present like a drug addict: patient and clinician perspectives on trust and trustworthiness in chronic pain management. *Pain Med.* 2016;17(8):1394–1406.

33. Merrill JO, Rhodes LA, Deyo RA, Marlatt GA, Bradley KA. Mutual mistrust in the medical care of drug users: the keys to the "narc" cabinet. *J Gen Int Med.* 2002;17(5):327–333.

34. Esquibel AY, Borkan J. Doctors and patients in pain: conflict and collaboration in opioid prescription in primary care. *Pain.* 2014;155(12):2575–2582.

35. Dowell D, Haegerich TM, Chou R. CDC guideline for prescribing opioids for chronic pain—United States, 2016. *JAMA*. 2016;315(15):1624—1645.

36. Brown R, Kraus C, Fleming M, Reddy S. Methadone: applied pharmacology and use as adjunctive treatment in chronic pain. *Postgrad Med J*. 2004;80(949):654—659.

37. Novick DM, Salsitz EA, Joseph H, Kreek MJ. Methadone medical maintenance: an early 21st-century perspective. *J Addict Dis*. 2015;34(2—3):226—237.

38. Saulle R, Vecchi S, Gowing L. Supervised dosing with a long-acting opioid medication in the management of opioid dependence. *Cochrane Database Syst Rev*. 2017;4: CD011983.

39. Mattick RP, Breen C, Kimber J, Davoli M. Methadone maintenance therapy versus no opioid replacement therapy for opioid dependence. *Cochrane Database Syst Rev*. 2009;(3):CD002209.

40. Mattick RP, Breen C, Kimber J, Davoli M. Buprenorphine maintenance versus placebo or methadone maintenance for opioid dependence. *Cochrane Database Syst Rev*. 2014; (2):CD002207.

41. Cherny N. Is oral methadone better than placebo or other oral/transdermal opioids in the management of pain? *Palliat Med*. 2011;25(5):488—493.

42. McNicol ED, Ferguson MC, Schumann R. Methadone for neuropathic pain in adults. *Cochrane Database Syst Rev*. 2017;5:CD012499.

43. Kao DP, Haigney MC, Mehler PS, Krantz MJ. Arrhythmia associated with buprenorphine and methadone reported to the Food and Drug Administration. *Addiction*. 2015; 110(9):1468—1475.

44. Kao D, Bucher Bartelson B, Khatri V, et al. Trends in reporting methadone-associated cardiac arrhythmia, 1997-2011: an analysis of registry data. *Ann Int Med*. 2013;158(10):735—740.

45. Florian J, Garnett CE, Nallani SC, Rappaport BA, Throckmorton DC. A modeling and simulation approach to characterize methadone QT prolongation using pooled data from five clinical trials in MMT patients. *Clin Pharmacol Ther*. 2012;91(4):666—672.

46. Chou R, Cruciani RA, Fiellin DA, et al. Methadone safety: a clinical practice guideline from the American Pain Society and College on Problems of Drug Dependence, in collaboration with the Heart Rhythm Society. *J Pain*. 2014;15(4):321—337.

47. Jones CM, Baldwin GT, Manocchio T, White JO, Mack KA. Trends in methadone distribution for pain treatment, methadone diversion, and overdose deaths - United States, 2002-2014. *MMWR Morb Mortal Wkly Rep*. 2016;65(26):667—671.

48. Katz NP, Paillard FC, Edwards RR. Review of the performance of quantitative sensory testing methods to detect hyperalgesia in chronic pain patients on long-term opioids. *Anesthesiology*. 2015;122(3):677—685.

49. Laboureyras E, Aubrun F, Monsaingeon M, Corcuff JB, Laulin JP, Simonnet G. Exogenous and endogenous opioid-induced pain hypersensitivity in different rat strains. *Pain Res Manag*. 2014;19(4):191—197.

50. Fletcher D, Martinez V. Opioid-induced hyperalgesia in patients after surgery: a systematic review and a meta-analysis. *Br J Anaesth*. 2014;112(6):991—1004.

51. Doverty M, White JM, Somogyi AA, Bochner F, Ali R, Ling W. Hyperalgesic responses in methadone maintenance patients. *Pain*. 2001;90(1—2):91—96.

52. Compton P, Charuvastra VC, Kintaudi K, Ling W. Pain responses in methadone-maintained opioid abusers. *J Pain Symptom Manage*. 2000;20(4):237—245.

53. Compton P, Charuvastra VC, Ling W. Pain intolerance in opioid-maintained former opiate addicts: effect of long-acting maintenance agent. *Drug Alcohol Depend*. 2001; 63(2):139—146.

54. Compton P, Geschwind DH, Alarcon M. Association between human mu-opioid receptor gene polymorphism, pain tolerance, and opioid addiction. *Am J Med Genet B Neuropsychiatr Genet*. 2003;121B(1):76—82.

55. Peles E, Schreiber S, Hetzroni T, Adelson M, Defrin R. The differential effect of methadone dose and of chronic pain on pain perception of former heroin addicts receiving methadone maintenance treatment. *J Pain*. 2011;12(1): 41—50.

56. Compton P, Canamar CP, Hillhouse M, Ling W. Hyperalgesia in heroin dependent patients and the effects of opioid substitution therapy. *J Pain*. 2012;13(4): 401—409.

57. Hay JL, White JM, Bochner F, Somogyi AA, Semple TJ, Rounsefell B. Hyperalgesia in opioid-managed chronic pain and opioid-dependent patients. *J Pain*. 2009; 10(3):316—322.

58. Liebmann PM, Lehofer M, Moser M, Legl T, Pernhaupt G, Schauenstein K. Nervousness and pain sensitivity: II. Changed relation in ex-addicts as a predictor for early relapse. *Psychiatry Res*. 1998;79(1):55—58.

59. Liebmann PM, Lehofer M, Moser M, et al. Persistent analgesia in former opiate addicts is resistant to blockade of endogenous opioids. *Biol Psychiatry*. 1997;42(10): 962—964.

60. Treister R, Eisenberg E, Lawental E, Pud D. Is opioid-induced hyperalgesia reversible? A study on active and former opioid addicts and drug naive controls. *J Opioid Manag*. 2012;8(6):343—349.

61. Liebmann PM, Lehofer M, Schonauercejpek M, et al. Pain sensitivity in former opioid addicts. *Lancet*. 1994; 344(8928):1031—1032.

62. Compton MA. Cold-pressor pain tolerance in opiate and cocaine abusers: correlates of drug type and use status. *J Pain Symptom Manage*. 1994;9(7):462—473.

63. Lee M, Silverman SM, Hansen H, Patel VB, Manchikanti L. A comprehensive review of opioid-induced hyperalgesia. *Pain Physician*. 2011;14(2): 145—161.

64. Inturrisi CE. Pharmacology of methadone and its isomers. *Minerva Anestesiol*. 2005;71(7—8):435—437.

65. Vadivelu N, Schermer E, Kodumudi V, Belani K, Urman RD, Kaye AD. Role of ketamine for analgesia in adults and children. *J Anaesthesiol Clin Pharmacol*. 2016; 32(3):298—306.

66. Compton PA, Ling W, Torrington MA. Lack of effect of chronic dextromethorphan on experimental pain tolerance in methadone-maintained patients. *Addict Biol.* 2008;13(3–4):393–402.

67. Compton P, Kehoe P, Sinha K, Torrington MA, Ling W. Gabapentin improves cold-pressor pain responses in methadone-maintained patients. *Drug Alcohol Depend.* 2010;109(1–3):213–219.

68. Yi P, Pryzbylkowski P. Opioid induced hyperalgesia. *Pain Med.* 2015;16(suppl 1):S32–S36.

69. Samuelsen PJ, Nielsen CS, Wilsgaard T, Stubhaug A, Svendsen K, Eggen AE. Pain sensitivity and analgesic use among 10,486 adults: the Tromso study. *BMC Pharmacol Toxicol.* 2017;18(1):45.

70. Blanco C, Wall MM, Okuda M, Wang S, Iza M, Olfson M. Pain as a predictor of opioid use disorder in a nationally representative sample. *Am J Psychiatry.* 2016;173(12):1189–1195.

71. Chu LF, D'Arcy N, Brady C, et al. Analgesic tolerance without demonstrable opioid-induced hyperalgesia: a double-blinded, randomized, placebo-controlled trial of sustained-release morphine for treatment of chronic nonradicular low-back pain. *Pain.* 2012;153(8):1583–1592.

72. Doverty M, Somogyi AA, White JM, et al. Methadone maintenance patients are cross-tolerant to the antinociceptive effects of morphine. *Pain.* 2001;93(2):155–163.

73. Gallagher RM, Welz-Bosna M, Gammaitoni A. Assessment of dosing frequency of sustained-release opioid preparations in patients with chronic nonmalignant pain. *Pain Med.* 2007;8(1):71–74.

74. Taveros MC, Chuang EJ. Pain management strategies for patients on methadone maintenance therapy: a systematic review of the literature. *BMJ Support Palliat Care.* 2017;7(4):383–389.

75. Blinderman CD, Sekine R, Zhang B, Nillson M, Shaiova L. Methadone as an analgesic for patients with chronic pain in methadone maintenance treatment programs (MMTPs). *J Opioid Manag.* 2009;5(2):107–114.

76. Beitel M, Oberleitner L, Kahn M, et al. Drug counselor responses to patients' pain reports: a qualitative investigation of barriers and facilitators to treating patients with chronic pain in methadone maintenance treatment. *Pain Med.* 2017;18(11):2152–2161.

77. Butner JL, Bone C, Martinez CCP, et al. Training addiction counselors to deliver a brief psychoeducational intervention for chronic pain among patients in opioid agonist treatment: a pilot investigation. *Subst Abuse.* 2018:1–18.

78. Sessler NE, Walker E, Chickballapur H, Kacholakalayil J, Coplan PM. Disproportionality analysis of buprenorphine transdermal system and cardiac arrhythmia using FDA and WHO postmarketing reporting system data. *Postgrad Med.* 2017;129(1):62–68.

79. Isbister GK, Brown AL, Gill A, Scott AJ, Calver L, Dunlop AJ. QT interval prolongation in opioid agonist treatment: analysis of continuous 12-lead electrocardiogram recordings. *Br J Clin Pharmacol.* 2017;83(10):2274–2282.

80. Aiyer R, Gulati A, Gungor S, Bhatia A, Mehta N. Treatment of chronic pain with various buprenorphine formulations: a systematic review of clinical studies. *Anesth Analg.* 2017. https://doi.org/10.1213/ANE.0000000000002718.

81. Weiss RD, Potter JS, Fiellin DA, et al. Adjunctive counseling during brief and extended buprenorphine-naloxone treatment for prescription opioid dependence: a 2-phase randomized controlled trial. *Arch Gen Psychiatry.* 2011;68(12):1238–1246.

82. Weiss RD, Potter JS, Griffin ML, et al. Long-term outcomes from the National drug abuse treatment clinical trials network prescription opioid addiction treatment study. *Drug Alcohol Depend.* 2015;150:112–119.

83. Chakrabarti A, Woody GE, Griffin ML, Subramaniam G, Weiss RD. Predictors of buprenorphine-naloxone dosing in a 12-week treatment trial for opioid-dependent youth: secondary analyses from a NIDA Clinical Trials Network study. *Drug Alcohol Depend.* 2010;107(2–3):253–256.

84. Griffin ML, McDermott KA, McHugh RK, Fitzmaurice GM, Jamison RN, Weiss RD. Longitudinal association between pain severity and subsequent opioid use in prescription opioid dependent patients with chronic pain. *Drug Alcohol Depend.* 2016;163:216–221.

85. Heit HA, Gourlay DL. Buprenorphine: new tricks with an old molecule for pain management. *Clin J Pain.* 2008;24(2):93–97.

86. Khanna IK, Pillarisetti S. Buprenorphine - an attractive opioid with underutilized potential in treatment of chronic pain. *J Pain Res.* 2015;8:859–870.

87. Boas RA, Villiger JW. Clinical actions of fentanyl and buprenorphine. The significance of receptor binding. *Br J Anaesth.* 1985;57(2):192–196.

88. Greenwald MK, Comer SD, Fiellin DA. Buprenorphine maintenance and mu-opioid receptor availability in the treatment of opioid use disorder: implications for clinical use and policy. *Drug Alcohol Depend.* 2014;144:1–11.

89. Jonan AB, Kaye AD, Urman RD. Buprenorphine formulations: clinical best practice strategies recommendations for perioperative management of patients undergoing surgical or interventional pain procedures. *Pain Physician.* 2018;21(1):E1–E12.

90. Leighton BL, Crock LW. Case series of successful postoperative pain management in buprenorphine maintenance therapy patients. *Anesth Analg.* 2017;125(5):1779–1783.

91. Silva MJ, Rubinstein A. Continuous perioperative sublingual buprenorphine. *J Pain Palliat Care Pharmacother.* 2016;30(4):289–293.

92. Wasserman RA, Hassett AL, Harte SE, et al. Pressure sensitivity and phenotypic changes in patients with suspected opioid-induced hyperalgesia being withdrawn from full mu agonists. *J Nat Sci.* 2017;3(2):e319.

93. Daitch D, Daitch J, Novinson D, Frey M, Mitnick C, Pergolizzi Jr J. Conversion from high-dose full-opioid agonists to sublingual buprenorphine reduces pain scores and improves quality of life for chronic pain patients. *Pain Med.* 2014;15(12):2087–2094.

94. Mercieri M, Palmisani S, De Blasi RA, et al. Low-dose buprenorphine infusion to prevent postoperative hyperalgesia in patients undergoing major lung surgery and remifentanil infusion: a double-blind, randomized, active-controlled trial. *Br J Anaesth*. 2017;119(4): 792–802.

95. Vanderah TW, Gardell LR, Burgess SE, et al. Dynorphin promotes abnormal pain and spinal opioid antinociceptive tolerance. *J Neurosci*. 2000;20(18):7074–7079.

96. Stanciu CN, Glass OM, Penders TM. Use of buprenorphine in treatment of refractory depression-A review of current literature. *Asian J Psychiatr*. 2017;26:94–98.

97. Upadhyay J, Anderson J, Baumgartner R, et al. Modulation of CNS pain circuitry by intravenous and sublingual doses of buprenorphine. *Neuroimage*. 2012;59(4): 3762–3773.

98. Kornfeld H, Reetz H. Transdermal buprenorphine, opioid rotation to sublingual buprenorphine, and the avoidance of precipitated withdrawal: a review of the literature and demonstration in three chronic pain patients treated with butrans. *Am J Ther*. 2015;22(3): 199–205.

99. Hammig R, Kemter A, Strasser J, et al. Use of microdoses for induction of buprenorphine treatment with overlapping full opioid agonist use: the Bernese method. *Subst Abuse Rehabi*. 2016;7:99–105.

100. Patten DK, Schultz BG, Berlau DJ. The safety and efficacy of low-dose naltrexone in the management of chronic pain and inflammation in multiple sclerosis, fibromyalgia, Crohn's disease, and other chronic pain disorders. *Pharmacotherapy*. 2018. https://doi.org/10.1002/phar.2086.

101. Pergolizzi Jr JV, Raffa RB, Taylor Jr R, Vacalis S. Abuse-deterrent opioids: an update on current approaches and considerations. *Curr Med Res Opin*. 2018;34(4):711–723.

102. Coplan PM, Kale H, Sandstrom L, Landau C, Chilcoat HD. Changes in oxycodone and heroin exposures in the National Poison Data System after introduction of extended-release oxycodone with abuse-deterrent characteristics. *Pharmacoepidemiol Drug Saf*. 2013;22(12): 1274–1282.

103. Coplan PM, Sessler NE, Harikrishnan V, Singh R, Perkel C. Comparison of abuse, suspected suicidal intent, and fatalities related to the 7-day buprenorphine transdermal patch versus other opioid analgesics in the National Poison Data System. *Postgrad Med*. 2017;129(1): 55–61.

104. Vosburg SK, Jones JD, Manubay JM, Ashworth JB, Shapiro DY, Comer SD. A comparison among tapentadol tamper-resistant formulations (TRF) and OxyContin(R) (non-TRF) in prescription opioid abusers. *Addiction*. 2013;108(6):1095–1106.

105. Vosburg SK, Severtson SG, Dart RC, et al. Assessment of tapentadol API abuse liability with the researched abuse, diversion and addiction-related surveillance (RADARS) system. *J Pain*. 2017. https://doi.org/10.1016/j.jpain.2017.11.007.

106. Dugosh K, Abraham A, Seymour B, McLoyd K, Chalk M, Festinger D. A systematic review on the use of psychosocial interventions in conjunction with medications for the treatment of opioid addiction. *J Addict Med*. 2016; 10(2):93–103.

107. Magill M, Kiluk BD, McCrady BS, Tonigan JS, Longabaugh R. Active ingredients of treatment and client mechanisms of change in behavioral treatments for alcohol use disorders: progress 10 years later. *Alcohol Clin Exp Res*. 2015;39(10):1852–1862.

108. McHugh RK, Hearon BA, Otto MW. Cognitive behavioral therapy for substance use disorders. *Psychiatr Clin North Am*. 2010;33(3):511–525.

109. Eccleston C, Crombez G. Advancing psychological therapies for chronic pain. *F1000Res*. 2017;6:461.

110. Kaiser RS, Mooreville M, Kannan K. Psychological interventions for the management of chronic pain: a review of current evidence. *Curr Pain Headache Rep*. 2015;19(9):43.

111. Schutze R, Rees C, Smith A, Slater H, Campbell JM, O'Sullivan P. How can we best reduce pain catastrophizing in adults with chronic noncancer pain? A systematic review and meta-analysis. *J Pain*. 2018;19(3):233–256.

112. Nicholls JL, Azam MA, Burns LC, et al. Psychological treatments for the management of postsurgical pain: a systematic review of randomized controlled trials. *Patient Relat Outcome Meas*. 2018;9:49–64.

113. Hilton L, Hempel S, Ewing BA, et al. Mindfulness meditation for chronic pain: systematic review and meta-analysis. *Ann Behav Med*. 2017;51(2):199–213.

114. Hughes LS, Clark J, Colclough JA, Dale E, McMillan D. Acceptance and commitment therapy (act) for chronic pain: a systematic review and meta-analyses. *Clin J Pain*. 2017;33(6):552–568.

115. Geneen LJ, Moore RA, Clarke C, Martin D, Colvin LA, Smith BH. Physical activity and exercise for chronic pain in adults: an overview of cochrane reviews. *Cochrane Database Syst Rev*. 2017;4:CD011279.

116. Chou R, Deyo R, Friedly J, et al. Nonpharmacologic therapies for low back pain: a systematic review for an American College of Physicians Clinical Practice Guideline. *Ann Int Med*. 2017;166(7):493–505.

117. Bidonde J, Busch AJ, Schachter CL, et al. Aerobic exercise training for adults with fibromyalgia. *Cochrane Database Syst Rev*. 2017;6:Cd012700.

118. Sosa-Reina MD, Nunez-Nagy S, Gallego-Izquierdo T, Pecos-Martin D, Monserrat J, Alvarez-Mon M. Effectiveness of therapeutic exercise in fibromyalgia syndrome: a systematic review and meta-analysis of randomized clinical trials. *BioMed Res Int*. 2017;2017:2356346.

119. Rawson RA, Chudzynski J, Mooney L, et al. Impact of an exercise intervention on methamphetamine use outcomes post-residential treatment care. *Drug Alcohol Depend*. 2015;156:21–28.

120. Robertson CL, Ishibashi K, Chudzynski J, et al. Effect of exercise training on striatal dopamine D2/D3 receptors in methamphetamine users during behavioral treatment. *Neuropsychopharmacology*. 2016;41(6):1629–1636.

121. Lin YC, Wan L, Jamison RN. Using integrative medicine in pain management: an evaluation of current evidence. *Anesth Analg.* 2017;125(6):2081–2093.

122. Vickers AJ, Vertosick EA, Lewith G, et al. Acupuncture for chronic pain: update of an individual patient data meta-analysis. *J Pain.* 2018;19(5):455–474.

123. Coulter ID, Crawford C, Hurwitz EL, et al. Manipulation and mobilization for treating chronic low back pain: a systematic review and meta-analysis. *Spine J.* 2018. https://doi.org/10.1016/j.spinee.2018.01.013.

124. Jamison RN, Ross EL, Michna E, Chen LQ, Holcomb C, Wasan AD. Substance misuse treatment for high-risk chronic pain patients on opioid therapy: a randomized trial. *Pain.* 2010;150(3):390–400.

125. Garland EL, Manusov EG, Froeliger B, Kelly A, Williams JM, Howard MO. Mindfulness-oriented recovery enhancement for chronic pain and prescription opioid misuse: results from an early-stage randomized controlled trial. *J Consult Clin Psychol.* 2014;82(3): 448–459.

126. Naylor MR, Keefe FJ, Brigidi B, Naud S, Helzer JE. Therapeutic interactive voice response for chronic pain reduction and relapse prevention. *Pain.* 2008;134(3): 335–345.

127. Naylor MR, Naud S, Keefe FJ, Helzer JE. Therapeutic interactive voice response (TIVR) to reduce analgesic medication use for chronic pain management. *J Pain.* 2010; 11(12):1410–1419.

128. Sullivan MD, Turner JA, DiLodovico C, D'Appollonio A, Stephens K, Chan YF. Prescription opioid taper support for outpatients with chronic pain: a randomized controlled trial. *J Pain.* 2017;18(3):308–318.

129. Stumbo SP, Yarborough BJ, McCarty D, Weisner C, Green CA. Patient-reported pathways to opioid use disorders and pain-related barriers to treatment engagement. *J Subst Abuse Treat.* 2017;73:47–54.

130. Moore RA, Derry S, Wiffen PJ, Straube S, Aldington DJ. Overview review: comparative efficacy of oral ibuprofen and paracetamol (acetaminophen) across acute and chronic pain conditions. *Eur J Pain.* 2015;19(9): 1213–1223.

131. Moore RA, Wiffen PJ, Derry S, Maguire T, Roy YM, Tyrrell L. Non-prescription (OTC) oral analgesics for acute pain - an overview of cochrane reviews. *Cochrane Database Syst Rev.* 2015;(11):CD010794.

132. Scherrer JF, Salas J, Schneider FD, et al. Characteristics of new depression diagnoses in patients with and without prior chronic opioid use. *J Affect Disord.* 2017;210: 125–129.

133. Grant BF, Saha TD, Ruan WJ, et al. Epidemiology of DSM-5 drug use disorder: results from the national epidemiologic survey on alcohol and related conditions-III. *JAMA Psychiatry.* 2016;73(1):39–47.

134. Grant BF, Goldstein RB, Saha TD, et al. Epidemiology of DSM-5 alcohol use disorder: results from the National Epidemiologic survey on alcohol and related conditions III. *JAMA Psychiatry.* 2015;72(8):757–766.

135. Racine M. Chronic pain and suicide risk: a comprehensive review. *Prog Neuropsychopharmacol Biol Psychiatry.* 2017. https://doi.org/10.1016/j.pnpbp.2017.08.020.

136. Goesling J, Henry MJ, Moser SE, et al. Symptoms of depression are associated with opioid use regardless of pain severity and physical functioning among treatment-seeking patients with chronic pain. *J Pain.* 2015;16(9):844–851.

137. Yovell Y, Bar G, Mashiah M, et al. Ultra-low-dose buprenorphine as a time-limited treatment for severe suicidal ideation: a randomized controlled trial. *Am J Psychiatry.* 2016;173(5):491–498.

138. Fava M, Memisoglu A, Thase ME, et al. Opioid modulation with buprenorphine/samidorphan as adjunctive treatment for inadequate response to antidepressants: a randomized double-blind placebo-controlled trial. *Am J Psychiatry.* 2016;173(5):499–508.

139. Scherrer JF, Salas J, Sullivan MD, et al. Impact of adherence to antidepressants on long-term prescription opioid use cessation. *Br J Psychiatry.* 2018;212(2):103–111.

140. Obata H. Analgesic mechanisms of antidepressants for neuropathic pain. *Int J Mol Sci.* 2017;18(11):2483.

141. Finnerup NB, Attal N, Haroutounian S, et al. Pharmacotherapy for neuropathic pain in adults: a systematic review and meta-analysis. *Lancet Neurol.* 2015;14(2):162–173.

142. Ford AC, Quigley EM, Lacy BE, et al. Effect of antidepressants and psychological therapies, including hypnotherapy, in irritable bowel syndrome: systematic review and meta-analysis. *Am J Gastroenterol.* 2014;109(9): 1350–1365; quiz 1366.

143. Rico-Villademoros F, Slim M, Calandre EP. Amitriptyline for the treatment of fibromyalgia: a comprehensive review. *Expert Rev Neurother.* 2015;15(10):1123–1150.

144. Walitt B, Urrutia G, Nishishinya MB, Cantrell SE, Hauser W. Selective serotonin reuptake inhibitors for fibromyalgia syndrome. *Cochrane Database Syst Rev.* 2015;(6):CD011735.

145. Lunn MP, Hughes RA, Wiffen PJ. Duloxetine for treating painful neuropathy, chronic pain or fibromyalgia. *Cochrane Database Syst Rev.* 2014;(1):CD007115.

146. Wiffen PJ, Derry S, Bell RF, et al. Gabapentin for chronic neuropathic pain in adults. *Cochrane Database Syst Rev.* 2017;6:CD007938.

147. Derry S, Cording M, Wiffen PJ, Law S, Phillips T, Moore RA. Pregabalin for pain in fibromyalgia in adults. *Cochrane Database Syst Rev.* 2016;9:CD011790.

148. Cooper TE, Derry S, Wiffen PJ, Moore RA. Gabapentin for fibromyalgia pain in adults. *Cochrane Database Syst Rev.* 2017;1:CD012188.

149. Shanthanna H, Gilron I, Rajarathinam M, et al. Benefits and safety of gabapentinoids in chronic low back pain: a systematic review and meta-analysis of randomized controlled trials. *PLoS Med.* 2017;14(8):e1002369.

150. Calandre EP, Rico-Villademoros F, Slim M. Alpha2delta ligands, gabapentin, pregabalin and mirogabalin: a review of their clinical pharmacology and therapeutic use. *Expert Rev Neurother.* 2016;16(11):1263–1277.

151. Buttram ME, Kurtz SP, Dart RC, Margolin ZR. Law enforcement-derived data on gabapentin diversion and misuse, 2002-2015: diversion rates and qualitative research findings. *Pharmacoepidemiol Drug Saf.* 2017; 26(9):1083–1086.

152. Smith RV, Lofwall MR, Havens JR. Abuse and diversion of gabapentin among nonmedical prescription opioid users in Appalachian Kentucky. *Am J Psychiatry.* 2015; 172(5):487–488.

153. Baird CR, Fox P, Colvin LA. Gabapentinoid abuse in order to potentiate the effect of methadone: a survey among substance misusers. *Eur Addict Res.* 2014;20(3):115–118.

154. Reeves RR, Ladner ME. Potentiation of the effect of buprenorphine/naloxone with gabapentin or quetiapine. *Am J Psychiatry.* 2014;171(6):691.

155. Bonnet U, Scherbaum N. How addictive are gabapentin and pregabalin? A systematic review. *Eur Neuropsychopharmacol.* 2017;27(12):1185–1215.

156. Gomes T, Juurlink DN, Antoniou T, Mamdani MM, Paterson JM, van den Brink W. Gabapentin, opioids, and the risk of opioid-related death: a population-based nested case-control study. *PLoS Med.* 2017; 14(10):e1002396.

157. Lyndon A, Audrey S, Wells C, et al. Risk to heroin users of polydrug use of pregabalin or gabapentin. *Addiction.* 2017;112(9):1580–1589.

158. Chou R, Peterson K, Helfand M. Comparative efficacy and safety of skeletal muscle relaxants for spasticity and musculoskeletal conditions: a systematic review. *J Pain Symptom Manage.* 2004;28(2):140–175.

159. Horsfall JT, Sprague JE. The pharmacology and toxicology of the 'holy Trinity'. *Basic Clin Pharmacol Toxicol.* 2017;120(2):115–119.

160. Reeves RR, Burke RS. Carisoprodol: abuse potential and withdrawal syndrome. *Curr Drug Abuse Rev.* 2010;3(1): 33–38.

161. Laskowski K, Stirling A, McKay WP, Lim HJ. A systematic review of intravenous ketamine for postoperative analgesia. *Can J Anaesth.* 2011;58(10):911–923.

162. Nielsen RV, Fomsgaard JS, Siegel H, et al. Intraoperative ketamine reduces immediate postoperative opioid consumption after spinal fusion surgery in chronic pain patients with opioid dependency: a randomized, blinded trial. *Pain.* 2017;158(3):463–470.

163. Loftus RW, Yeager MP, Clark JA, et al. Intraoperative ketamine reduces perioperative opiate consumption in opiate-dependent patients with chronic back pain undergoing back surgery. *Anesthesiology.* 2010;113(3): 639–646.

164. Andrade C. Ketamine for depression, 1: clinical summary of issues related to efficacy, adverse effects, and mechanism of action. *J Clin Psychiatry.* 2017;78(4): e415–e419.

165. Pourmand A, Mazer-Amirshahi M, Royall C, Alhawas R, Shesser R. Low dose ketamine use in the emergency department, a new direction in pain management. *Am J Emerg Med.* 2017;35(6):918–921.

166. Bowers KJ, McAllister KB, Ray M, Heitz C. Ketamine as an adjunct to opioids for acute pain in the emergency department: a randomized controlled trial. *Acad Emerg Med.* 2017;24(6):676–685.

167. Michelet D, Brasher C, Horlin AL, et al. Ketamine for chronic non-cancer pain: a meta-analysis and trial sequential analysis of randomized controlled trials. *Eur J Pain.* 2018;22(4):632–646.

168. Zekry O, Gibson SB, Aggarwal A. Subanesthetic, subcutaneous ketamine infusion therapy in the treatment of chronic nonmalignant pain. *J Pain Palliat Care Pharmacother.* 2016;30(2):91–98.

169. Strickler EM, Schwenk ES, Cohen MJ, Viscusi ER. Use of ketamine in a multimodal analgesia setting for rapid opioid tapering in a profoundly opioid-tolerant patient: a case report. *A A Case Rep.* 2018;10(7):179–181.

170. Lalanne L, Nicot C, Lang JP, Bertschy G, Salvat E. Experience of the use of ketamine to manage opioid withdrawal in an addicted woman: a case report. *BMC Psychiatry.* 2016;16(1):395.

171. Sassano-Higgins S, Baron D, Juarez G, Esmaili N, Gold M. A review of ketamine abuse and diversion. *Depress Anxiety.* 2016;33(8):718–727.

172. Ivan Ezquerra-Romano I, Lawn W, Krupitsky E, Morgan CJA. Ketamine for the treatment of addiction: evidence and potential mechanisms. *Neuropharmacology.* 2018. https://doi.org/10.1016/j.neuropharm.2018.01.017.

173. Dakwar E, Nunes EV, Hart CL, Hu MC, Foltin RW, Levin FR. A sub-set of psychoactive effects may be critical to the behavioral impact of ketamine on cocaine use disorder: results from a randomized, controlled laboratory study. *Neuropharmacology.* 2018. https://doi.org/10.1016/j.neuropharm.2018.01.005.

174. Kerr WC, Lui C, Ye Y. Trends and age, period and cohort effects for marijuana use prevalence in the 1984-2015 US National Alcohol Surveys. *Addiction.* 2018;113(3): 473–481.

175. National Academies of Sciences E, Medicine, Health. The National Academies Collection: reports funded by National Institutes of Health. In: *The Health Effects of Cannabis and Cannabinoids: The Current State of Evidence and Recommendations for Research.* Washington (DC): National Academies Press (US); 2017. Copyright 2017 by the National Academy of Sciences. All rights reserved.

176. MacCallum CA, Russo EB. Practical considerations in medical cannabis administration and dosing. *Eur J Int Med.* 2018;49:12–19.

177. Abuhasira R, Shbiro L, Landschaft Y. Medical use of cannabis and cannabinoids containing products - regulations in Europe and North America. *Eur J Int Med.* 2018;49:2–6.

178. O'Connell BK, Gloss D, Devinsky O. Cannabinoids in treatment-resistant epilepsy: a review. *Epilepsy Behav.* 2017;70(pt B):341–348.

179. Aviram J, Samuelly-Leichtag G. Efficacy of cannabis-based medicines for pain management: a systematic review and meta-analysis of randomized controlled trials. *Pain Physician.* 2017;20(6):E755–E796.

180. Whiting PF, Wolff RF, Deshpande S, et al. Cannabinoids for medical use: a systematic review and meta-analysis. *JAMA*. 2015;313(24):2456–2473.

181. Powell D, Pacula RL, Jacobson M. Do medical marijuana laws reduce addictions and deaths related to pain killers? *J Health Econ*. 2018;58:29–42.

182. Bachhuber MA, Saloner B, Cunningham CO, Barry CL. Medical cannabis laws and opioid analgesic overdose mortality in the United States, 1999-2010. *JAMA Intern Med*. 2014;174(10):1668–1673.

183. Wang GS, Le Lait MC, Deakyne SJ, Bronstein AC, Bajaj L, Roosevelt G. Unintentional pediatric exposures to marijuana in Colorado, 2009-2015. *JAMA Pediatr*. 2016; 170(9):e160971.

184. Williams AR, Santaella-Tenorio J, Mauro CM, Levin FR, Martins SS. Loose regulation of medical marijuana programs associated with higher rates of adult marijuana use but not cannabis use disorder. *Addiction*. 2017; 112(11):1985–1991.

185. Sarvet AL, Wall MM, Fink DS, et al. Medical marijuana laws and adolescent marijuana use in the United States: a systematic review and meta-analysis. *Addiction*. 2018. https://doi.org/10.1111/add.14136.

186. Santaella-Tenorio J, Mauro CM, Wall MM, et al. US traffic fatalities, 1985-2014, and their relationship to medical marijuana laws. *Am J Public Health*. 2017;107(2): 336–342.

187. Kim JH, Santaella-Tenorio J, Mauro C, et al. State medical marijuana laws and the prevalence of opioids detected among fatally injured drivers. *Am J Public Health*. 2016; 106(11):2032–2037.

188. Cooper ZD, Bedi G, Ramesh D, Balter R, Comer SD, Haney M. Impact of co-administration of oxycodone and smoked cannabis on analgesia and abuse liability. *Neuropsychopharmacology*. 2018. https://doi.org/10.1038/s41386-018-0011-2.

189. Mahajan G. Role of urine drug testing in the current opioid epidemic. *Anesth Analg*. 2017;125(6):2094–2104.

190. Moeller KE, Kissack JC, Atayee RS, Lee KC. Clinical interpretation of urine drug tests: what clinicians need to know about urine drug screens. *Mayo Clin Proc*. 2017; 92(5):774–796.

191. Melanson SE, Ptolemy AS, Wasan AD. Optimizing urine drug testing for monitoring medication compliance in pain management. *Pain Med*. 2013;14(12):1813–1820.

192. Manchikanti L, Kaye AM, Knezevic NN, et al. Responsible, safe, and effective prescription of opioids for chronic non-cancer pain: American Society of Interventional Pain Physicians (ASIPP) guidelines. *Pain Physician*. 2017;20(2S):S3–S92.

193. Deyo RA, Hallvik SE, Hildebran C, et al. Association of prescription drug monitoring program use with opioid prescribing and health outcomes: a comparison of program users and nonusers. *J Pain*. 2018;19(2):166–177.

194. Chang HY, Murimi I, Faul M, Rutkow L, Alexander GC. Impact of Florida's prescription drug monitoring program and pill mill law on high-risk patients: a comparative interrupted time series analysis. *Pharmacoepidemiol Drug Saf*. 2018. https://doi.org/10.1002/pds.4404.

195. Nam YH, Shea DG, Shi Y, Moran JR. State prescription drug monitoring programs and fatal drug overdoses. *Am J Manag Care*. 2017;23(5):297–303.

196. Brown R, Riley MR, Ulrich L, et al. Impact of New York prescription drug monitoring program, I-STOP, on statewide overdose morbidity. *Drug Alcohol Depend*. 2017;178: 348–354.

197. Ali MM, Dowd WN, Classen T, Mutter R, Novak SP. Prescription drug monitoring programs, nonmedical use of prescription drugs, and heroin use: evidence from the National Survey of Drug Use and Health. *Addict Behav*. 2017;69:65–77.

198. Schuchat A, Guy Jr GP, Dowell D. Prescription drug monitoring programs and opioid death rates-Reply. *JAMA*. 2017;318(20):2045.

199. DiPrinzio D, Sethi R. Will adding methadone to controlled substance monitoring programs help psychiatrists prevent prescription drug overdoses? *Prim Care Companion CNS Disord*. 2016;18(2); 10.4088/PCC.4015l01871.

200. Krebs EE, Lorenz KA, Bair MJ, et al. Development and initial validation of the PEG, a three-item scale assessing pain intensity and interference. *J Gen Int Med*. 2009; 24(6):733–738.

201. Ostelo RW, Deyo RA, Stratford P, et al. Interpreting change scores for pain and functional status in low back pain: towards international consensus regarding minimal important change. *Spine*. 2008;33(1):90–94.

202. Fellows SE, Coppola AJ, Gandhi MA. Comparing methods of naloxone administration: a narrative review. *J Opioid Manag*. 2017;13(4):253–260.

203. Lewis CR, Vo HT, Fishman M. Intranasal naloxone and related strategies for opioid overdose intervention by nonmedical personnel: a review. *Subst Abuse Rehabi*. 2017;8:79–95.

204. Banta-Green CJ, Coffin PO, Merrill JO, et al. Impacts of an opioid overdose prevention intervention delivered subsequent to acute care. *Inj Prev*. 2018. https://doi.org/10.1136/injuryprev-2017-042676.

205. Frank RG, Pollack HA. Addressing the fentanyl threat to public health. *N Engl J Med*. 2017;376(7):605–607.

206. Fairbairn N, Coffin PO, Walley AY. Naloxone for heroin, prescription opioid, and illicitly made fentanyl overdoses: challenges and innovations responding to a dynamic epidemic. *Int J Drug Policy*. 2017;46:172–179.

207. Somerville NJ, O'Donnell J, Gladden RM, et al. Characteristics of fentanyl overdose - Massachusetts, 2014-2016. *MMWR Morb Mortal Wkly Rep*. 2017;66(14): 382–386.

208. Mueller SR, Koester S, Glanz JM, Gardner EM, Binswanger IA. Attitudes toward naloxone prescribing in clinical settings: a qualitative study of patients prescribed high dose opioids for chronic non-cancer pain. *J Gen Int Med*. 2017;32(3):277–283.

209. Takeda MY, Katzman JG, Dole E, et al. Co-prescription of naloxone as a Universal Precautions model for patients on chronic opioid therapy-Observational study. *Subst Abuse*. 2016;37(4):591–596.

210. Coffin PO, Behar E, Rowe C, et al. Nonrandomized intervention study of naloxone coprescription for primary care patients receiving long-term opioid therapy for pain. *Ann Int Med*. 2016;165(4):245–252.

211. Spelman JF, Peglow S, Schwartz AR, Burgo-Black L, McNamara K, Becker WC. Group visits for overdose education and naloxone distribution in primary care: a pilot quality improvement initiative. *Pain Med*. 2017;18(12):2325–2330.

212. Miller M, Barber CW, Leatherman S, et al. Prescription opioid duration of action and the risk of unintentional overdose among patients receiving opioid therapy. *JAMA Intern Med*. 2015;175(4):608–615.

213. Garg RK, Fulton-Kehoe D, Franklin GM. Patterns of opioid use and risk of opioid overdose death among medicaid patients. *Med Care*. 2017;55(7):661–668.

214. Tedesco D, Asch SM, Curtin C, et al. Opioid abuse and poisoning: trends in inpatient and emergency department discharges. *Health Aff (Millwood)*. 2017;36(10):1748–1753.

215. Cormier S, Lavigne GL, Choiniere M, Rainville P. Expectations predict chronic pain treatment outcomes. *Pain*. 2016;157(2):329–338.

216. Matthias MS, Krebs EE, Bergman AA, Coffing JM, Bair MJ. Communicating about opioids for chronic pain: a qualitative study of patient attributions and the influence of the patient-physician relationship. *Eur J Pain*. 2014;18(6):835–843.

217. Loeser JD. Pain and suffering. *Clin J Pain*. 2000;16(suppl 2):S2–S6.

CHAPTER 10

Evidence-based Behavioral Treatments for Substance Use Disorders

SUZETTE GLASNER, PHD • TESS K. DRAZDOWSKI, PHD

There are a variety of behavioral treatments with established evidence for treating substance use disorders (SUDs). These include cognitive behavioral therapy (CBT)-based approaches, contingency management, motivational interventions, mindfulness-based treatments, and marital and family therapies. Additionally, self-help organizations/mutual help groups can play an integral role in a comprehensive recovery plan and can be a useful adjunct to evidence-based psychotherapies for SUDs. Each of these approaches will be reviewed below with an overview of the treatment protocol, populations for which it has been found to be effective and/or efficacious, and known limitations of the intervention. While many of these strategies can be used in a "stand alone" fashion, particularly with clients in the early stages of recovery from SUDs, many of these approaches have been used and studied as part of comprehensive treatment programs (e.g., Project COMBINE).[1]

COGNITIVE BEHAVIORAL THERAPY-BASED APPROACHES

While different variations of cognitive behavioral therapy (CBT) interventions have been developed for SUDs, the common theoretically based thread of each of these approaches is that our thought processes, emotional responses, and behaviors are all interconnected. Marlatt's cognitive-behavioral model,[2,3] grounded in social learning theory and the tenets of operant conditioning,[4] forms the basis of this approach, which can be offered in both individual and group treatment modalities. Length of treatment using CBT is variable, with protocols ranging from six to 12 weeks in duration (e.g.[5]).

Using CBT, clients learn to understand their substance use within a functional analysis framework. As part of the functional analysis, clients explore the antecedents and consequences of their substance use. Subsequently, clients build the necessary skills to recognize different situations or states (antecedents) that are associated with their specific substance use patterns. Next, clients learn to identify and avoid high-risk situations (i.e., those that increase the likelihood of relapse). The treatment also focuses on teaching a variety of behavioral and cognitive coping skills for when high-risk situations cannot be avoided.[4] These include techniques including distraction, recall of negative consequences, and positive thought substitution. Additionally, some approaches include social skills training (e.g.,[6]). Specifically, assertiveness training and role-playing skills (e.g., how to refuse substance when offered) are methods used to facilitate adoption of new coping strategies.

Clients are educated about the treatment model at the initiation of therapy and collaboration between the client and therapist is encouraged through the selection of treatment goals. Further, treatment includes "homework" (i.e., structured practice outside of sessions), which can include scheduling activities, thought recording and challenging, self-monitoring, and interpersonal skills practice (e.g.,[7,8]). Sessions typically follow a structure that includes reviewing homework from the previous session, discussing new information or a new skill, practice of the skill in session, and assignment of homework for the following week. These treatments are concentrated primarily on the client's present and future experiences. A potential advantage of CBT approaches is that the client learns skills that can be helpful to reduce problems in areas beyond substance use, such as management of anxiety and depressive symptoms, although these symptoms are not directly targeted.

According to a recent review of the literature in the Clinical Practice Guideline for the Management of Substance Use Disorders by the U.S. Department of

The Assessment and Treatment of Addiction. https://doi.org/10.1016/B978-0-323-54856-4.00010-9

Veterans Affairs (VA) and Department of Defense (DoD[9]), CBT approaches have been found to be as effective as other active interventions and treatment as usual for individuals with alcohol, stimulant, and cannabis use disorders. Additionally, evidence supports using CBT in combination with pharmacotherapy and/or other evidence-based psychosocial interventions for individuals with alcohol, opioid, and cannabis use disorders. Of note, while CBT was found to have additional benefits for individuals in methadone treatment, its added benefit for office-based buprenorphine is unclear. Additionally, CBT approaches have been modified for tobacco cessation and are recommended to be included in treatment, based on clinical practice guidelines.[10] Importantly, CBT approaches are well supported empirically; nevertheless, a systematic review indicated that outcomes may vary as a function of different aspects of the interventions and populations for which they are targeted.[11]

CONTINGENCY MANAGEMENT

Contingency management (CM) uses positive reinforcement for clients who abstain from substance use or for successfully meeting another predetermined treatment goal (e.g., treatment attendance). Based on operant conditioning principles, CM clients receive incentives for attaining treatment goals, thereby improving the likelihood that these behaviors will be repeated in the future. This intervention approach aims to increase the positive consequences from reduced and discontinued substance use, providing incentives in the face of some of the difficulties that are typically experienced in early recovery (e.g., clients may suffer from withdrawal symptoms, loss of peer groups, etc.). Additionally, to increase effectiveness, the rewards provided are delivered frequently and immediately after the desired behavior is objectively observed (e.g., drug-free urine sample) and consistently over time.[12] CM is not considered a stand-alone treatment, rather it is used in conjunction with other behavioral treatments, such as CBT or the community reinforcement approach (CRA, see more details below[13]).

Incentives may comprise a variety of items, and since they need to be effective for each individual, they can be customized to appeal to diverse clients. However, the vast majority of CM programs use vouchers or some type of item with monetary value given that it is generally universally rewarding.[14] Some techniques used to increase treatment attendance and reduce client drop out include providing a "priming" reward and

explanation of the process at intake that is not contingent on a treatment goal to introduce clients to the program, giving a bonus for attending the first session after the initial intake, and providing client successive rewards with escalating values as they continue to meet treatment goals.[15] It is important that the incentives are of sufficient magnitude for CM to be successful. Generally, research indicates that the higher the monetary value of the incentive, the more likely treatment goals will be met,[16–18] although there is emerging evidence of a potential limit of higher monetary values leading to improved treatment outcomes (e.g.,[19]).

If the treatment goal is abstinence, urine samples frequently serve as the objective measure of compliance. At the beginning of the program, urine samples should be collected at least twice a week, with the frequency decreased as the client demonstrates continued success in the program.[20,21] Alternatively, urine samples can be collected randomly to decrease the likelihood that clients can plan for an upcoming test.[15] Urine or saliva samples can also be used to detect nicotine over a several-day period, but are not useful if the client is using nicotine replacement products as part of treatment.[15] Detection of alcohol can be more difficult to ascertain given that is quickly exits the body. Typically, breath alcohol level is the most commonly used means of acute alcohol consumption. However, there are new methods for detecting alcohol consumption that may improve treatment compliance as consumption can be monitored across longer periods of time (e.g., testing for ethyl-glucuronide[22] and transdermal alcohol sensors [e.g., Secure Continuous Remote Alcohol Monitor [SCRAM] bracelets]).[23] Both breath alcohol and breath carbon monoxide can be used to test for these substances within the past few hours and can be monitored remotely using a camera on a computer or cell phone (e.g.,[24,25]). The testing for cannabis can additionally be a limitation of this method as it has slow clearance in urine[9]; giving rewards for just providing urine samples at first may be a good treatment approach until the urine samples are clear of cannabis if abstinence is the treatment goal.

Empirical evidence supporting the efficacy of CM programs is robust (e.g.,[26]) with strong support for its effectiveness for the treatment of opioid, stimulant, and cannabis users.[9] However, a meta-analysis found that once the incentives of CM have discontinued the treatment effects begin to fade,[27] a finding that has been documented with clinical trials including long-term follow-up (e.g., up to 52 weeks of treatment[28]). Additionally, in light of the fact that the longer clients are abstinent during CM treatment the better their outcomes, it is recommended that clients remain in CM for an extended period of time (e.g., 6–12 months[29]). CM is effective both as an individual and group treatment[30] and has been found to be effective in populations that historically have been difficult to treat (e.g., clients diagnosed with antisocial personality disorder and homeless populations with co-occurring psychiatric conditions).[31,32] A limitation of CM can be the cost of the treatment; however, intermittent reinforcement schedules, where clients receive rewards only sometimes after goals have been met, have also been found to be effective.[33]

Community Reinforcement Approach (CRA). CRA is a multidimensional treatment based on CBT principles, but with a focus on the environmental contingencies that influence the client's behavior. CRA is most effective when including CM.[9] The objective of this approach is to create a sober living environment that is more rewarding than the context in which the client actively uses substances. To do so, CRA targets familial, social, occupational, and recreational events. CRA combines approaches in that it uses techniques to increase the client's motivation to abstain from substance use, assesses the client's substance use pattern, puts in place positive reinforcement for sobriety, teaches new coping skills, and involves significant others in the treatment process.[34,35] CRA is considered a first-line treatment for alcohol and stimulants.[9]

MOTIVATIONAL INTERVENTIONS

Motivational interventions are a powerful tool for the treatment of SUDs. Motivational interviewing (MI) is a collaborative, client-centered approach in which the clinician helps clients explore and resolve their ambivalences about changing unhealthy behaviors. In regard to substance use, clients typically report both positive (e.g., I feel good while intoxicated) and negative aspects (e.g., causes problems at work and in my relationships) related to their use. Clinicians using MI encourage their clients to explore these dichotomies in efforts to move them toward change. MI is a nonconfrontational approach that is delivered in a nonjudgmental atmosphere. Clinicians allow the clients to select their own goals and priorities, while guiding them through explaining how their current behaviors fit with their values. MI typically takes place within one to four sessions, with 15 min having been found as the "minimum dose" necessary to facilitate effectiveness.[36] However, attending more than one MI session increased the efficacy of the treatment.[36]

MI uses specific techniques both in clinician communication and style. The acronym OARS provides a framework for clinicians in regard to how best to communicate with clients: O—open-ended questions, A—affirmations, R—reflective listening, and S—summary statements. The acronym DEARS highlights the five principles of MI: D-develop discrepancy, E—express empathy, A—amplify ambivalence, R—roll with resistance, and S—support self-efficacy. A key component in MI is "change talk," where the clinician highlights for the client statements he or she makes about desire to change, ability to change, reasons for change, need to change, and commitment to change (acronym: DARN-C). Likewise, clinicians practicing MI follow the therapeutic processes of engaging, focusing, evoking, and planning.[37] Often the use of client ratings is used to prompt change talk (e.g., "On a scale of 1–10 how important is changing this behavior to you?"). According to a review of the MI literature, eliciting "change talk" and the client's experience of discrepancy between their current actions (i.e., substance use) and their goals predicts better client outcomes, while approaches inconsistent with MI (e.g., giving advice without permission) have been found to be related to poorer client outcomes.[38]

A specific type of MI treatment that has been investigated in large clinical trials for SUDs is motivational enhancement therapy [MET] (e.g.,[39]). This is a manualized four-session MI approach. MET includes specific assessment of the client's substance use in a structured approach and personalized risk feedback.[40] Within the MI framework, MET prompts for clients' reactions to their assessment feedback, commitment to changing behaviors, and collaboration with the clinician on developing an individualized change plan. Further, clients are encouraged to bring a significant other to at least one of the MET sessions.[40] MET was found to reduce drinking outcomes at similar levels to CBT and 12-step facilitation approaches.[39] It is considered a first-line treatment for alcohol and cannabis use disorders, and an effective adjunctive intervention for alcohol, and possibly for stimulant and cannabis users.[9]

Additionally, brief forms of motivational interventions have been evaluated for efficacy and effectiveness in SUD treatment and prevention. Screening, brief intervention, and referral to treatment (SBIRT) is considered an evidence-based practice used to identify, reduce, and prevent problematic substance use and SUDs US.[41] SBIRT consists of three major components: (1) screening, (2) brief intervention, and (3) referral to treatment. It was developed as a public health initiative to identify people at risk for substance misuse, to perform brief interventions with those at-risk, and to refer those with more severe difficulties to specialized treatment. The adoption of SBIRT has been widely endorsed, with multiple programs across the nation funded by SAMHSA to promote its adoption and sustained implementation.[42,43] Similarly, the World Health Organization (WHO) supported a large multi-center cross-national trial of SBIRT.[44] Findings from these large-scale implementation studies have found overall reductions in drug use, though more research is needed.

An advantage of motivational approaches is that they can be implemented with clients across the spectrum of substance use, ranging from those at-risk for developing unhealthy substance use behaviors to individuals who have been diagnosed with SUDs. Indeed, a meta-analysis found that clients who received MI had significantly lower levels of substance use at the end of treatment, and for up to a year following the intervention, as compared to clients who received no treatment.[45] However, MI was found to be no more effective when compared to treatment as usual, other active treatments (e.g., alcohol education, medications, CM, etc.), and receiving substance use focused assessment and feedback. MI also has support for effectively reducing drinking in college students[46] and substance use in adolescents.[47] The support for using MI approaches in criminal justice systems has been more mixed.[48] Often, MI approaches have been used in settings where longer, more traditional approaches may not work well logistically, such as primary care and emergency rooms, facilitating the potential to reach individuals who may not be actively seeking treatment (e.g.,[49]).

MINDFULNESS-BASED INTERVENTIONS

Given that stress and negative affect are well-established relapse precipitants, mindfulness-based treatment, through a focus on reducing stress reactivity and improving affect regulation, has recently emerged as a promising approach to improving outcomes among addicted populations.[49a,50,51] The adaptation of mindfulness-based stress reduction techniques to individuals with substance use disorders focuses on skills training for coping with cravings and tolerating other forms of psychological discomfort that heighten relapse vulnerability (e.g., anxiety, dysphoria, and other affective states that may trigger the urge or desire to use substances).[52,53] By promoting awareness and acceptance of one's immediate experience, the practice of

mindfulness may interrupt the automatic conditioned behavioral sequence that characterizes addicted individuals' tendency to relapse in response to urges or temptations to use substances. Mindfulness-based techniques, while overlapping with some commonly used CBT skills such as "urge surfing," are distinct and complementary to CBT techniques in their focus on alternating automatic cognitive *processes* (e.g., the tendency to shift one's attentional focus away from the present), relative to the emphasis in CBT on challenging cognitive *content* (e.g., by challenging dysfunctional cognitions).

The Mindfulness Based Relapse Prevention (MBRP) approach, an 8-week, manualized therapy program combining principles of relapse prevention therapy with mindfulness practices, combines CBT-based techniques for identifying identify relapse triggers with mindfulness-based strategies for processing situational cues and monitoring internal reactions to such cues.[54] Using the skill of "mindful awareness," MBRP promotes positive behavioral choices consistent with treatment goals. A growing body of literature suggests that meditation-based interventions effectively reduce substance use, relative to wait list and supportive or educational control conditions, an effect that has been reported across a variety of substances, including alcohol, stimulants, cannabis, nicotine, and opiates.[55] An accumulating evidence base for MBRP suggests that this approach effectively reduces negative affect, stress reactivity, substance use, and cravings.[55a,56,57,58,59] Glasner-Edwards and colleagues found that MBRP, when implemented as an adjunct to contingency management, effectively reduced stress reactivity and negative affect among stimulant users, and importantly, was particularly efficacious in reducing stimulant use among stimulant-addicted individuals with comorbid mood and anxiety disorders. Likewise, in the largest study of MBRP targeting addictive disorders to date, depression and anxiety symptoms were found to moderate the efficacy of MBRP, with significant and large effects on substance use outcomes among those with severe substance use and depressive and anxiety symptoms.[60,61] Moreover, a recent review and meta-analysis of mindfulness studies targeting substance misuse found a range of small-to-large effects of mindfulness-based interventions in reducing substance use frequency and severity, craving intensity, and stress severity.[51] In light of the accumulating literature supporting this approach to the treatment of addiction, coupled with the emerging evidence of selective effects on depressed and anxious substance users, further research on efficacy and implementation of meditation-based interventions for substance using and psychiatrically comorbid populations is warranted.

MARITAL AND FAMILY-BASED INTERVENTIONS

While most treatments for SUDs focus on the individual, there is also evidence that including significant others and family members in treatment can improve client outcomes. One of the most well-studied interventions is Behavioral Couples Therapy (BCT, also referred to as Behavioral Marital Therapy and Learning Sobriety Together[62]). This treatment is designed for people seeking SUD treatment and who are married or cohabiting. Abstinence from substances and improving the couple's relationship are the typical goals of treatment. Treatment characteristically lasts for 12 to 20 weekly sessions over a 3–6-month period. Couples typically have been living together for at least a year without current psychosis. However, BCT has expanded to also include significant others beyond traditional partners (e.g., parents, siblings, roommates). BCT can be offered as a standalone SUD treatment or provided in conjunction with individual drug counseling treatment.[63]

Achieving abstinence and regular attendance is recommended as the initial focus of treatment. An important part of BCT is the daily "Recovery Contract." As part of the contract, the client states his or her intention to not use substances that day and the partner expresses his or her support. Additional parts of the contract can include daily medication verification (e.g., naltrexone and disulfiram), not discussing past substance use or fears of future substance use outside of treatment sessions, attendance at twelve-step or other self-help meetings, and urine drug screens. Discussing thoughts, feelings, and situations associated with substance use along with potential coping strategies also occurs in treatment. Relapse is seen as likely to occur and early intervention is stressed as a critical component. Also, the discussion of maintenance and relapse prevention is part of the treatment protocol.

The next phase of treatment focuses on increasing positive feelings and commitment to the relationship and teaching appropriate communication skills. In reference to increasing positive feelings, clients are encouraged to increase positive activities by catching their partner doing something nice, sharing rewarding activities, and "Caring Day" assignments (i.e., perform special acts to show caring toward one's partner). In order to improve communication, clients are taught listening skills, expressing feelings directly, negotiating

for requests, and communication sessions (i.e., planned, structured face-to-face conversations without distractions or interruptions). Similar to other behavioral approaches, these skills are typically taught through therapist instruction/modeling, practicing under therapist supervision in session and at home through homework assignments, and review of homework in session with more practice.

BCT is considered a first-line, and potential adjunctive, treatment for alcohol for both male and female clients and their partners, based on the research to date.[9] Results from a meta-analysis revealed that clients receiving BCT had less substance use, less negative consequences as a result of their use, and more relationship satisfaction as compared to those in individual-based treatment.[64] Results from intervention trials have also found that BCT results in fewer separations and divorces, has a benefit cost ratio greater than 5 to 1, reduces domestic violence, is helpful to couples' children, and improves compliance with medications targeting addiction (see O'Farrell & Schein[63] for a review). BCT is not considered an appropriate treatment for couples with active restraining orders or severe domestic violence (i.e., resulting in medical attention in the past 2 years).

There are a variety of other marital and/or family-based treatments that have been developed to help treat SUDs (for a review see[65]). Many focus on the treatment of the individual client within the family or other larger systems (e.g., Wegscheider-Cruse's Theory[66]; Stanton's Therapeutic Techniques[67]; Behavioral Contracting[68]; Solution-Focused Therapy [SFT][69]; Network Therapy[70]; Multisystemic Family Therapy [MFT]),[71] while others focus on prevention of SUDs by focusing on the parent–child relationship, typically for children ages 3–14 (e.g., Preparing for the Drug-Free Years,[72] Family Effectiveness Training,[73] Focus on Families Project,[74] the Strengthening Families Program).[75] Alternatively, different approaches have been developed to help individuals with SUDs recognize and initiate change (e.g., Community Reinforcement and Family Training [CRAFT[76]; the Johnson Institute Intervention[77]]).

SELF-HELP ORGANIZATIONS AND MUTUAL HELP GROUPS

While distinct from professionally led behavioral treatments, involvement in peer-led self-help groups, for many, is an integral component of a comprehensive addiction recovery plan. Participation in self-help groups, which are often facilitated by peers who have successfully maintained a program of addiction recovery, can provide benefits that augment the clinical impact of evidence-based treatments such as psychotherapy (e.g., relapse prevention/CBT) and addiction pharmacotherapy. Self-help organizations and mutual help groups are based on importance of creating supportive peer and mentoring relationships during SUD recovery. Self-help groups center around a common problem, are free of charge, use self-directed leadership, outline specific goals for change, focus on experiential learning, and encourage mutual helping. The group dynamic itself is seen as fundamental to the recovery process, with giving and receiving help seen as critical components to promote change. Purported mechanisms of action underlying the effects of self-help groups on substance use include providing structure, teaching coping strategies, improving social networks, strengthening self-efficacy, and encouraging a new identity (for a review see[78]). The majority of self-help group meetings in the United States focus on substance use.[79]

One of the most popular self-help groups in relation to SUDs is Alcoholic Anonymous (AA), which laid the foundation for other 12-step self-help groups (e.g., Narcotics Anonymous, Overeaters Anonymous, etc.). Founded by two alcoholics, AA meetings consist of an opening and closing ritual and members' sharing their personal narratives. There are 12 steps of AA which include[80]:

1. We admitted we were powerless over alcohol—that our lives had become unmanageable.
2. Came to believe that a Power greater than ourselves could restore us to sanity.
3. Made a decision to turn our will and our lives over to the care of God as we understood Him.
4. Made a searching and fearless moral inventory of ourselves.
5. Admitted to God, to ourselves, and to another human being the exact nature of our wrongs.
6. Were entirely ready to have God remove all these defects of character.
7. Humbly asked Him to remove our shortcomings.
8. Made a list of all persons we had harmed, and became willing to make amends to them all.
9. Made direct amends to such people wherever possible, except when to do so would injure them or others.
10. Continued to take personal inventory and when we were wrong promptly admit it.
11. Sought through prayer and meditation to improve our conscious contact with God as we understood Him, praying only for knowledge of His will for us and power to carry that out.

12. Having had a spiritual awakening as the result of these steps, we tried to carry this message to alcoholics and to practice these principles in all our affairs.

As noted in the steps, a core belief of AA is that individuals do not have the power within themselves to maintain sobriety. Instead, they need to surrender to a "Higher Power," which can be defined to fit a range of beliefs from a deity, to nature, to the support of group fellowship.[78] Additionally, members are expected to select a sponsor, who is a more senior group member, to provide them with support and guidance as they work their way through the steps. AA encourages humility, responsibility, and honesty in all relationships. AA also includes behavioral techniques such as stimulus control (e.g., avoiding peers with alcohol problems), counterconditioning (e.g., calling sponsor instead of using substances), and reinforcement (e.g., use of tokens to mark number of days sober[78,81]). Some limitations to AA and other 12-step programs can be that not all individuals are comfortable with many of the main tenets. Specifically, it can be difficult for people who do not accept the concept of a Higher Power or agree with the label of lifelong alcoholic. Further, those who do not identify abstinence as their goal may have difficulty identifying with the fundamental objectives of AA.

Twelve-step Facilitation (TSF) therapy is a manualized approach used to increase a client's engagement in 12-step mutual help groups that was established as part of Project MATCH.[82] Designed as a 12-session course of individual therapy, the clinician encourages participation in 12-step groups and guides the client through the first four steps. The message the clinician conveys to the client is that addiction is a serious, chronic, and progressive disease in which abstinence is the goal, focusing on 1 day at a time. Each session is divided into three sections: (1) reviewing events from the previous week (e.g., urges to use, recovery-oriented activities), (2) introduction of new 12-step material, and (3) assigning homework and planning recovery-oriented activities (e.g., attending 12-step meeting, contacting sponsor). TSF is considered an effective first line of treatment, and adjunctive intervention, for alcohol problems.[9]

Moderation Management (MM) has evolved from the traditional 12-step self-help groups and differs in important ways to AA. Rather than an abstinence goal, the objective of MM is based on harm reduction, with goals of reducing alcohol use. Additionally, there is no mention of a Higher Power and the steps are framed within a behavioral change program. The nine steps of MM are[83]:

1. Attend meetings or online groups and learn about the program of Moderation Management.
2. Abstain from alcoholic beverages for 30 days and complete steps three through six during this time.
3. Examine how drinking has affected your life.
4. Write down your life priorities.
5. Take a look at how much, how often, and under what circumstances you had been drinking.
6. Learn the MM guidelines and limits for moderate drinking.
7. Set moderate drinking limits and start weekly "small steps" toward balance and moderation in other areas of your life.
8. Review your progress and update your goals.
9. Continue to make positive lifestyle changes and attend meetings whenever you need ongoing support or would like to help newcomers.

MM is targeted for individuals who are able to complete a 30-day period of abstinence before attending group meetings as noted in Step 2. The organization suggests that those with more severe alcohol problems, indicated by loss of control over drinking, seek alternative methods of help. MM has a large presence online, as well as in face-to-face modalities.[84] Of note, positive treatment outcomes are unlikely to result from MM among those with a moderate to severe alcohol use disorder; as such, this approach would not be recommended for this subgroup but rather those with relatively mild alcohol-related problems.

CONCLUSION

To date, there is no evidence that one type of treatment approach is the most appropriate or effective for people with SUDs in general. In fact, in a large multisite randomized control study of individuals with alcohol problems, all three treatments investigated (cognitive-behavioral coping skills training, motivational enhancement therapy, and 12-step facilitation therapy) were found to be beneficial, but none had better outcomes than any other treatment.[39] Therefore, it is suggested that clients be provided with the possible treatment options and allowed to decide which may work best for them.[8] In this chapter, we highlighted the most well-studied approaches to addiction treatment to date, including motivational interventions, CBT, CM, CRA, mindfulness-based treatments, and couples and family therapy. In addition, adjunctive recovery-oriented activities such as self-help groups were described and reviewed. Both research and clinical experience suggest

that individualizing a plan of behavioral treatment to the individual's treatment needs and preferences is the means of optimizing outcomes.

RESOURCES FOR CLINICIANS

Below is a list of resources for individuals interested in learning more about different psychosocial treatment options for substance use disorders.

- Manuals (TSF, MET, CBT, etc.): http://pubs.niaaa. nih.gov/publications/ProjectMatch/matchIntro.htm
- A free computer software program for the implementation of contingency management as well as online training: *Motivational Incentives: A proven approach to treatment.* National Institute of Drug Abuse. http://www.bettertxoutcomes.org
- A free online SBIRT course through Medscape: http://www.medscape.org/viewarticle/830331
- A free SBIRT App, developed at Baylor College of Medicine to support the use of SBIRT by physicians, other health workers, and mental health professionals: sbirtapp.org/
- A web-based distance learning course on BCT: www. ireta.org/ireta_main/distance_learning.html

REFERENCES

1. Pettinati HM, Anton RF, Willenbring ML. The COMBINE study: an overview of the largest pharmacotherapy study to date for treating alcohol dependence. *Psychiatry.* 2006; 3(10):36−39.
2. Marlatt GA, Donovan DM, eds. *Relapse prevention: Maintenance strategies in the Treatment of Addictive Behaviors.* 2nd ed. New York: Guilford Press; 2005.
3. Marlatt GA, Gordon JR. *Relapse Prevention: Maintenance Strategies in the Treatment of Addictive Behaviors.* New York: Guilford; 1985.
4. Carroll KM, Onken LS. Behavioral therapies for drug abuse. *Am J Psychiatry.* 2005;162(8):1452−1460.
5. Kadden R, Carroll KM, Donovan D, et al. *Cognitive-Behavioral Coping Skills Therapy Manual: A Clinical Research Guide for Therapists Treating Individuals With Alcohol Abuse and Dependence.* Vol 3. Rockville, MD: National Institute on Alcohol Abuse and Alcoholism; 1995. DHHS No. 94−3724.
6. Chaney EF. Social skills training. In: Hester RK, Miller WR, eds. *Handbook of Alcoholism Treatment Approaches: Effective Alternatives.* New York: Pergamon; 1989.
7. Carroll KM. *A Cognitive-behavioral Approach: Treating Cocaine Addiction. Therapy Manuals for Drug Addiction.* Rockville, MD: National Institute of Drug Abuse; 1998.
8. Daley DC, Marlett GA. *Overcoming Your Alcohol or Drug Problem: Effective Recovery Strategies: Therapist Guide, Treatments that Work.* 2nd ed. New York, NY: Oxford University Press; 2006.

9. Drexler K, Kivlahan D, Perry C. *(Co-Chairs). VHA/DoD Clinical Practice Guideline for the Management of Substance Use Disorders (Version 3.0).* Washington, DC: Veteran's Health Administration; 2015. Retrieved from http://www.healthquality.va.gov/guidelines/mh/sud/index.asp.

10. U.S. Department of Health, Human Services (USDHHS). *Treating Tobacco Use and Dependence: 2008 Update: Clinical Practice Guideline.* Rockville, MD: U.S. Department of Health and Human Services; 2008.

11. Miller WR, Willbourne PL, Hettema JE. What works? A summary of alcohol treatment outcome research. In: Hester RK, Miller WR, eds. *Handbook of Alcoholism Treatment Approaches: Effective Alternatives.* 3nd ed. Boston: Allyn & Bacon; 2003:13–63.

12. Griffith JD, Rowan-Szal GA, Roark RR, Simpson DD. Contingency management in outpatient methadone treatment: a meta-analysis. *Drug Alcohol Dependence.* 2000;58:55–66.

13. Higgins ST, Alessi SM, Dantona RL. Voucher-based incentives: a substance abuse treatment innovation. *Addict Behav.* 2002;27(6):887–910.

14. Petry NM. *Contingency Management for Substance Abuse Treatment: A Guide to Implementing This Evidence-based Practice.* New York: Routledge; 2012.

15. Stitzer M, Cunningham CS, Sweeney MM. Contingency management for substance use disorders: theoretical foundation, principles, assessment, and components. In: Post TW, Saxon AJ, Hermann R, eds. *UpToDate.* Waltham, MA: UpToDate; 2017. Retrieved from https://www.uptodate.com/contents/contingency-management-for-substance-use-disorders-theoretical-foundation-principles-assessment-and-components.

16. Higgins ST, Heil SH, Dantona R, Donham R, Matthews M, Badger GJ. Effects of varying the monetary value of voucher-based incentives on abstinence achieved during and following treatment among cocaine-dependent outpatients. *Addiction.* 2007;102(2):271–281.

17. Lussier JP, Heil SH, Mongeon JA, Badger GJ, Higgins ST. A meta-analysis of voucher-based reinforcement therapy for substance use disorders. *Addiction.* 2006;101(2):192–203.

18. Petry NM, Barry D, Alessi SM, Rounsaville BJ, Carroll KM. A randomized trial adapting contingency management targets based on initial abstinence status of cocaine-dependent patients. *J Consult Clin Psychol.* 2012;80(2):276–285.

19. Petry NM, Alessi SM, Barry D, Carroll KM. Standard magnitude prize reinforcers can be as efficacious as larger magnitude reinforcers in cocaine-dependent methadone patients. *J Consult Clin Psychol.* 2015;83(3):464–472.

20. Petry NM, Alessi SM, Carroll KM, et al. Contingency management treatments: reinforcing abstinence versus adherence with goal-related activities. *J Consult Clin Psychol.* 2006;74(3):592–601.

21. Petry NM, Tedford J, Austin M, Nich C, Carroll KM, Rounsaville BJ. Prize reinforcement contingency management for treating cocaine users: how low can we go, and with whom? *Addiction.* 2004;99(3):349–360.

22. McDonell MG, Leickly E, McPherson S, et al. A randomized controlled trial of ethyl glucuronide-based contingency management for outpatients with co-occurring alcohol use disorders and serious mental illness. *Am J Psychiatry.* 2017;174(4):370–377.

23. Barnett NP, Celio MA, Tidey JW, Murphy JG, Colby SM, Swift RM. A preliminary randomized controlled trial of contingency management for alcohol use reduction using a transdermal alcohol sensor. *Addiction.* 2017;112(6):1025–1035.

24. Alessi SM, Petry NM. A randomized study of cellphone technology to reinforce alcohol abstinence in the natural environment. *Addiction.* 2013;108(5):900–909.

25. Dallery J, Raiff BR, Kim SJ, Marsch LA, Stitzer M, Grabinski MJ. Nationwide access to an internet-based contingency management intervention to promote smoking cessation: a randomized controlled trial. *Addiction.* 2017;112(5):875–883.

26. Dutra L, Stathopoulou G, Basden SL, Leyro TM, Powers MB, Otto MW. A meta-analytic review of psychosocial interventions for substance use disorders. *Am J Psychiatry.* 2008;165:179–187.

27. Prendergast M, Podus D, Finney J, Greenwell L, Roll J. Contingency management for treatment of substance use disorders: a meta-analysis. *Addiction.* 2006;101(11):1546–1560.

28. Silverman K, Robles E, Mudric T, Bigelow GE, Stitzer ML. A randomized trial of long-term reinforcement of cocaine abstinence in methadone-maintained patients who inject drugs. *J Consult Clin Psychol.* 2004;72(5):839–854.

29. Stitzer M, Cunningham CS. Contingency management for substance use disorders: efficacy, implementation, and training. In: Post TW, Saxon AJ, Hermann R, eds. *UpToDate.* Waltham, MA: UpToDate; 2017. Retrieved from https://www.uptodate.com/contents/contingency-management-for-substance-use-disorders-efficacy-implementation-and-training?source=see_link.

30. Petry NM, Martin B, Simcic F. Prize reinforcement contingency management for cocaine dependence: integration with group therapy in a methadone clinic. *J Consult Clin Psychol.* 2005;73:354–359.

31. Messina N, Farabee D, Rawson R. Treatment responsivity of cocaine-dependent patients with antisocial personality disorder to cognitive-behavioral and contingency management interventions. *J Consult Clin Psychol.* 2003;71:320–329.

32. Tracy K, Babuscio T, Nich C, et al. Contingency management to reduce substance use in individuals who are homeless with co-occurring psychiatric disorders. *The Am J Drug Alcohol Abuse.* 2007;33:253–258.

33. Petry NM, Martin B, Cooney JL, Kranzler HR. Give them prizes and they will come: contingency management for treatment of alcohol dependence. *J Consult Clin Psychol.* 2000;68(2):250–257.

34. Budney AJ, Higgins ST. *National Institute on Drug Abuse Therapy Manuals for Drug Addiction: Manual 2. A Community Reinforcement Approach: Treating Cocaine Addiction (NIH Publication No. 98–4309).* Rockville, MD: US Department of Health and Human Services; 1998.

35. Meyers RJ, Smith JE. *Clinical Guide to Alcohol Treatment: The Community Reinforcement Approach*. New York: Guilford Press; 1995.

36. Rubak S, Sandbæk A, Lauritzen T, Christensen B. Motivational interviewing: a systematic review and meta-analysis. *Br J Gen Pract*. 2005;55(513):305–312.

37. Miller WR, Rollnick S. *Motivational Interviewing: Helping People Change*. New York: Guilford; 2013.

38. Apodaca TR, Longabaugh R. Mechanisms of change in motivational interviewing: a review and preliminary evaluation of the evidence. *Addiction*. 2009;104(5):705–715.

39. Project MATCH. Matching alcoholism treatments to client heterogeneity: Project MATCH three- year drinking outcomes. *Alcohol Clin Exp Res*. 1998;22(6):1300–1311.

40. Miller WR, Zweben A, DiClemente CC, Rychtarik RG. *Motivational Enhancement Therapy Manual: A Clinical Research Guide for Therapists Treating Individuals with Alcohol Abuse and Dependence (NIH Publication No. 94-3723)*. Vol 2. Rockville, MD: National Institute on Alcohol Abuse and Alcoholism; 1999.

41. Substance Abuse, Mental health Services Administration (SAMHSA)-Health Resources and Services Administration (HRSA). *SBIRT: Screening, Brief Intervention, and Referral to Treatment*; 2017. Retrieved from https://www.integration.samhsa.gov/clinical-practice/sbirt.

42. Babor TF, Del Boca F, Bray JW. Screening, Brief Intervention and Referral to Treatment: implications of SAMHSA's SBIRT initiative for substance abuse policy and practice. *Addiction*. 2017;112(S2):110–117.

43. Bray JW, Del Boca FK, McRee BG, Hayashi SW, Babor TF. Screening, brief intervention and referral to treatment (SBIRT): rationale, program overview and cross-site evaluation. *Addiction*. 2017;112(S2):3–11.

44. Humeniuk R, Ali R, Babor T, et al. A randomized controlled trial of a brief intervention for illicit drugs linked to the Alcohol, Smoking and Substance Involvement Screening Test (ASSIST) in clients recruited from primary health-care settings in four countries. *Addiction*. 2012;107(5):957–966.

45. Smedslund G, Berg Rigmor C, Hammerstrom Karianne T, et al. Motivational interviewing for substance abuse. *Cochrane Database Syst Rev*. 2011;5:CD008063.

46. Carey KB, Scott-Sheldon LA, Carey MP, DeMartini KS. Individual-level interventions to reduce college student drinking: a meta-analytic review. *Addict Behav*. 2007; 32(11):2469–2494.

47. Tait RJ, Hulse GK. A systematic review of the effectiveness of brief interventions with substance using adolescents by type of drug. *Drug Alcohol Rev*. 2003;22(3):337–346.

48. Prendergast ML, McCollister K, Warda U. A randomized study of the use of screening, brief intervention, and referral to treatment (SBIRT) for drug and alcohol use with jail inmates. *J Subst Abuse Treat*. 2017;74:54–64.

49. VanBuskirk KA, Wetherell JL. Motivational interviewing with primary care populations: a systematic review and meta-analysis. *J Behav Med*. 2014;37(4):768–780.

49a. Marlatt GA. Taxonomy of high-risk situations for alcohol relapse: evolution and development of a cognitive-behavioral model. *Addiction*. 1996;91 Suppl: S37–49.

50. Breslin FC, Zack M, McMain S. An information-processing analysis of mindfulness: implications for relapse prevention in the treatment of substance abuse. *Clin Psychol*. 2002;9(3):275–299.

51. Li W, Howard MO, Garland EL, McGovern P, Lazar M. Mindfulness treatment for substance misuse: a systematic review and meta-analysis. *J Subst Abuse Treat*. 2017;75: 62–96.

52. Kabat-Zinn J. *Full Catastrophe Living: Using the Wisdom of Your Mind to Face Stress, Pain and Illness*. New York: Dell; 1990.

53. Marlatt GA, Chawla N. Meditation and alcohol use. *South Med J*. 2007;100(4):451–454.

54. Witkiewitz K, Marlatt GA, Walker D. Mindfulness-based relapse prevention for alcohol and substance use disorders. *J Cogn Psychother*. 2005;19(3):211–228.

55. Chiesa A, Serretti A. Are mindfulness-based interventions effective for substance use disorders? A systematic review of the evidence. *Subst Use Misuse*. 2014;49(5): 492–512.

55a. Brewer JA, Sinha R, Chen JA, Michalsen RN, Babuscio TA, Nich C. Mindfulness training and stress reactivity in substance abuse: results from a randomized, controlled stage I pilot study. *Subst Abus*. 2009;30(4): 306–317.

56. Brewer JA, Sinha R, Chen JA, et al. Mindfulness training and stress reactivity in substance abuse: results from a randomized, controlled stage I pilot study. *Subst Abus*. 2009; 30(4):306–317.

57. Bowen S, Chawla N, Collins SE, et al. Mindfulness-based relapse prevention for substance use disorders: a pilot efficacy trial. *Subst Abus*. 2009;30(4):295–305.

58. Glasner-Edwards S, Mooney L, Ang A, et al. Mindfulness Based Relapse Prevention improves stimulant use among adults with major depression and generalized anxiety disorder. *Drug Alcohol Depend*. 2015;156:e80.

59. Glasner S, Mooney LJ, Ang A, et al. Mindfulness-based relapse prevention for stimulant dependent adults: a pilot randomized clinical trial. *Mindfulness*. 2017;8(1): 126–135.

60. Bowen S, Witkiewitz K, Clifasefi SL, et al. Relative efficacy of mindfulness-based relapse prevention, standard relapse prevention, and treatment as usual for substance use disorders: a randomized clinical trial. *JAMA Psychiatry*. 2014; 71(5):547–556.

61. Roos CR, Bowen S, Witkiewitz K. Baseline patterns of substance use disorder severity and depression and anxiety symptoms moderate the efficacy of mindfulness-based relapse prevention. *J Consult Clin Psychol*. 2017;85(11): 1041–1051.

62. O'Farrell TJ, Fals-Stewart W. *Behavioral Couples Therapy for Alcoholism and Drug Abuse*. New York: Guilford Press; 2006.

63. O'Farrell TJ, Schein AZ. Behavioral couples therapy for alcoholism and drug abuse. *J Fam Psychotherapy*. 2011; 22(3):193–215.

64. Powers MB, Vedel E, Emmelkamp PM. Behavioral couples therapy (BCT) for alcohol and drug use disorders: a meta-analysis. *Clin Psychol Rev*. 2008;28(6):952–962.

65. Klostermann K. Marital and family approaches. In: Sher KJ, ed. *The Oxford Handbook of Substance Use and Substance Use Disorders*. Vol 2. Oxford, UK: Oxford University Press; 2016. Retrieved from http://www.oxfordhandbooks.com/view/10.1093/oxfordhb/9780199381708.001.0001/oxfordhb-9780199381708-e-11.

66. Wegscheider S. *Another Chance: Hope and Health for the Alcoholic Family*. Palo Alto, CA: Science and Behavior Books; 1981.

67. Stanton MD, Todd TC, Associates. *The Family Therapy of Drug Abuse and Addiction*. New York: Guilford; 1982.

68. Steinglass P, Bennett LA, Wolin SJ, Reiss D. *The Alcoholic Family*. New York: BasicBooks; 1987.

69. Berg IK, Miller SD. *Working with the Problem Drinker: A Solution-focused Approach*. New York: W.W. Norton; 1992.

70. Galanter M. Network therapy for addiction: a model for office practice. *Am J Psychiatry*. 1993;150:28–36.

71. Cunningham PB, Henggeler SW. Engaging multiproblem families in treatment: lessons learned throughout the development of multisystemic therapy. *Fam Process*. 1999;38:265–281.

72. Hawkins JD, Catalano RF, Brown EO, et al. *Preparing for the Drug (Free) Years: A Family Activity Book*. Seattle, WA: Comprehensive Health Education Foundation; 1988.

73. Szapocznik J, Santisteban D, Rio A, Perez-Vidal A, Santisteban D, Kurtines WM. Family effectiveness training: an intervention to prevent drug abuse and problem behaviors in Hispanic adolescents. *Hispanic J Behav Sci*. 1989;11:4–27.

74. Catalano RF, Gainey RR, Fleming CB, Haggerty KP, Johnson NO. An experimental intervention with families of substance abusers: one-year follow-up of the Focus on Families Project. *Addiction*. 1999;94(2):241–254.

75. Kumpfer K, Magalhães C, Greene JA. Strengthening families program. In: Ponzetti Jr JJ, ed. *Evidence-based Parenting Education: A Global Perspective*. New York: Routledge; 2015: 277–292.

76. Smith JE, Meyers RJ. Community reinforcement and family training. In: Fisher GL, Roget NA, eds. *Encyclopedia of Substance Abuse Prevention, Treatment, and Recovery*. Thousand Oaks, CA: Sage; 2009.

77. Johnson VE. *Intervention: How to Help Someone Who Doesn't Want Help*. Center City, MN: Hazelden; 1986.

78. Lembke A, Humphreys K. Self-help organizations for substance use disorders. In: Sher KJ, ed. *The Oxford Handbook of Substance Use and Substance Use Disorders*. Vol 2. Oxford, UK: Oxford University Press; 2016. Retrieved from http://www.oxfordhandbooks.com/view/10.1093/oxfordhb/9780199381708.001.0001/oxfordhb-9780199381708-e-16#oxfordhb-9780199381708-e-16-bibItem-11.

79. Humphreys K. *Circles of Recovery: Self-help Organizations for Addictions*. Cambridge, UK: Cambridge University Press; 2004.

80. Alcoholics Anonymous. *Twelve Steps and Twelve Traditions*. New York: Alcoholics Anonymous World Services; 2012.

81. DiClemente CC. Alcoholics Anonymous and the structure of change. In: McCrady BS, Miller WR, eds. *Research on Alcoholics Anonymous: Opportunities and Alternatives*. Piscataway, NJ: Rutgers Center of Alcohol Studies; 1993:79–97.

82. Nowinski J, Baker S, Carroll K. *Twelve-step Facilitation Therapy Manual: A Clinical Research Guide for Therapists Treating Individuals with Alcohol Abuse and Dependence (NIH Publication No. 94–3722)*. Rockville, MD: National Institute on Alcohol Abuse and Alcoholism; 1999.

83. Kishline A. *Moderate Drinking: The Moderation Management Guide for People Who Want to Reduce Their Drinking*. New York: Crown; 1994.

84. Klaw E, Huebsch PD, Humphreys K. Communication patterns in an on-line mutual help group for problem drinkers. *J Community Psychol*. 2000;28:535–546.

CHAPTER 11

Substance Use in Adolescents Chapter

SETH AMMERMAN, MD, FAAP, FSAHM, DABAM

INTRODUCTION

The use of intoxicating addictive substances by adolescents may lead to serious adverse cognitive, mental health, psychosocial, and medical consequences, as well as negatively impact normal adolescent brain development. Thus, substance use among adolescents is a major health concern.

One of the most important tasks of adolescence is called "identity formation," ideally leading to a healthy, happy, and productive adulthood. There are numerous aspects of an individual's identity, including social, sexual, gender, moral, cultural, religious/spiritual, and racial/ethnic identity. In this chapter, the definition of adolescence will be that of the World Health Organization, which combines "adolescence" and "youth," as ages 10–24 years of age.[1] Adolescence is typically divided into three stages of development, based on physical/physiologic, psychosocial, and cognitive development. The average ages of these stages are: Early Adolescence 10–13 years; Middle Adolescence 14–17 years; and Late Adolescence (also called Young Adulthood or Emerging Adulthood) 18–24 years. It is in Middle Adolescence that adolescents significantly expand behavioral experimentation and engage in what are usually labeled as "exploratory" behaviors (healthy and positive) or "risk-taking" behaviors, which can often result in unhealthy or negative outcomes.[2]

Many factors influence whether an adolescent tries addictive substances,[3] including their availability within the neighborhood, community, and school, and whether the adolescent's friends are using them. A best friend who uses, or having a user peer group, is highly predictive of an individual using. The family environment is also important: violence, physical or emotional abuse, mental health issues, or substance use in the household increase the likelihood that the adolescent will use addictive substances (Adverse Childhood Experiences Score[4]). Genetic vulnerability also plays a role, with personality traits like poor impulse control or a high need for excitement; mental health

conditions such as depression, anxiety, and attention deficit with hyperactivity disorder (ADHD). Beliefs such as that drugs are "cool" or harmless make it more likely that an adolescent will use drugs.

Adolescents meeting criteria for a severe substance use disorder, sometimes referred to as addiction, suggests that the individual has lost control over substance use. Addiction is a chronic, neurological condition associated with changes in the brain's reward center. Effective treatments, including medication and psychosocial support, are available, though addiction is not curable and long-term treatment is recommended.

DIFFERENCES BETWEEN RISKY SUBSTANCE USE, PROBLEM USE, AND ADDICTION

Risky substance use in adolescence is different than problem use or having a substance use disorder (addiction). See Table 11.1 for specific definitions. Use of addictive substances by adolescents can lead them to engage in risky behaviors that they otherwise would not engage in.[5] Examples of these risky behaviors include having unsafe sex (e.g., not using condoms when otherwise they would), which can result in an unintended pregnancy or acquiring sexually transmitted infections including Chlamydia, Gonorrhea, Human Papilloma Virus (genital warts and cervical cancer), Syphilis, and/or HIV; riding in a car as a passenger with an impaired driver, or driving when impaired, leading to injuries and accidents (including fatal motor vehicle accidents); "shooting up" with dirty needles, leading to HIV, Hepatitis C, or endocarditis; and getting into fights when under the influence of alcohol. Adolescents have a tendency to act impulsively (see brain development above), and risky substance use will often increase this impulsive behavior.

On the other hand, a hallmark of addiction is its compulsive aspect, which is not true of risky use. Risky use can lead to problem use or addiction, so again, early

The Assessment and Treatment of Addiction. https://doi.org/10.1016/B978-0-323-54856-4.00011-0

TABLE 11.1
Definitions of Types of Substance Use
Risky Substance Use: Use of addictive substances by adolescents can lead them to engage in risky behaviors that they otherwise wouldn't engage in.
Problem Substance Use: psycho-social, mental health, medical, or legal problems as a result of the substance use.
Substance Use Disorder/Addiction: The Diagnostic and Statistical Manual of Mental Disorders, Fifth Edition (DSM-5), no longer uses the terms substance abuse and substance dependence. Rather, it refers to substance use disorders, which are defined by level of severity as mild, moderate, or severe. Degree of severity is determined by the number of diagnostic criteria—11 total—met by an individual. Substance use disorders occur when the recurrent use of alcohol and/or drugs causes clinically and functionally significant impairment, such as health problems, disability, and failure to meet major responsibilities at work, school, or home. According to the DSM-5, a diagnosis of substance use disorder is based on evidence of impaired control, social impairment, risky use, and pharmacological criteria.

intervention is a key component of helping adolescents not become problem users or addicts.

Note that evidence for use of "soft drugs," i.e., alcohol, marijuana, and tobacco, being "gateways" to the use of hard drugs (e.g., cocaine, heroin) is very weak. Although most hard drug users do start with use of soft drugs, the vast majority of soft drug users do not go on to hard drug use. The vast majority of users start with soft drugs because they are the most widely available and easily obtainable.

ADOLESCENT BRAIN DEVELOPMENT

Research on adolescent brain development has demonstrated that maturational brain changes, particularly myelination (the ability of brain nerves to communicate more quickly) and synaptic pruning (the ability of brain nerves to communicate more efficiently), occur throughout adolescence, well into the early-mid 20s. These changes are ultimately responsible for optimal neurocognitive performance.[6] The last part of the brain to develop is the prefrontal cortex, which is responsible for executive function and impulse control. Use of addictive substances may alter the developing brain itself, in ways that are not yet fully understood but are different than usual development, leading to the adverse cognitive and other consequences noted above.[7] Use of addictive substances—including the three most commonly used addictive substances by adolescents—nicotine, alcohol, and marijuana—may alter normal brain development, although not all studies show consistent findings.[8–13] Various social determinants of health may also predispose adolescents to using addictive substances and in and of themselves significantly impact brain development, including childhood poverty, abuse, and neglect.[14,15]

The younger an adolescent starts using addictive substances, whether nicotine, alcohol, or other drugs, the more likely problem use, or substance use disorder, will occur.[16] Starting use at age 14 is a greater risk than starting at age 16, which is a greater risk than starting age 18, which is a greater risk than age 21. Threshold ages for decreasing risk seem to be ages 18 and 21. Thus, adolescents who do not start using addictive substances until age 18 are less likely to develop problem use than those who started before age 18, and those who do not use addictive substances until age 21 are at even less risk. Frequency of use is also correlated with problem use. Regular Users (defined as using 10–19 times/month) and Heavy Users (defined as using $>= 20$ times a month)[17] are at particular risk of developing problem use.

Having a family history of a substance use disorder (SUD) may put an adolescent at higher risk, but otherwise it is difficult to predict who will develop problems. Thus, prevention and early intervention strategies are key to preventing the development of a SUD and all the associated adverse consequences.

Adverse Consequences of Adolescent Substance Use

When an adolescent gets into a pattern of repeated use, it can pose serious social and health risks,[5] including:
- School failure and/or poor job performance
- Problems with family and other relationships
- Loss of interest in normal healthy activities
- Impaired memory
- Mental health problems, including anxiety, depression, psychosis, and substance use disorders of varying severity.

Accidents; Violence; Assaults
- Morbidity and mortality due to substance use overdose

EPIDEMIOLOGY

There are three longitudinal databases in the United States tracking adolescent substance use: Monitoring The Future (MTF), through the University of Michigan and the National Institute of Drug Abuse[18]; the Youth Risk Behavior Survey (YRBS), through individual states and the Centers for Disease Control and Prevention[19]; and the National Survey of Drug Use and Health (NSDUH), through the Substance Abuse and Mental Health Services Administration (SAMHSA).[20] Looking at Monitoring The Future 2016, rates of *current use* (defined as using the substance at least once in the last 30 days) by 12th graders for the three most commonly used addictive substances are: alcohol 33.2%; marijuana 22.5%; nicotine (electronic vaporizers) 12.5%. Current users are at risk for becoming regular or heavy users and developing problem use, so this is an important intervention point to help adolescents cut back or discontinue use. For more detailed data

on MTF current substance use rates nationally for 8th, 10th, and 12th graders, see Table 11.2. Note that MTF has additional data on both lifetime and daily use rates.

For the 2016 NSDUH adolescent past month misuse of prescription pain relievers, tranquilizers, stimulants, and sedatives, see Table 11.3.

Increasing use of marijuana, nicotine, and opioids is of major concern in the adolescent population and will be briefly discussed below.

MARIJUANA

Use of marijuana for both medical and recreational purposes is becoming more normalized. In 2017, 29 states and Washington, D.C. have legalized medical marijuana, and eight states have legalized recreational marijuana for adults ages 21 and older. Medical marijuana is portrayed as having numerous benefits, and recreational use is portrayed as benign. Concurrently, surveys

TABLE 11.2
Current Substance Use

MTF 2016 Data: <u>Current Use</u> (Used At Least Once In The Past 30 Days), 2 of 2

ANY ILLICIT DRUG	ALCOHOL	MARIJUANA	ELECTRONIC VAPORIZERS	ANY RX DRUGS	AMPHETA-MINES
	33.2%	22.5%	12.5%	18%	10%
Most commonly used, ranked, 12ᵗʰ grade (at least 10%)					
8ᵀᴴ: 6.9%	Flavored Alcoholic		Cigarettes		
10ᵀᴴ: 15.9%	Drinks		10.5%		
12ᵀᴴ: 24.4%	18.3%				
	Been Drunk				
	20.4%				

Adapted from Monitoring the Future (MTF) 2016.

TABLE 11.3
Past-month Misuse of Prescription Medications

NSDUH 2015 Adolescents/Young Adults:
Past Month Misuse of Prescription Pain Relievers,
Tranquilizers, Stimulants, and Sedatives

	Ages 12-17	Ages 18-25
Pain Relievers:	276,000 = 1.1%	829,000 = 2.4%
Tranquilizers:	162,000 = 0.7%	582,000 = 1.7%
Stimulants:	117,000 = 0.5%	757,000 = 2.2%
Sedatives:	21,000 = 0.1%	86,000 = 0.2%

Adapted from the National Survey of Drug Use and Health (NSDUH) 2016

have shown that adolescents' perception of possible harm of marijuana use is decreasing. One consequence of this may be more likelihood to drive under the influence, or ride with a driver under the influence, leading to more motor vehicle accidents and associated morbidity and mortality.[21] It should be noted that there are no published clinical trials on the use of medical marijuana in children and adolescents, and that although occasional use of recreational marijuana by adults may not be harmful, no safe quantity has been established for adolescents.[22] Frequent marijuana use throughout adolescence and into young adulthood appears linked to worsened cognitive performance. Earlier age of onset also appears to be associated with poorer neurocognitive outcomes that emerge by young adulthood, providing further support for the notion that the brain may be uniquely sensitive to frequent marijuana exposure during the adolescent phase of neurodevelopment. Additionally, there may be gender differences, with adolescent female users possibly more prone to anxiety and depression. Limited data

in recreational marijuana states have not shown a significant increase in use in younger adolescents, though in Colorado use among college students has increased. More research and data are needed to know the impact of these legalization trends.

Counseling tips for parents and adolescents are included in a recently published American Academy of Pediatrics Clinical Report.[23]

NICOTINE

Electronic cigarettes (E-cigarettes or Electronic vaporizers) are electronic devices that vaporize liquid nicotine, and are often promoted for smoking cessation. However, they are sold in flavors such as bubble gum and cotton candy that are attractive to adolescents, who may initiate their "smoking careers" with these devices. E-cigarettes are now more commonly used by adolescents than traditional cigarettes and can be highly addictive. Use of nicotine products often precedes use of other addictive substances.[24] Youth who smoke cigarettes are 5 times more likely than adolescent non-smokers to use alcohol, 13 times more likely to use marijuana, and 7 times more likely to use cocaine or heroin.

OPIOIDS

The opioid epidemic in the USA has significantly affected adolescents.[25] Between 1991 and 2012, the rate of "nonmedical use" of opioid medication, i.e., use without a prescription or using more than prescribed, by adolescents more than doubled. NIDA reported in 2014 that 6% of teens had misused prescription opioids in the past year ($\sim$2.4 million). The rate of opioid use disorders, including heroin addiction, has increased in parallel. NSDUH reported in 2014 that an estimated 467,000 adolescents (1.9%) aged 12 to 17 were current nonmedical users of pain relievers, and 16,000 were currently using heroin.[26]

Co-occurring Disorders

Co-occurring disorders are common in adolescence, with those ages 18–25 with the highest rates by the National Survey of Drug Use and Health[20]: adolescents having both a SUD and any mental health issues: 27.2%; adolescents having both a SUD and a serious mental health issues: 33.8%. Co-occurring disorders can include learning problems or disabilities; depression; anxiety; psychosis; and/or attention deficit hyperactivity disorder (ADHD). The evaluation and treatment of ADHD in adolescents with a SUD is a particularly common and challenging issue to diagnose and treat and is further discussed below.

Thus, patients with a mental health issue should be assessed for substance use issues, and those with problem substance use should be assessed for mental health issues.[27]

ADHD AND SUD

There is an increased prevalence of ADHD in patients with a SUD. ADHD may increase risk for the development of a SUD, and untreated ADHD may worsen SUD outcomes.[28–30] Using validated screening tools for the diagnosis of ADHD is necessary to make an accurate diagnosis.

There are a number of validated screening tools for ADHD; two of the more commonly used are the Connors Rating Scale and the National Institute for Children's Health Quality (NICHQ) Vanderbilt Assessment Scales. Both scales have questionnaires for parents and teachers; the Connors also includes a patient self-assessment component.

Other validated screening tools important to use for comorbid symptoms, e.g., for anxiety, are the Screen for Anxiety Related Emotional Disorders (SCARED), and for depression, the Patient Health Questionnaire–9 (PHQ-9).

Evidence-based pharmacologic treatments for ADHD are well established, especially in patients without co-occurring disorders. Appropriate treatment of ADHD can help improve SUD outcomes.[30] However, studies have overall shown less favorable outcomes in patients diagnosed with both ADHD and SUD. Effective treatment of ADHD can make SUD easier to treat. Typically, stimulant medications are first-line treatment for ADHD. There is no evidence that stimulant treatment increases risk of developing a substance use disorder. However, stimulant medications do have addictive potential. If a patient with a SUD meets ADHD criteria using a validated screening tool, use of a stimulant medication is usually indicated. Besides screening and medication, family and patient education, and counseling concerning substance use need to be part of the treatment plan. It is important to explicitly address with patients signs of possible misuse or diversion of the stimulant medication prescribed, including missed appointments, repeated requests for higher doses, and/or a pattern of "lost" prescriptions. With a specific stimulant SUD, nonstimulant medications, e.g., atomoxetine, a selective norepinephrine reuptake inhibitor, may be a helpful substitution therapy.

In terms of outcome measures, it is important to formally assess improvements for both the ADHD and the SUD. For ADHD, improvement in targeted symptoms and functioning is assessed; for SUD, self-reported abstinence and urine screens are most helpful.

One key point of ADHD diagnosis in the DSM-5 is that "several inattentive or hyperactive-impulsive symptoms were present prior to age 12 years."

Treatment Needs of SUD Among Adolescents in General

Treatment should address the needs of the whole person, rather than just focusing on his or her drug use. Treatment needs to adolescent-focused; the components necessary for successful treatment of adolescent substance use[31] are noted in Fig. 11.1 and Table 11.4.

Evidenced-Based Treatment: Behavioral Therapies[32–37]

Behavioral therapies need to be delivered by clinicians trained not only in the specific behavior therapies noted below, but also trained in adolescent development and adolescent substance use issues. A major focus is

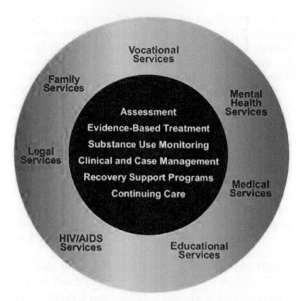

FIG. 11.1 Evidenced-based treatment components for adolescents. (https://www.drugabuse.gov/publications/principles-adolescent-substance-use-disorder-treatment-research-based-guide/principles-adolescent-substance-use-disorder-treatment.)

strengthening the patient's motivation to change. This can be done by:

- Providing incentives for abstinence
- Building skills to resist and refuse addictive substances and deal with triggers or craving
- Replacing drug use with constructive and rewarding activities
- Improving problem-solving skills
- Facilitating better interpersonal relationships.

Specific evidence-based behavioral therapies for adolescents are listed in Table 11.5. Note that no one single therapy has been shown to be superior for all adolescents with problem substance use, and that more than one therapy may be utilized for best results for a given adolescent patient.

Underserved and homeless adolescents, who tend to have higher rates of substance use and problem use, may still benefit from some of the above treatments,[38] with additional support for stable housing, vocational training, and life skills training.

SAFE PRESCRIBING PRACTICES FOR ADOLESCENT DETOX/TREATMENT

Both pharmacologic and nonpharmacologic treatments are indicated for adolescent detox and treatment.[31,39]

TABLE 11.4
Successful Treatment Components of Adolescent Substance Use

1. Adolescent substance use needs to be identified and addressed as soon as possible.
2. Adolescents can benefit from a drug abuse intervention even if they are not addicted to a drug.
3. Routine annual medical visits are an opportunity to ask adolescents about drug use.
4. Legal interventions and sanctions or family pressure may play an important role in getting adolescents to enter, stay in, and complete treatment. Adolescents with substance use disorders rarely feel they need treatment and almost never seek it on their own. Research shows that treatment can work even if it is mandated or entered into unwillingly.
5. Substance use disorder treatment should be tailored to the unique needs of the adolescent.
6. Treatment should address the needs of the whole person, rather than just focusing on his or her drug use.
7. Behavioral therapies are effective in addressing adolescent drug use.
8. Families and the community are important aspects of treatment.
9. Effectively treating substance use disorders in adolescents requires also identifying and treating any other mental health conditions they may have.
10. Sensitive issues such as violence and child abuse or risk of suicide should be identified and addressed.
11. It is important to monitor drug use during treatment.
12. Staying in treatment for an adequate period of time and continuity of care afterward are important.
13. Testing adolescents for sexually transmitted diseases like HIV, as well as hepatitis B and C, is an important part of drug treatment.

TABLE 11.5
Behavioral Therapies for Adolescent Substance Use

- Adolescent Community Reinforcement Approach (A-CRA) replaces influences that had reinforced substance use with healthier family, social, and educational or vocational reinforcers.
- Cognitive Behavioral Therapy (CBT) seeks to help patients recognize, avoid, and cope with the situations in which they are most likely to abuse drugs.
- Contingency Management (CM) uses positive reinforcement such as providing rewards or privileges for remaining drug free, for attending and participating in counseling sessions, or for taking treatment medications as prescribed.
- Motivational Enhancement Therapy (MET) uses strategies to evoke rapid and internally motivated behavior change to stop drug use and facilitate treatment entry.
- Family Therapy (FT) approaches a person's drug problems in the context of family interactions and dynamics that may contribute to drug use and other risky behaviors.
- Complementary Medicine Techniques address stress and triggers for substance use, e.g., Mindfulness-based relapse prevention (MBRP) (Ref. 38)

Nonpharmacologic treatments include:
- Outpatient individual or group.
- Intensive Outpatient (IOP)/Partial Hospitalization Program (PHP).
- Family Therapy and Parent Support.
- Recovery High School: a high school specifically for adolescents in recovery from problem use or addiction, and from which students can graduate with a high school diploma.
- Acute or Long-term Residential.
- Sober Home/Half-Way House: Sober Homes/ Halfway Houses are alcohol and drug free living environments, with a focus on continuing abstinence, until the adolescent seems ready to re-enter a regular living situation.

Pharmacologic Treatments

Three pharmacologic treatments are currently indicated for treating severe opioid use disorder: methadone, buprenorphine, and naltrexone.

Methadone is a full opioid agonist with a long half-life that can ameliorate the cycle of intense euphoria followed by intense withdrawal associated with opioid use. Methadone is mainly for patients >=18 years, although use is allowed for 16–18 year olds if they have twice-failed two opioid detox treatments, and parents give written permission.

Buprenorphine is a partial opioid agonist used to treat opioid use disorders in general medical/office settings for patients 16 and older. Physicians can complete 8 h of training (online or in-person) and apply for a federal government waiver to prescribe buprenorphine. For example, the American Academy of Pediatrics offers this online training at:
https://www.aap.org/en-us/my-aap/Pages/Pediatric-Online-Waiver-Training.aspx

Naltrexone is an opioid antagonist with high affinity for the opioid receptor. Unlike opioid agonists, naltrexone has a very limited potential for misuse or diversion. The extended-release formulation may improve patient adherence. Naltrexone is for patients >=18 years. Naltrexone may also reduce alcohol cravings.

NEEDS OF ADOLESCENTS WHOSE PARENTS OR GUARDIANS ARE ADDICTS

Adolescents need accurate information about addiction, and how it affects the addicted individual, the child/adolescent, and family. The ACES, as previously noted, can be utilized, which focuses on Trauma-Informed Care.[40] A focus on learning new skills and strength-based interventions[41] is important. Treatment needs to be developmentally based, with consideration of age, gender, and cultural background.

Relapse Prevention

Relapse rates for adults with addiction and other substance use disorders (40%–60%) are similar to relapse rates for other well-understood chronic medical illnesses such as diabetes (30%–50%), hypertension (50%–70%), and asthma (50%–70%). For adolescents, relapse rates are as high as or higher than above, in part due to frequency of use, intensity of use, substance used, and psychosocial and developmental factors, as noted previously. Relapse should not be seen as a sign that treatment failed, but as an occasion to engage in additional or different treatment.[31,32,42]

Although there are few approved medications for relapse prevention in adolescents, use of approved medications (e.g., buprenorphine, methadone, and naltrexone for opioid use disorders as discussed above) can be very helpful. For tobacco use disorder, limited research has confirmed that over the counter nicotine replacement treatments, and prescription bupropion, are safe and can be effective in teens <18 years old, though none are FDA approved for minors.

PREVENTION AND POLICY

There are three widely used substance use prevention strategies.[43–45] Primary Prevention (Universal): prevent the problem before it occurs. An example of primary prevention is general substance use education for all youth who are in sixth grade. Secondary Prevention (Selected): targets those who are at-risk of, or starting to have, the problem. An example of secondary prevention is focused substance use education for youth who have gotten in minor trouble for substance use. Tertiary Prevention (Indicated): helps those with problem use get back to good health. An example of tertiary prevention is ongoing treatment and relapse prevention for those with substance use disorders.

Policy strategies utilize individual and environmental intervention approaches as two primary methods for preventing substance use disorders. The most effective prevention interventions incorporate both approaches. Policy strategies are multilevel, including approaches by schools, the local community, and at the state and federal level. An example of a successful policy strategy is Student Assistant Programs (SAPs) in school.[46] SAPs help students stay in school and ultimately do well. These are counter to "Zero-Tolerance" policies, which suspend or expel any student caught using addictive substances at school. SAPs focus on both prevention (universal, selected, and indicated) and intervention (ranging from early to late). Privacy/confidentiality protections for students are necessary, and formal family engagement is crucial. Additionally, regular testing of students for substance use in SAPs is part of successful treatment. SAP staff need to have training in substance use counseling and treatment, cognitive/learning issues, and adolescent development. Relapses during SAP treatment do not equal intervention failures, but need to be explicitly addressed. Community-based referrals for support systems and/or professional care are part of SAPs. Stable funding for long-term outcomes evaluations and standardization of outcomes metrics is important.

OFFICE-BASED SCREENING

Since almost all substance use starts during adolescence, office-based screening is of key importance in prevention and early intervention. Indications for this kind of substance use screening include:

- Adolescent visits for preventive services
- Any youth undergoing mental health treatment
- School dropouts
- Youth demonstrating behavioral changes
- School problems—grades dropping, absences, etc.
- Acute medical problems (GI disturbances, trauma)

The HEADSSSSS Assessment[47] is a commonly used psycho-social assessment for adolescent well-being, including substance use. There are nine components to the latest HEADSSSSS (see Appendices). SBIRT, which stands for Screening, Brief Intervention, and Referral for Treatment, is a simple and straightforward way to assess adolescents for substance use [48–50] (see Appendices). There are three simple yes/no screening questions. For any "yes" answer, the CRAFFT is then utilized (see Appendices). SBIRT utilizes a counseling method of a Brief Intervention (BI), which is a provider—patient interaction whose primary impact is motivational. The BI is used to increase motivation to continue healthy behavior or change unhealthy behavior. The BI ranges from a couple positive feedback statements (e.g., "You're making smart choices not using drugs. Good going.") to 3–5 min of discussion addressing use frequency and intensity; circumstances around use; perceived benefits and risks of use; and patient motivation to change. The provider suggests healthy alternatives to current use. BIs can be more intensive, with 15–30 min of counseling using in-depth Motivational Interviewing techniques,[51] building on the 3–5 min of discussion. See Appendices for the details of these screening tools.

PRIMARY CARE PROVIDER (PCP) MANAGEMENT

Although there are no clear referral guidelines for adolescents with a SUD, unless there are co-occurring mental health issues, those with a mild SUD can likely be managed in primary care.[52] Patients with a moderate SUD may not require a referral to subspecialty care; the referral decision can be left to the discretion of the PCP and his or her comfort with managing SUDs.

Patients with a severe SUD should be referred to subspecialty addiction care. However, since many adolescents with a severe SUD will not accept a referral to treatment, PCPs should be prepared to manage these patients in primary care while trying to facilitate completion of the referral.

CONFIDENTIALITY AND SUBSTANCE USE

Given that substance use is one of a number of sensitive topics that may come up in the course of adolescent care, PCPs should have a systematic way to establish "limits" of confidentiality with both youth and parents in the practice.[52] This is particularly important before a pediatrician begins taking the medical history and screening for drug use. Discussions between the pediatrician and patient should remain confidential unless the pediatrician determines that the reported behaviors are putting either the patient or someone else at acute risk of harm. Determining whether a behavior requires breach of confidentiality is a matter of clinical judgment; in most cases, reports of occasional tobacco, alcohol, or marijuana use can be kept confidential, though a physician may decide to involve parents if a child is very young or being treated for a medical condition that could be dangerously impacted by substance use. Even when there is no reason to breach confidentiality, it is often best to request permission from the youth to engage with parents for their support. In situations where a parent is already aware of use the youth may be willing to share information, particularly if s/he has agreed to a quit attempt or to engage in further treatment.

LABORATORY TESTING

Laboratory testing may be a useful part of a complete assessment for a substance use disorder. As with any laboratory test, this procedure yields limited information and should be used only as an adjunct to the history and physical examination. The use of drug testing in general populations, e.g., school drug testing programs, has less utility and many associated ethical and legal concerns. Drug testing is a complex laboratory procedure with significant potential for false-positive and false-negative results; the American Academy of Pediatrics (AAP) has produced a clinical report to help guide clinicians on how to use this procedure most effectively.[53]

COUNSELING TIPS FOR ADOLESCENTS

I have found the following counseling tips useful for adolescents:

- Brain Development: I say; "Your brain is developing, and will continue to do so into your 20s. Regular substance use may alter normal brain development. That's likely not good." Note that showing fMRI photos of the normal brain and the drug-affected brain can be particularly interesting to adolescents, along with the counseling tip.

- Knowing an alcoholic or an addict: "Do you know anyone who is an alcoholic or a drug addict?" Almost always the answer is "Yes." I say: "Do you think that person started drinking or using drugs to become an alcoholic or an addict? Of course not. But the alcohol or drug took over slowly but surely."

- Control: no adolescent likes to feel controlled by anyone or anything. I say: "Who's in control: you or the drug?" Usually the adolescent says "I am." I say: "If you are, you can cut back or quit anytime, right? So let's do a brief test—try cutting back or quitting for X amount of time. It's your choice to either cut back or quit, and to decide for how long." The adolescent says what he or she is comfortable with, and that will be the plan. Then I say: "I'll see you back in a few weeks, and we'll see how it went." At the follow-up visit, if the adolescent was able to cut back or quit, we discuss how it went, how it felt, and can he or she continue on that path. If the adolescent wasn't able to cut back or quit, then we discuss how the drug may actually be in more control than the adolescent thought, and next steps.

- Goals: I say: "Write down some short- and long-term goals. I'm concerned your drug use may interfere with you reaching them. I'll check in with you every few weeks and we can see how they're going."

- Problem use: I say: "So you don't feel like you have problem use. Great. But, if you were to develop problem use, and hopefully you won't, what would that be like?"

- Cultural norming: "I know your friends use substance X regularly, but actually most kids your age don't. And if they're really your friends, they won't care if you don't use substance X."

SUMMARY

Almost all substance use begins during adolescence. Regular and heavy use of addictive substances may alter normal brain development and cause serious adverse medical, mental health, psychosocial, and cognitive consequences. Prevention and early intervention are key aspects for preventing the development of a substance use disorder. There are successful evidence-based approaches for prevention, early intervention, and treatment of problem substance use in adolescents. Due to the prevalence of co-occurring disorders, adolescents with problem substance use should be evaluated for mental illness and adolescents with mental illness should be evaluated for substance use issues.

APPENDICES
Appendix 1: SBIRT Screen

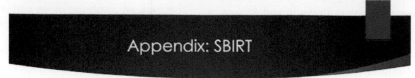

Appendix: SBIRT

SBIRT OPENING SCREENING QUESTIONS:

3 opening screening questions.

▶ In the past 12 months have you:

1. Drunk any alcohol (more than a few sips)?

2. Smoked any marijuana?

3. Used any other drugs to get high (including illegal drugs, non-prescription drugs, prescription drugs, or things you sniff or "huff")?

If "No" to Opening Screening Questions:

▶ No need to perform the CRAFFT

▶ Praise patient for making smart choices: "You have made some very good decisions in your choice not to use drugs and alcohol. I hope you keep it up."

If "Yes" to Opening Screening Questions:

▶ Perform the CRAFFT

Appendix 2: CRAFFT: 2 or More + (Positive)
Answers Likely Indicate An SUD

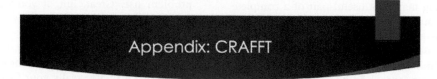

Appendix: CRAFFT

The CRAFFT is a validated and reliable tool to screen for adolescent substance use

▶ Similar to the adult "CAGE" screening tool, but applies to all alcohol and drug use in adolescents

CRAFFT Elements

▶ C Have you ever ridden in a CAR driven by someone (including yourself) who was "high" or had been using alcohol or drugs?

▶ R Do you ever use alcohol or drugs to RELAX, feel better about yourself, or fit in?

▶ A Do you ever use alcohol or drugs while you are by yourself, ALONE?

▶ F Do you ever FORGET things you did while using alcohol or drugs?

▶ F Do your FAMILY or FRIENDS ever tell you that you should cut down on your drinking or drug use?

▶ T Have you ever gotten into TROUBLE while you were using alcohol or drugs?

Appendix 3: HEADSS Screen

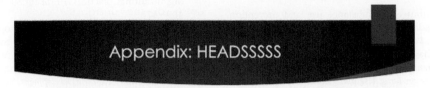

Appendix: HEADSSSSS

9 components, assessing the following aspects of an adolescent's psychosocial situation:

▶ Home
▶ Education
▶ Activities
▶ Drugs* (can use SBIRT here)
▶ Suicidality/Mood
▶ Sexual Activity
▶ Safety
▶ Spirituality
▶ Strengths

REFERENCES

1. http://apps.who.int/adolescent/second-decade/section2/page1/recognizing-adolescence.html.
2. Sanders RA. Adolescent psychosocial, social, and cognitive development. *Pediatr Rev.* 2013;34(8):354–358.
3. https://www.drugabuse.gov/publications/principles-adolescent-substance-use-disorder-treatment-research-based-guide/introduction.
4. LeTendre ML, Reed MB. The effect of adverse childhood experience on clinical diagnosis of a substance use disorder: results of a nationally representative study. *Subst Use Misuse.* 2017;52(6):689–697.
5. Levy S, Bagley S. Substance use: initial approach in primary care. In: McInerny TK, Adam HM, Campbell DE, DeWitt TG, Foy JM, Kamat DM, eds. *American Academy of Pediatrics Textbook of Pediatric Care.* 2nd ed. Elk Grove Village, IL: American Academy of Pediatrics; 2017:1620–1627.
6. Toga AW, Thompson PM, Sowell ER. Mapping brain maturation. *Trends Neurosci.* 2006;29:148–159.
7. Tau G, Peterson BS. Normal development of brain circuits. *Neuropsychopharmacol Rev.* 2010;35:147–168.
8. Jacobus J, Squeglia LM, Alejandra Infante M, et al. Neuropsychological performance in adolescent marijuana users with co-occurring alcohol use: a three-year longitudinal study. *Neuropsychology.* 2015;29(6):829–843.
9. Squeglia1 LM, Gray KM. Alcohol and drug use and the developing brain. *Curr Psychiatry Rep.* 2016;18:46.
10. McQueenya T, Padulaa CB, Pricea J, et al. Gender effects on amygdala morphometry in adolescent marijuana users. *Behav Brain Res.* 2011.
11. Camchong J, Lim KO, Kumra S. Adverse effects of cannabis on adolescent brain development: a longitudinal study. *Cereb Cortex.* 2017;27:1922–1930.
12. Weiland BJ, Thayer RE, Depue BE, et al. Daily marijuana use is not associated with brain morphometric measures in adolescents or adults. *J Neurosci.* 2015;35(4):1505–1512.
13. Morales AM, Ghahremani D, Kohno M, et al. Cigarette exposure, dependence, and craving are related to insula thickness in young adult smokers. *Neuropsychopharmacology.* 2014;39(8):1816–1822.
14. Notterman DA, Mitchell C. Epigenetics and understanding the impact of social determinants of health. *Pediatr Clin N Am.* 2015;62:1227–1240.
15. Baera TE, Gottliebb L, Sandel M. Addressing social determinants of health in the adolescent medical home. *Pediatr Clin N Am.* 2015;62:1227–1240.
16. Chen CU, Storr CL, Anthony JC. Early-onset drug use and risk for drug dependence problems. *Addict Behav.* 2009;34:319–322.
17. http://surveydata.wested.org/resources/Biennial_State_1315.pdf.
18. Monitoring the Future. www.monitoringthefuture.org.
19. Youth Risk Behavior Survey. https://www.cdc.gov/healthyYouth/data/yrbs/index.htm.
20. National Survey of Drug Use and Health. https://nsduhweb.rti.org/respweb/homepage.cfm.
21. Ewing BA, Tucker JS, Miles JNV, et al. Early substance use and subsequent DUI in adolescents. *Pediatrics.* 2015;136(5).
22. Ammerman S, Tau G. Weeding out the truth: adolescents and cannabis. *J Addict Med.* 2016;10:75–82.
23. Ryan S, Ammerman S, the Committee On Substance Abuse. Clinical report: counseling parents and teens about marijuana use in the era of legalization of marijuana. *Am Acad Pediatr;* February 27, 2017. http://pediatrics.aappublications.org/content/early/2017/02/23/peds.2016-4069.

24. NCoAaS A. *Tobacco: The Smoking Gun. Prepared for the Citizen's Commission to Protect the Truth*. Columbia University; 2007.

25. Levy S. Committee on substance use and prevention. Medication-assisted treatment of adolescents with opioid use disorders. *Pediatrics*. 2016;138(3).

26. Center for Behavioral Health Statistics and Quality. *Behavioral Health Trends in the United States: Results from the 2014 National Survey on Drug Use and Health (HHS Publication No. SMA 15–4927, NSDUH Series H-50)*; 2015. http://www.samhsa.gov/data/.

27. Brewer S, Godley MD, Hulvershorn LA. Treating mental health and substance use disorders in adolescents: what is on the menu? *Curr Psychiatry Rep*. 2017;19(5).

28. Casperson S, Tau G, Ammerman S. Weeding out the truth: adolescents and cannabis: case and discussion. *J Addict Med*. 2016;10:83–88.

29. Nelson A, Galon P. Exploring the relationship among ADHD, stimulants, and substance abuse. *J Child Adolesc Psychiatric Nurs*. 2012;25:113–118.

30. Harstad E, Levy S, Committee on Substance Abuse. Attention-deficit/hyperactivity disorder and substance abuse. *Pediatrics*. 2014;134(1).

31. National Institute of Drug Abuse. National Institutes of Health Publication Number 14-7953. *Principles of Adolescent Substance Use Disorder Treatment: A Research-based Guide*. January 2014.

32. *Drugs, Brains, and Behavior: The Science of Addiction*. NIDA. NIH Pub No. 14-5605; 2014.

33. Winters KC, Tanner-Smith EE, Bresani E. Current advances in the treatment of adolescent drug use. *Adolesc Health Med Ther*. 2014;5:199–210.

34. Gray K, Squeglia L. Research Review: what have we learned about adolescent substance use? *J Child Psychol Psychiatry*. 2017:PMID: 28714184.

35. Sussman S, Skara S, Ames SL. Substance abuse among adolescents. *Subst Use Misuse*. 2008;43(12–13):1802–1828.

36. Principles of drug addiction treatment. *A Research-based Guide*. 3rd ed. National Institute on Drug Abuse National Institutes of Health U.S. Department of Health and Human Services; 2012.

37. Bowen S, Witkiewitz K, Clifasefi SL, et al. Relative efficacy of mindfulness-based relapse prevention, standard relapse prevention, and treatment as usual for substance use disorders: a randomized clinical trial. *JAMA Psychiat*. 2014; 71(5):547–556.

38. Slesnick N, Guo X, Brakenhoff B, et al. A comparison of three interventions for homeless youth evidencing substance use disorders: results of a randomized clinical trial. *J Subst Abuse Treat*. 2015;54:1–13.

39. Simkin DR, Grenoble s. Pharmacotherapies for adolescent substance use disorders. *Child Adolesc Psychiatr Clin N Am*. 2010;19:591–608.

40. Lucio R, Nelson TL. Effective practices in the treatment of trauma in children and adolescents: from guidelines to organizational practices. *J Evid Inf Soc Work*. 2016;13(5): 469–478.

41. Black JM, Hoeft F. Utilizing Biopsychosocial and Strengths-based Approaches within the Field of Child Health: What We Know and where We Can Grow. In: Grigorenko EL, ed. *The Global Context for New Directions for Child and Adolescent Development*. Vol. 147. New Directions for Child and Adolescent Development; 2015: 13–20.

42. Catalano RF, Hawkins JD, Wells EA, et al. Evaluation of the effectiveness of adolescent drug abuse treatment, assessment of risks for relapse, and promising approaches for relapse prevention. *Intl J Addict*. 1991;25(9):1085–1140.

43. Harrop E, Catalano RF. Evidence-based prevention for adolescent substance use. *Child Adolesc Psychiatr Clin N Am*. 2016;25:387–410.

44. Stockings E, Hall WD, Lynskey M, et al. Prevention, early intervention, harm reduction, and treatment of substance use in young people. *Lancet Psychiatry*. 2016;3:280–296.

45. https://www.samhsa.gov/capt/practicing-effective-prevention/prevention-approaches.

46. Banys P, Cermak T. Student assistance programs (SAPs): aligning prevention services with need. *A Brief Pap Submitt Calif Blue Ribb Comm Marijuana Policy*; 2015. https://www.safeandsmartpolicy.org/wp-content/uploads/2015/05/Student-Assistance-Programs-authored-and-submitted-by-T-Cermak-MD-and-P-....pdf.

47. Klein D, Goldenring J, Adelman W. HEEADSSS 3.0. The psychosocial interview for adolescents: updated for a new century fueled by media. *Contemp Pediatr*. 2014: 16–28.

48. D'Amico EJ, Parast L, Meredith LS, et al. Screening in primary care: what is the best way to identify at-risk youth for substance use? *Pediatrics*. 2016;138(6): e2 0161717.

49. Levy SJ, Williams JF, COSUP. Policy statement. Substance use screening, brief intervention, and referral to treatment. *Pediatrics*. 2016;(1):138.

50. Levy SJ, Williams JF, COSUP. Clinical report. Substance use screening, brief intervention, and referral to treatment. *Pediatrics*. 2016;(1):138.

51. Barnett E, Sussman S, Smith C. Motivational interviewing for adolescent substance use: A review of the literature. *Addict Behav*. 2012;37:1325–1334.

52. Bagley S, Shrier L, Levy S. Talking to adolescents about alcohol, drugs and sexuality. *Minerva Pediatr*. 2014;66:77.

53. Levy S, Siqueira LM, Committee On Substance Abuse. Clinical report. Testing for drugs of abuse in children and adolescents. *Pediatrics*. 2014;133(6).

CHAPTER 12

How Healers Became Dealers*

ANNA LEMBKE, MD

INTRODUCTION

How did doctors become complicit in the worst opioid epidemic in US history, and why are they continuing to prescribe copious opioids despite increased national awareness of the dangers associated with these drugs? In other words, how did healers become dealers?

To understand the origins, evolution, and persistence of this massive public health debacle, it is essential to understand that opioids never were the solution to patients' problems. They have been and continue to be the solution to doctors' problems. Doctors' problems arise from four invisible forces shaping modern medical practice: the "Toyota-ization" of medicine, the co-optation of medicine by Big Pharma, the medicalization of poverty, and the demonization of pain.

Finding a solution to the current opioid epidemic, an epidemic which is likely to continue for the foreseeable future, will depend upon elucidating how these invisible forces driving overprescribing impact the doctor–patient relationship. We begin by examining what motivates the compassionate doctor. We then explore what motivates the drug-seeking patient. Finally, we examine the complex dance between the compassionate doctor and the drug-seeking patient, when it comes to writing a prescription for a potentially addictive drug. A deeper understanding of the factors contributing to overprescribing offers potential solutions to the current opioid crisis.

WHO IS THE COMPASSIONATE DOCTOR?

To begin, let's first examine this person we call the "compassionate doctor". Why? Because this opioid epidemic is not the result of a few prolific prescribers, otherwise known as "pill mill doctors." The problem of overprescribing is rampant across all medical

specialties all over the nation.[1] We have all become pill mill doctors.

Doctors are by and large pleasers. They make it through the complex maze of schooling all the way to medical school by figuring out early on what other people want and providing it. They are temperamentally anxious, obsessional types, preferring structure and certainty to loose boundaries and uncertainty.

Doctors are motivated by a higher calling. When they graduate from college, usually near or at the top of their class, they can choose to go into any number of professions, from business to law to computer science. They choose medicine, however, because they are looking for a chance to make a real difference in the most tangible sense, by saving lives and alleviating suffering.

Once in medical school, doctors are called upon to empathize with patients and imagine their suffering as their own without judgment. They are socialized to believe their patients, without second-guessing the veracity of their stories. The relationship between doctor and patients is founded on an assumption of trust and mutual cooperation.

Once they enter practice, these perennial A-students are intensely invested in being the best doctor they can be. They are, in other words, narcissistically invested in being successful doctors. This is not to say that doctors are narcissists.

Narcissism is not the exclusive domain of pathological self-involvement. The psychoanalytic conception of narcissism leaves room for "healthy narcissism." Freud described early childhood self-involvement as a normal and healthy part of development. The psychoanalyst Heinz Kohut believed that when the narcissistic demands of early childhood are adequately met by available caregivers, then childhood narcissism evolves into healthy adult self-esteem.[2] Healthy narcissism of adulthood is what allows us to invest our energy and creativity into the things we care about to achieve success, however we define it, whether that activity is bird-watching, parenting, or doctoring.

*This chapter was excerpted and adapted from the book Drug Dealer, MD. *How Doctors Were Duped, Patients Got Hooked, and Why It's So Hard to Stop*. Johns Hopkins University Press; 2016, with the permission of the publisher.

The Assessment and Treatment of Addiction. https://doi.org/10.1016/B978-0-323-54856-4.00012-2

So how do doctors define success? By mutually affectionate interactions with patients. These mutually affectionate interactions are often characterized by a patient's expression of gratitude. What balm to a doctor's soul when the patient says, "Thank-you, doctor, you have really helped me," or "Thank-you, doctor, I don't know what I would have done without you." More objective measures of doctoring-success matter too—a chemotherapy regimen that has eliminated a cancer, or a knee replacement which allows a patient to walk again. But for doctors working day in and day out treating patients, many of whom are chronically ill and will never get better but can only hope not to get worse, the most essential measure of success is a positive, trusting, mutually affectionate interaction.

At its most professionally satisfying, the interaction between doctor and patient can even approach the spiritual, or what philosopher and theologian Martin Buber called an "I and Thou" moment: "Man wishes to be confirmed in his being by man, and wishes to have a presence in the being of the other…. Secretly and bashfully he watches for a YES which allows him to be and which can come to him only from one human person to another."[3]

When these kinds of moments occur between doctor and patient, and thankfully they occur often enough, all the years of schooling, all the exams, all the nights on-call, all the petty bureaucratic demands (which only seem to get worse with each passing day) are worth it for those moments of deeply shared humanity.

WHO IS THE DRUG-SEEKING PATIENT?

Now let's turn our attention to the drug-seeking patient. For the purposes of this discussion, the drug-seeking patient is the patient who attempts to obtain a medication from a doctor for their own, nontherapeutic/addictive use, not the drug-seeking patient who plans to give or sell the medication to others (drug diversion).

The prevailing explanation for drug-seeking is malingering. According to the Diagnostic and Statistical Manual of Mental Disorders (DSM), malingering is "feigning illness with the conscious intent of obtaining some tangible good not related to illness recovery."[4] Malingerers are often seeking a hot meal and shelter (referred to in medical slang as "three hots and a cot"), a disability payment, and/or prescription drugs for nontherapeutic use. Patients who are malingering represent one of the very few instances in medicine in which doctors can refuse care.

But malingering does not fully capture the phenomenon of drug-seeking. Yes drug-seeking patients lie and

manipulate their doctors, and they do so knowingly. But if drugs were really all that mattered, they could obtain them with greater ease from a street dealer or an Internet pharmacy in less time and often less money.

The drug-seeking patient is better understood through the lens of addiction. Addiction is an altered brain state in which motivation for basic survival has been "hijacked" by the drive to obtain and use substances.

Patients use many different strategies to manipulate doctors to get the drugs they want. The myriad ways drug-seeking patients effectively manipulate doctors can be codified into distinct categories, or personas, as follows. These labels are not intended to denigrate drug-seeking patients, but to capture complex behavior in memorable ways.

Sycophants: Sycophants are patients who flatter and cajole, assuring their doctor of their competence and compassion, especially as compared to every other doctor they've seen. The patient satisfaction surveys give this technique additional leverage, because the communication goes beyond just the doctor and the patient. It is unveiled for the larger institution to see, and sometimes the whole Internet world, as in the case of Web-based doctor rating platforms who use patient ratings as the only measure.

Senators: Senators are patients who use the filibuster technique, taking most of the allotted time with the doctor to talk about issues unrelated to the prescription, intentionally waiting until the last few minutes of the encounter to bring it up. In doing so, they are relying on the time pressures they know the doctor is under, to tip the doctor over into prescribing because it is the expedient thing to do. Saying yes to a prescription and ordering it takes less than 1 min. Saying no could take 30 min or more, much less time than the doctor has to stay on schedule.

Exhibitionists: Exhibitionists are patients who display intense emotions and dramatic gestures associated with refill requests. Sometimes they writhe in pain. Other times they achieve various stages of undress to reveal colostomy bags, surgical scars, congenital deformities. The heightened theatrics are intended to illustrate a sense of dire need. As one patient said to me regarding my ability to prescribe him the drugs he was requesting, "I'm on fire, and you've got the hose."

Losers: Losers are patients who exhibit a remarkable tendency to misplace medications. With astonishing regularity, these patients run their medication in the wash cycle, drop them over the side of the fishing boat, flush them down the toilet—water seems to be a common theme. There's also leaving them in a hotel room, being parted from them as a result of lost luggage during a weekend getaway, and yes, I have even heard eaten by the family pet.

Weekenders: Weekenders call for early refills or an increased doses when their regular doctors, the ones who know them best, are least likely to be around. Academic medical centers, where less experienced trainees are most likely to get calls off-hours, are particularly vulnerable to this technique. But large healthcare conglomerates where shift work is the norm also fall prey.

Doctor-Shoppers: Doctor-shoppers are patients who go to multiple doctors simultaneously for the same or similar prescriptions. These patients seek out clinics where drop-in visits are welcome, and where doctors are accustomed to seeing a patient once and possibly never again. Emergency rooms are the ultimate one-stop shopping, because they are staffed by many different doctors. According to one study, doctor-shoppers seeking prescription opioids are more likely to be between 26 and 35 years of age, to pay for prescriptions with cash, and to obtain oxycodone formulations (2.8%), followed by oxymorphone (2.3%), followed by tramadol (2.0%).

Impersonators: Impersonators are patients who assume different identities at different clinics or hospitals—the inverse of doctor shopping. Instead of searching around for different doctors, they become different people.

Dynamic Duos: The Dynamic Duos is patients who present in teams of two, usually the patient and the patient's mother, the most natural codependent. While the patient is writhing in pain, the patient's mother is crying. Together they make a formidable and persuasive team.

Twins: Twins are the patients who are also healthcare providers or occupy a professional and social class that the doctor relates to. These patients know how to create a sense of affiliation with the doctor by talking about the schools they went to, the high-level jobs they've had or have, the people they may know in common. The ones who are healthcare providers use their intimate knowledge of the healthcare system to encourage their doctors to prescribe for them.

Country Mice and City Mice: Country mice and city mice are patients who situate themselves on the opposite ends of the savvy spectrum. The country mouse is the faux-naïve, and the city mouse the slicker. The country mouse pretends to know nothing about prescription medication and gently persuades the doctor to suggest the drugs. The city mouse, by contrast, saunters into the emergency room and announces she is allergic to all pain medications except intravenous Dilaudid push (the "push" meaning the syringe with the opioid

medication is emptied into the bloodstream all at once to create an immediate high) with a Benadryl chaser (Benadryl is an antihistamine known to augment the high of opioids). A nurse practitioner I interviewed told me that she once treated a city mouse who was so resistant to transitioning from intravenous Dilaudid push, given to him in the emergency room, to the oral or rectal opioid she offered him once he was admitted to the floor, that he left the hospital without further treatment.

Bullies: Bullies are patients who use emotional or even physical intimidation to coerce doctors to prescribe. Bullying may represent one of the most effective techniques. These patients have a deep understanding of the fears that plague doctors—the fear of a negative review, the fear of litigation. Patients exploit these fears to serve their own agenda.

Internet Copy-Cats: Internet copy-cats use the Internet to obtain information on how to get drugs from doctors. A Google query of "How to trick dr's to give u pain medicine" gives the following result. "The trick—seriously—is to visit a poor doctor in a poor area of town. Get your textbook list of requirements, pay cash for your appointment, and be the perfect patient. Each time, ask for a little bit more painkillers for a little bit more pain. The doctors want to cover their asses legally and not go to jail or get sued, but it's no hair off their back if you're a lifetime pain mgmt candidate." And "Just look up bullsh_t medical problems like fibromyalgia symptoms and go to the doctor and tell him/her that is how you feel. Fibromyalgia is just a made up medical term for people that want pain killers."

Little Engines that Could: Little engines are patients who plod along, always communicating enough improvement to convince the doctor they're almost there, almost over the hump, while endorsing enough ongoing distress to continue to receive the desired prescription. These are the same patients who say "I really want to get off these meds," but never take the necessary steps to make that happen.

WHAT ARE THE FOUR INVISIBLE FORCES DRIVING OVERPRESCRIBING?

Neither the compassionate doctor nor the drug-seeking patient functions in a vacuum. Both are affected by contextual factors. Let us examine four fundamental changes in healthcare delivery in the past 4 decades, which in sum have conspired to fuel overprescribing, particularly prescribing of addictive drugs like opioid analgesics.

The Toyota-ization of Medicine

In 2002, more than 70% of medical practices were physician owned. Today, more than 70% of doctors work as salaried employees for large hospital conglomerates.[5] In little over 2 decades, a new industrialized approach to medicine on a massive scale has transformed healthcare delivery and contributed to the current prescription drug epidemic.

Physicians today experience growing pressures to see patients quickly, prescribe pills or perform procedures (because that's what pays), palliate pain, protect privacy, and please patients (the P-Paradigm). Doctors resort to prescribing pills because it is fast and pays better than other types of care. Most patients have a different doctor for every body part, making it hard for the right hand to know what the left hand is prescribing. Privacy laws, such as 42CFR, forbid doctors from communicating with other doctors except in cases of emergency, which means the doctor prescribing Vicodin might work right across the hall from the doctor trying to get the patient off. The shift work inherent in industrialized medicine leads to decreased continuity of care, which in turn weakens the therapeutic alliance which is necessary to have those difficult conversations about cutting back or stopping opioids.

Doctors are terrified of negative evaluations or low satisfaction survey rating from a patient and for good reason. A negative review can affect not only reputation, but also salary and professional advancement. Opioids in the short term are an almost guaranteed way to produce a satisfied customer, even with a 5-min visit. They work well short-term for pain, and patients who take them describe feeling "cradled" or "covered by a warm blanket." Patients return a month later and express gratitude, and the prescriber experiences a warm glow. Both patient and doctor are vulnerable to getting addicted to this reinforcing cycle. In short, in this new era of assembly line care, opioids have become proxy for the doctor patient relationship.

The Co-optation of Medicine by Big Pharma

Beginning in the 1980s, there was a movement from within medicine to improve the care of patients with pain; a movement which advocated for, albeit cautiously at first, more liberal use of opioids in the treatment of pain, especially at the end of life. (Prior to 1980, doctors were reluctant to prescribe opioids for fear their patients could get addicted.) The makers of opioid analgesics such as Purdue Pharma (Oxycontin) sensed an opportunity. Taking advantage of the so-called "evidence-based medicine" movement, Purdue and others infiltrated medicine's watch-dog organizations—professional pain societies, continuing medical education meetings, The Joint Commission, the Federation of State Medical Boards, even the Food and Drug Administration—to convince doctors that prescribing opioids for chronic and minor pain was both compassionate and "evidence-based."

Big Pharma enlisted the help of academic "thought leaders" to promote a few small observational studies[6,7] to support the use of opioids in the treatment of chronic pain and to advertise opioids as minimally addictive as long as prescribed by a doctor for a medical condition. They paid these thought leaders to weave a narrative on the benefits of using opioids for chronic pain, despite the absence of evidence.[8] These data were presented at continuing education meetings, which doctors are mandated to attend.

The Joint Commission's job is to accredit hospitals based on performance standards (quality measures) which it creates. According to The Joint Commission's own literature, new standards can only be implemented if they "can be accurately and readily measured."[9] A Joint Commission seal of approval is vital to maintaining cash inflow from third-party payers, like the Center for Medicare and Medicaid Services. In 2001, The Joint Commission made assessment and treatment of pain a "quality measure," echoing the American Pain Society's promulgation of pain as the "fifth vital sign", alongside heart rate, temperature, respiratory rate, and blood pressure.

Pain, however, unlike the original vital signs, cannot be objectively measured. To overcome this barrier, The Joint Commission encouraged use of the Visual Analog Scale of pain assessment: a series of happy and sad faces corresponding to degrees of pain. By assigning pain, a number on a scale from one to ten, with 10 out of 10 pain being the worst pain a human being could endure, and 1 the pain equivalent of, let's say, a stubbed toe, The Joint Commission standardized a process across the country for measuring pain and gave this process the trappings of science by numerizing it. No scientific studies support the use of the Pain Scale to improve pain outcomes. Data do show, however, that use of the Pain Scale increases opioid prescribing and opioid use.

According to a 2003 Government Accountability Office Report, The Joint Commission also disseminated teaching tools (videos, hand-outs) that it received for free from Purdue Pharma, the makers of the opioid Oxycontin, and sold to hospitals nationwide. These educational materials encouraged prescribers to overcome their "opioi-phobia" and use opioids more liberally to target pain.[10]

Today, The Joint Commission denies that it ever promoted opioid prescribing. But by disguising a qualitative and subjective experience, pain, as an objectively measurable data point, and by disseminating material made by Purdue Pharma which encouraged opioid prescribing, The Joint Commission played an important role in opioid overprescribing in the 1990s and early 2000.

Big Pharma's Trojan horse approach was very effective in propagating four myths about opioid prescribing: (1) Opioids work long term for chronic pain, (2) Less than 1% of patients taking opioids prescribed by a doctor will become addicted, (3) No dose is too high, and (4) Patients displaying signs and symptoms of addiction are in fact experiencing "pseudoaddiction" and are actually in pain, the remedy for which is to increase the opioids.

In 2007, Purdue Pharma, the makers of Oxycontin, pleaded guilty to misbranding Oxycontin as less addictive and paid $634 million in fines. But by then, the damage had already been done.

The Medicalization of Poverty

Doctors and other healthcare providers are increasingly asked to care for patients with complex psycho-socio-economic problems, in addition to biomedical problems. At the same time, doctors are not being given the resources needed to tackle problems like chronic pain, chronic depression, addiction, multigenerational trauma, underemployment, malnutrition, or homelessness, nor is the healthcare delivery system designed to manage chronic conditions effectively. A mechanized medical system modeled on the Toyota car-making company is better suited to one-time replacement repair of body parts, such as knee replacement surgery or cataract removal.

As a result, doctors have been forced to medicalize social problems. They use opioids as a desperate attempt to provide short-term relief and comfort to patients struggling with multilayered problems. People receiving Medicaid, federal insurance for poor and indigent populations, are prescribed opioid painkillers at twice the rate of non-Medicaid patients and die from prescription overdoses at six times the rate of non-Medicaid patients.[11] Twenty-percent of pregnant women on Medicaid fill an opioid prescription during pregnancy.[12]

At the same time that doctors are ill equipped to handle the social and economic problems of their patients, patients themselves have been incentivized to seek out and maintain the sick role as a way to procure an income. A subset of disability seekers and holders take medications in part to validate their sick-role status. Getting well threatens their only income. This phenomenon has created a generation of professional patients, consuming pills not to treat an illness, but to pay the bills.

In the early 1980s, the monetary value of Social Security Disability Insurance (SSDI, federally funded support for those who cannot work due to illness and have paid Social Security taxes through prior employment) began steadily rising, especially for lower income wage earners, making disability more attractive than available employment options. Changes in disability laws in the mid 1980s made it easier to get disability for pain and mental illness.[13]

In 1957, 150,000 American were receiving SSDI, and the most common disability diagnoses were cancer and cardiac disease. Today, over 8 million people are receiving SSDI, and the most common disability diagnoses are mental illness and musculoskeletal disorders, i.e., chronic pain. According to the US Census Bureau 2006, 40 million American receive disability compensation through one of the three federally funded agencies that provide disability compensation (SSDI, SSI, VDC). Most are poor and undereducated.

Although much of the media attention to date has been focused on the ways in which the current opioid epidemic has crossed socioeconomic and racial boundaries, i.e., it has penetrated into the white middle class, it is still true that the poor have been disproportionately affected by this epidemic, and disability status has contributed to the problem.

Karl Marx once quipped "Religion is the opium of the masses." Today, sadly, opium has become the religion of the masses.

New Illness Narratives Promote Pills as Quick-Fixes for Pain

Autobiographical narratives are the stories we tell about our lives, and they are as fundamental to human existence as breathing. Our life stories connect us to others, organize experience, and shape time. Autobiographical narratives are deeply influenced by the prevailing culture, e.g., religious affiliation, ethnic background, and contemporaneous historical events. Just like a fish does not recognize water, we are seldom aware of the way implied cultural narratives filter our own experiences and in turn influence future actions: culture shapes narrative, and narrative shapes experience.

One hundred and 50 years ago, doctors viewed pain as salutary, believing it boosted the immune and cardiovascular systems.[14] When modern forms of analgesia and anesthesia were introduced around 1850, leading surgeons were reluctant to adopt these practices, convinced that experiencing some degree of pain abetted the healing process.

Contrast that view of pain with today's contemporary view, in which hurt in any form is tantamount to harm, and any doctor who does not work to eliminate all pain is fundamentally lacking in compassion. Indeed, we now believe pain can leave a psychic scar that causes future pain in the form of post-traumatic stress disorder (PTSD) or a centralized pain syndrome. In other words, pain is dangerous. Other contemporary narratives that have contributed to overprescribing include: "People are fragile and the body cannot heal itself," "Doctors have infinite ability to heal," and "Illness is identity and victimhood a right to be compensated."

The Upshot

These four invisible forces—the Toyota-ization of medicine, Big Pharma's infiltration of medicine's watch-dog organizations under the guise of "science," the medicalization of poverty, and new illness narratives which conceptualize all pain as dangerous and every patient as a potential victim—have fundamentally altered the doctor–patient relationship.

No longer are doctors and patients alone in the exam room. They are accompanied by a host of invisible partners with demands that may have little to do with treating illness: Patient Relations stands gazing into the mirror, a patient satisfaction survey on a clipboard in her hand; Billing is standing on the scale, the numbers on display never far from her mind; Disability Claims sits with one leg in a cast, propped on the empty chair; The Joint Commission is digging through a file cabinet, a magnifying glass in hand; Private Insurance is occupying the chair intended for the patient, distracted and encumbered by a stack of prior authorization forms; the Centers for Medicare and Medicaid Services, morbidly obese, is leaning precariously on the edge of the exam table; Big Pharma hides in the corner, just out of sight, confidently spinning a drug company pen; The State Medical Board is hovering behind the doctor, looking stern and unyielding; and two lawyers, the hospital's legal council and the patient's lawyer, are facing off, fists raised, ready to do battle. Time personified is there, ticking steadily, reminding the doctor that time is short and other patients are waiting.

The impact of this transformation on healthcare delivery, and its contribution to the prescription drug epidemic, cannot be underestimated. With awareness of this larger context, we can now drill down to the specific interactions between the compassionate doctor and the drug-seeking patient, to explore the dynamic which leads to overprescribing.

WHAT HAPPENS WHEN THE COMPASSIONATE DOCTOR AND THE DRUG-SEEKING PATIENT MEET?

When the compassionate doctor and the drug-seeking patient enter an exam room, what the doctor experiences is anxiety. Maybe not consciously, but anxiety nonetheless. If the doctor mistrusts the patient or questions the patient's story, then the doctor is not living up to the principles of empathy and compassion. If the doctor openly challenges the patient, she risks the mutually affectionate interaction which is key to measuring her day-to-day success as a "good doctor." On the other hand, if she doesn't challenge the drug-seeking patient, then she is also not living up to the ideal of the compassionate healer. In short, the doctor is stuck between a prescription and a hard place, and the result is anxiety.

What does the doctor do with this anxiety? She buries it by turning to primitive, largely unconscious defense mechanisms. First described by Freud, defense mechanisms are automatic, unconscious psychological maneuvers human beings employ to avoid having to cope with or even acknowledge uncomfortable emotions.

The psychiatrist George Vaillant classified defense mechanisms into four levels, from pathological defenses such as denial, to immature defenses such as wishful thinking, to neurotic defenses such as rationalization, to mature defenses such as humor.[15] The important implication of Vaillant's classification is that we all employ unconscious defense mechanisms all the time to defend against all types of anxiety; and in times of acute distress, defenses mechanisms, even primitive ones, are adaptive. However, in our everyday lives, defense mechanisms tend to be maladaptive and should not be confused with coping strategies, which are adaptive and conscious. Typical defense mechanisms that doctors use with drug-seeking patients include passive aggression, projection, splitting, and denial, as follows.

Passive aggression is defined as aggression toward others expressed indirectly or passively, most often through avoidance and procrastination. Examples include finding reasons to cancel visits with such patients, rounding quickly on them in the hospital, or not at all, writing extended refills to minimize contact, not returning their phone calls, etc.

Projection is attributing a moral or psychological deficiency in ourselves to another individual or group. Doctors often project the contempt they feel for themselves around lax prescribing, onto their patients. It is easier for doctors to see patients as morally deficient than to acknowledge the ways in which they have abdicated their responsibilities to the patient in prescribing medications that may be harming rather than helping them. In this scenario, the doctor thinks "What is wrong with this patient? Can't she get it together and take the medicine like she's supposed to?!" instead of "What is wrong with me, and with the system, that I would prescribe a medication I know is not helping?"

The "splitting" defense involves segregating experience into all good and all bad categories, with no room for ambiguity or ambivalence. Doctors typically engage in splitting by mentally segregating drug-seeking patients into the category of "bad patients," as distinct from "good patients." A good patient takes many forms depending on the doctor, but is often the patient who expresses gratitude, gets better, and/or can be seen quickly. Bad patients are those who threaten the doctor's sense of competence as healer, or trigger negative emotions like anxiety, impatience, and anger.

Of all the primitive defenses doctors employ against drug-seeking patients, the most common and insidious is probably denial. Denial is the refusal to accept a threatening reality by simply believing it doesn't exist. This includes refusing even to perceive or acknowledge certain truths, like the fact that we are in the midst of a national prescription drug epidemic. For the past 2 decades, even very good doctors have ignored suspicious patterns of medication use, dispensed early refills, disregarded escalating doses, and failed to access data that would give them the information they need to make a more accurate assessment of current medication use, such as their state's prescription drug monitoring program (PDMP).

Despite a major public health campaign to encourage doctors to register for and utilize their states' PDMP, only 35% of doctors practicing in America today access their state's PDMP.[16] Time constraints hinder doctors' ability and willingness to gain access to and utilize the database. But without checking the PDMP, responsible prescribing of controlled drugs in the modern healthcare system borders on impossible.

New legislation in some states mandates that doctors gain access to their states' PDMP. Some states have even gone further, requiring that doctors check the PDMP before writing a prescription for any scheduled medication.

What happens when primitive defenses like denial no longer work, for example when the prescription drug monitoring database shows overt drug-seeking and the doctor is forced to acknowledge that she has been supplying drugs to an individual who has been misusing them. At this point, the doctor is unmasked

as nothing more than a gatekeeper of goods and services, or worse yet, a drug dealer, and she experiences a narcissistic injury. A narcissistic injury strikes at the heart of our sense of competence and self-esteem. It is extremely painful to experience, and the reaction is primordial, reflexive, and hostile. The idealized response, by contrast, is compassion and professionalism even in the face of these challenges.

In the last 5 years, the entire medical profession has experienced a narcissistic injury as a result of the media spotlight highlighting the harm done to patients from drugs obtained from doctors, tarnishing doctors' reputations and publicly shaming them. As a result, some doctors have not merely become more cautious about prescribing opioids to patients in pain, they have gone so far as to refuse to treat pain, declaring this out of their scope of practice. Dr. Steven Passik coined a phrase to describe these patients: "opioid refugees."

The term is apt, as one imagines these patients wandering from clinic to clinic trying to find a doctor to treat their pain. The rejection of these patients is furthermore not likely due to the stigma of addiction. Doctors don't throw patients out for misusing alcohol, smoking cigarettes, or even being addicted to heroin. It is the doctors' complicity in the patient's addiction which triggers the narcissistic injury and the retaliatory response.

This kind of permanent retaliation has created more problems than it has solved. Some patients may be turning to illicit sources of opioids, namely heroin, since doctors are no longer willing to prescribe for them. There are as yet no definitive data to support this hypothesis, outside of the remarkable statistic that three-quarters of people who use heroin today began with a prescription opioid.[17] Heroin use may be fueled by the search for cheaper and more readily accessible alternatives, rather than a crackdown on prescribing per se.

CONCLUSION—HOW CAN WE MOVE FORWARD?

The silver lining of the opioid epidemic—if a silver lining can be found for a public health tragedy which has killed more people than the Iraq and Vietnam wars combined—is that the medical profession is finally forced to consider the problem of addiction. Our complicity through egregious overprescribing, and the sheer scale of drug overdose deaths (an estimated 64,000 in 2016 alone) has meant we can no longer turn a blind eye.

I, like many of my colleagues in the field of addiction medicine, believe that tackling this epidemic will require a paradigm shift in the way medicine is practiced: *We must embrace addiction as a disease and treat it as such in the House of Medicine.* Patients should be able to walk into any primary care clinic, perinatal birthing center, or emergency department in the country and say "I have addiction, will you help me?" followed by a resounding "Yes!"

We need to embrace addiction as a disease not because science proves it is one (I believe reasonable people can disagree on that point), but because it is the best response to a public health crisis that shows no signs of abating. It is the model for our time.

Diseasifying problems is how contemporary society solves them. If we fail to diseasify addiction, especially as we continue to biologize and medicate other disorders with no objectively verifiable pathology, overprescribing will continue unchecked. The disease model allows physicians to rekindle compassion for the drug-seeking and addicted patient, a reframe which is as important for healthcare providers as it is for patients. The disease model decreases stigma, promoting access to treatment and research funding. The disease model works. When treatment for addiction is integrated into mainstream medical care, patients show similar rates of recovery, adherence to treatment, and recurrence (relapse), as patients being treated for type II diabetes, asthma, and certain types of heart disease (other chronic disorders with a behavioral component).[18] Healthcare systems also save money.

To make this vision a reality, we need to build a robust addiction treatment infrastructure integrated and colocated within the rest of medicine. Third-party payers must reimburse addiction treatment on par with treatment for other medical disorders, already law through the Mental Health Parity and Addiction Equity Act of 2008, but infrequently and inconsistently enforced. Doctors (and other healthcare providers) need to be trained from the first day of medical school to screen and intervene for substance use problems.

Our current assembly line approach to medical care creates perverse incentives that encourage overprescribing and will not work for the treatment of addiction (just as it does not work for the treatment of chronic pain). We need a chronic care model that incentivizes providers to talk to patients, educate patients, and spend time with patients, not just prescribe pills and perform procedures. Outcomes should be based not *only* on whether patients get well, but also on the effectiveness of the doctor—patient relationship to encourage effortful engagement in getting well, and judicious consumption of medical care in the context of chronic poor health. Patients and providers need time to engage in meaningful discussions about what it means to suffer, and how to define recovery in the midst of suffering.

If medicine is to be the social safety net to take care of this country's social, economic, and spiritual problems, then let's give healthcare providers the training, resources, and infrastructure they need to target the problems patients really have. Otherwise, we continue to run the risk that psycho-spiritual and socioeconomic problems will be treated as biomedical problems, and dangerous overprescribing will continue.

REFERENCES

1. Chen JH, Humphreys K, Shah NH, Lembke A. Distribution of opioids by different types of Medicare prescribers. *JAMA Intern Med.* December 2015:1—3. https://doi.org/10.1001/jamainternmed.2015.6662.
2. Kohut H. *The Kohut Seminars: On Self Psychology and Psychotherapy with Adolescents and Young Adults.* Vol (Elson M, ed.). New York: W.W. Norton and Company; 1987.
3. Buber M. *I and Thou.* Charles Scribner's Sons; 1937.
4. *Diagnostic and Statistical Manual of Mental Disorders.* Washington, DC: American Psychiatric Association; 2013.
5. Kocher R, Sahni N. Hospitals' race to employ physicians—the logic behind a money losing proposition. *N Engl J Med.* 2011:1790—1793.
6. Portenoy RK, Foley KM. Chronic use of opioid analgesics in non-malignant pain: report of 38 cases. *Pain.* 1986; 25(2):171—186.
7. Porter J, Jick H. Addiction rare in patients treated with narcotics. *N Engl J Med.* 1980;302(2):123.
8. Live interview with Dr. Russel Portenoy. *Physicians Responsible Opioid Prescr.* https://www.youtube.com/watch?v=DgyuBWN9D4w.
9. The Joint Commission. http://www.jointcommission.org/.
10. GAO. Prescription OxyContin abuse and diversion and efforts to address the problem. *J Pain Palliat Care Pharmacother.* 2003;18(3):109—113. https://doi.org/10.1300/J354v18n03_12.
11. Mack KA, Zhang K, Paulozzi L, Jones C. Prescription practices involving opioid analgesics among Americans with Medicaid, 2010. *J Health Care Poor Underserved.* 2015; 26(1):182—198. https://doi.org/10.1353/hpu.2015.0009.
12. Desai RJ, Hernandez-Diaz S, Bateman BT, Huybrechts KF. Increase in prescription opioid use during pregnancy among Medicaid-enrolled women. *Obstet Gynecol.* 2014; 123(5):997—1002.
13. Autor DH, Duggan MG. The growth in the social security disability rolls: a fiscal crisis unfolding. *J Econ Perspect.* 2006;20(3):71—96.
14. Meldrum ML. A capsule history of pain management. *JAMA.* 2003;290(18):2470—2475. https://doi.org/10.1001/jama.290.18.2470.

15. Vaillant GE, Bond M, Vaillant CO. AN empirically validated hierarchy of defense mechanisms. *Arch Gen Psychiatry*. 1986;43(8):786–794.

16. Perrone J, Nelson LS. Medication reconciliation for controlled substances — an "ideal" prescription-drug monitoring program. *N Engl J Med*. 2012;366(25): 2341–2343. https://doi.org/10.1056/NEJMp1204493.

17. Lankenau SE, Teti M, Silva K, Jackson Bloom J, Harocopos A, Treese M. Initiation into prescription opioid misuse amongst young injection drug users. *J Drug Policy*. 2012;23(1):37–44.

18. McLellan AT, Lewis DC, O'Brien CP, Kleber HD. Drug dependence, a chronic medical illness: implications for treatment, insurance, and outcomes evaluation. *JAMA*. 2000;284:1689–1695. https://doi.org/10.1097/00132586-200108000-00061.

CHAPTER 13

Trauma and Addiction—How to Treat Co-occurring PTSD and Substance Use Disorders

DOLORES VOJVODA, MD • ISMENE PETRAKIS, MD

Posttraumatic stress disorder (PTSD) is a disabling psychiatric disorder that develops after an exposure to a severe traumatic event. According to Diagnostic and Statistical Manual of Mental Disorders (DSM)-5 diagnostic criteria, a traumatic event is defined as exposure to actual or threatened death, serious injury, or sexual violence. Exposure to a traumatic event is very common; up to 90% of population has experienced a qualifying traumatic event[1,2] but only 7.8% develop PTSD over a lifetime.[3] In at-risk populations (such as women, younger persons, military personnel, police officers), its prevalence is much higher.[4] For example, PTSD affects up to 38% of Vietnam War veterans and up to 65% of rape victims over a lifetime.[3] The DSM-5 diagnosis of PTSD consists of four symptom clusters: (1) Intrusion symptoms; (2) Avoidance of stimuli associated with the traumatic event; (3) Negative alterations in cognitions and mood and; (4) Marked alterations in arousal and reactivity. Exposure to multiple traumatic events is associated with more severe PTSD symptomatology, higher functional impairment, and higher comorbidity with mood and anxiety disorders.[4] In addition, many individuals suffer from posttraumatic symptoms that do not meet full criteria for PTSD, such as intrusive and distressing recollections or thoughts, hypervigilance, distressing dreams of the trauma, and psychological reactions to trauma cues.[5]

Individuals with PTSD have elevated rates of comorbid disorders, notably substance use disorders. One large study of general population found alcohol dependence to be the most common co-occurring disorder in men with PTSD, followed by depressive disorder, anxiety disorders, conduct disorder, and drug use disorder.[3] In this study, 51.9% of men and 27.9% of women with PTSD met criteria for substance use disorder (SUD) and the most common substance used (other than nicotine) was alcohol. The National Vietnam Veterans Readjustment Study of Vietnam Veterans found that 74% of combat Vietnam Veterans with lifetime PTSD had comorbid SUD.[6] A more recent study[7] found that among individuals with PTSD, nearly half (46.4%) met criteria for SUD. Looking at it from another perspective, specifically treatment-seeking populations with SUD, there are higher rates of comorbidity with PTSD compared to the general population. For example, in a study of Operation Enduring Freedom/OEF and Operation Iraqi Freedom/OIF veterans seeking care at the Veterans Administration (VA), 63% veterans diagnosed with substance use disorder had comorbid PTSD.[8]

When PTSD and SUD co-occur, this has important clinical implications because individuals who have both disorders have worse outcomes, including higher rates of comorbid mental health disorders and medical problems, more functional impairments across multiple domains, higher rates of hospitalizations, as well as underemployment and homelessness.[9–11] Patients with PTSD and SUD often suffer from more severe PTSD symptoms than do patients with PTSD alone.[12] Heavy drinkers have been found to report more severe PTSD symptoms than moderate drinkers or nondrinkers.[13]

Given the high rates of comorbidity, accurately screening at risk populations is of great importance. In substance use specialty clinics, screening tools that can be used include the PTSD checklist (PCL).[14] PCL is a 20-item self-report measure that assesses the 20 DSM-5 symptoms of PTSD. It is easy to administer and provides a provisional PTSD diagnosis. In specialty PTSD clinics, screening for substance and alcohol use disorder is similarly important and there are several commonly used and validated screening tools. These include

The Assessment and Treatment of Addiction. https://doi.org/10.1016/B978-0-323-54856-4.00013-4

CAGE questionnaire[15] and the Alcohol Use Disorders Identification Test (AUDIT-C).[16] The CAGE questionnaire is a combination of four simple screening questions, with two or more positive answers indicating a positive history of alcoholism; however, it is nonspecific for current use. The AUDIT-C is a 3-item alcohol screen that can help identify patients who are hazardous drinkers or have active alcohol use disorders.

There are several strategies that can be used to treat comorbidity, and they include pharmacotherapy interventions and behavioral treatments. While there are other reviews that have been published reviewing pharmacotherapy approaches,[17–22] this review will focus on practical information for clinicians as well provide insight into future directions. Since there is a growing literature specifically evaluating medications to treat these disorders, clinicians can make evidence-based decisions on the best treatment strategies to address these issues. A review of the behavioral treatments is beyond the scope of this chapter, but for a recent review see Simpson et al.[23]

TREATMENT

Historically, treatment of SUD and PTSD comorbidity has been separate rather than integrated, provided by different clinicians and in even within different treatment settings. Many treatment settings specializing in PTSD would not treat PTSD in individuals who were active substance users; conversely, substance use disorder specialty clinics did not screen or recognize PTSD. There was also the perception that treatment to address trauma in comorbidity might actually make substance use worse. Recently, there is a better appreciation that postponing treatment of either disorder can lead to poorer outcomes; for example, ongoing and untreated symptoms of PTSD may be associated with relapse so it is important to treat the two disorders simultaneously, as that approach leads to best treatment outcomes. Nevertheless, there is still some question about how to best integrate the treatments, both in terms of pharmacotherapy and behavioral treatments, but there are some clear clinical considerations that are well established. For example, in cases of a substance use disorder, withdrawal management (i.e., "detoxification") might be medically indicated and as such would be the first step in the treatment process. It is important to remember that PTSD can intensify the severity of withdrawal symptoms (and vice versa), so in this group of individuals a supervised withdrawal management in a medical facility might be necessary. Conversely, for acute suicidality or other psychiatric

emergencies, adequate psychiatric treatment would be the first step of treatment and may even require inpatient psychiatric treatment before initiating outpatient treatment. The review will focus on nonemergent care in an outpatient setting.

Pharmacotherapies
Medications used to treat SUD (see Table 13.1)
Naltrexone and disulfiram have been successfully used in treatment of AUD for several decades in noncomorbid populations and are approved by the Food and Drug Administration (FDA) to treat alcohol us.[24] Several studies have evaluated medications to treat alcohol use disorders in patients with comorbidity. In 2006, a large (N = 254), randomized, double-blind clinical trial of AUD and comorbid Axis I psychiatric disorders examined effectiveness of naltrexone and disulfiram in veteran population.[25] Four treatment groups were compared: naltrexone, disulfiram, naltrexone and disulfiram and placebo. Those treated with any medication, or medication combination, had better alcohol use outcomes than placebo, although

TABLE 13.1
Summary of Evidence for Pharmacological Treatment of Comorbid AUD and PTSD

	AUD Symptoms	PTSD Symptoms
MEDICATIONS TO TREAT SUD (AUD)		
naltrexone	↓ ↔	↓ ↔
Naltrexone and Prolonged exposure	↓	↓
disulfiram	↓	↓
topiramate	↓ ↓	↓ ↓
MEDICATIONS TO TREAT PTSD		
sertraline	↓ ↔	↓ ?
sertraline and Seeking Safety	↔	↓
paroxetine	↔	↓
desipramine	↓	↓
prazosin	↓ ↔	↔ ↓
FUTURE DIRECTIONS		
N-acetylcysteine (NAC)[a]	↓	↓

↓, decrease in symptoms; ↔, no change in symptoms; ?, unclear results.
[a] In SUD.

there was no advantage to the combination. The PTSD subgroup (N = 87) had good outcomes, with even more robust reduction in alcohol use and an overall improvement in symptoms of PTSD in individuals who abstained from alcohol. Disulfiram was more effective than naltrexone in lowering overall PTSD and hyperarousal symptoms, while naltrexone and disulfiram lowered re-experiencing symptoms and were better than the combination. The study found that both naltrexone and disulfiram were safe and effective for patients with comorbid AUD and PTSD. Clinically, since neither medication was superior, prescriber and patient preference should be taken into account when prescribing medication.[17]

A more recent study evaluated the efficacy of adjunctive naltrexone to antidepressant medication (paroxetine and desipramine) in male veterans (N = 88) with AUD and PTSD.[26] Naltrexone was associated with a significant reduction in alcohol craving relative to placebo, but it showed no advantage to drinking use outcomes or PTSD symptoms. Foa et al.[27] examined the efficacy of naltrexone combined with an evidence-based treatment for PTSD—prolonged exposure therapy (PE). Participants (N = 165) were randomized into four treatment groups: PE and naltrexone, PE alone, supportive counseling and naltrexone and supportive counseling alone. Post-treatment, there was a reduction in PTSD symptoms in all four groups. However, the participants who received naltrexone had a lower percentage of days drinking than those who received placebo. At the 6-month follow-up, there was an increase in percentage of days drinking in all four groups, but in the PE and naltrexone group that increase was the smallest.

There is considerable evidence for the anticonvulsant topiramate as a treatment option for individuals with AUD as it seems to be effective in decreasing heavy drinking.[28,29] There is some evidence of its efficacy in those with comorbid PTSD: for example, an open-label pilot study[30] evaluated the efficacy of topiramate as an add-on therapy in male combat veterans with PTSD, the majority of whom (82.1%) were drinkers. After 8 weeks of treatment, veterans showed an improvement in PTSD symptoms (e.g., nightmares) and a reduction in alcohol intake. A more recent, randomized, double-blind, placebo-controlled pilot trial of flexible-dose topiramate in 30 veterans with PTSD and AUD[31] showed that topiramate treatment resulted in significant reduction in alcohol craving and frequency and amount of alcohol use. It also decreased severity of PTSD symptoms, especially those in the

hyperarousal cluster. Batki et al.[31] postulated that topiramate might be especially useful in treatment of patients with comorbid AUD and PTSD and particularly severe hyperarousal symptoms. The latter is an interesting finding because earlier studies of topiramate in treatment of PTSD without comorbidity[32,33] showed reductions in re-experiencing and avoidance symptoms, leading open the question of whether there are different effects in those with comorbid AUD and those without.

Topiramate is significantly associated with cognitive side effects (e.g., a decrease in verbal learning and memory), and this was empirically evaluated in the Batki comorbidity study. In that study, topiramate was significantly associated with cognitive side effects, which did improve after discontinuation.[31] This, combined with a long titration somewhat limits its clinical use—particularly in those with comorbidity.[19]

Medications used to treat PTSD (see Table 13.1)

Several selective serotonin reuptake inhibitors (SSRIs) and serotonin and norepinephrine reuptake inhibitors (SNRIs) have shown efficacy in reduction of PTSD symptoms severity including paroxetine,[34] sertraline,[35,36] fluoxetine,[37,38] and venlafaxine.[39] At this time, paroxetine and sertraline are the only medications approved by the FDA for the treatment of PTSD. However, their effects are modest and they seem to be less effective in veteran populations.[40,41] An early small open-label study of sertraline in the treatment of comorbid SUD and PTSD was encouraging,[42] with findings of a decrease in the number in standard drinks and an increase in the days of abstinence, and a decrease in PTSD symptom severity across all three PTSD symptoms clusters. These findings, however, were not supported by a larger trial.[43] In this randomized, placebo-controlled, 12-week trial of sertraline in 94 individuals with comorbid AUD and PTSD, sertraline was not superior to placebo in reducing alcohol use or PTSD outcomes. However, sertraline was more effective for a subgroup of patients with less severe AUD and early-onset PTSD.

A study by Hein et al.[44] evaluated the benefit of combining Seeking Safety, a cognitive-behavioral therapy for co-occurring PTSD and AUD, with sertraline. All 69 participants received the Seeking Safety therapy and were randomized to either sertraline or placebo during the 12-week trial. Both groups reported significant improvements in PTSD symptoms, with the Seeking Safety plus sertraline group demonstrating a significantly greater reduction in PTSD symptoms than Seeking Safety plus placebo group, even though the magnitude of effect was small (d = 0.19). There was a significant reduction in AUD outcomes overall, with no difference between sertraline and placebo groups.

In the previously mentioned study by Petrakis et al,[26] 88 veterans with AUD and PTSD were enrolled in a trial in which paroxetine, an SSRI, was compared to desipramine, a norepinephrine reuptake inhibitor, and also evaluated for adjunctive effects of naltrexone. Participants were randomly assigned to four groups: paroxetine and naltrexone, paroxetine and placebo, desipramine and naltrexone, and desipramine and placebo. Paroxetine and desipramine were equally effective in treatment of PTSD; however, desipramine was more effective in reduction of alcohol use.

Overall, these studies suggest that the serotonergic medications to treat PTSD are somewhat effective even in comorbidity, but there is no evidence to support their use in decreasing alcohol use. This suggests that while they may be safe and effective, they should be combined with other treatment modalities designed to treat the AUD. There are, however, some encouraging data that support further research of the noradrenergic antidepressant desipramine for patients with comorbid AUD and PTSD.

Several recent studies of prazosin have shown great promise in treatment of PTSD symptoms, especially in reduction of nightmares and sleep disturbance.[45–48] Disappointingly, the most recent and largest study,[49] however, found prazosin to be ineffective in alleviating nightmares or improving sleep quality in veterans with PTSD. In animal studies, prazosin suppressed ethanol consumption in rats.[50,51] Two randomized placebo-controlled trials evaluated its efficacy in decreasing alcohol consumption in individuals with PTSD. In the first study[52] of 30 subjects, results showed a reduction in the severity and frequency of heavy drinking in prazosin-treated subjects after 6 weeks of treatment. There was, however, no difference in the PTSD symptoms in the prazosin and placebo group. In the second, larger study (N = 98) of veteran population, prazosin was not superior to placebo in either reducing PTSD symptoms or alcohol consumption.[53] Together, prazosin does not seem to be effective in treating symptoms of PTSD in comorbidity, but its effects on alcohol are contradictory and further study would be indicated to evaluate these findings.

CANNABIS AND PTSD

A growing number of states have legalized medical use of cannabis for a number of medical and psychiatric conditions, including PTSD. The approval for cannabis use has come through state legislative process or popular vote.[54] It remains illegal under federal law and continues to be a Schedule I substance. Cannabis, or any cannabinoid, has not been approved by the FDA for the treatment of any psychiatric disorder. Nevertheless, it has been approved legally for a PTSD "indication" in several states and psychiatrists and other physicians are frequently asked to prescribe cannabis to patients with PTSD. There are still many questions about whether cannabis is helpful in decreasing symptoms of PTSD. A recent publication[55] reviewed existing studies of cannabis or other cannabinoids in individuals with PTSD. Two retrospective chart reviews[56,57] and an open-label study[58] reported improvement in sleep and reduction in nightmares after administration of a synthetic cannabinoid nabilone. In a longitudinal, observational study[54] of veterans with PTSD, cannabis use was associated with worsening of PTSD symptoms, violent behavior, and misuse of alcohol and drugs. However, to date, there are no randomized clinical trials (RTCs) examining the efficacy or safety of cannabis in PTSD.

It should be noted that the potential risks of cannabis use include tolerance, dependence, withdrawal, and cognitive effects. Long-term cannabis use is associated with cognitive decline, with, among other effects, a decline in IQ,[59] especially in adolescents, and risk for emergence or worsening of psychosis.[60] There is evidence that, in some individuals, cannabinoids worsen anxiety.[61] A recent review article[62] examined evidence for and against use of cannabis and cannabinoids in individuals with PTSD and called for the slowing in the pace of legalization of cannabis for therapeutic use until we have better scientific data about the risks and benefits of this substance in individuals with PTSD. This is particularly important for those with comorbid substance use disorder, since cannabis may exacerbate the substance abuse, or individuals with SUD may be more prone to abuse of cannabis. Certifying physicians should be aware of the lack of clear evidence for use of cannabis in PTSD and its potential of worsening of the existing substance use disorder.

FUTURE DIRECTIONS

Several agents have been evaluated in pilot work for efficacy in PTSD and comorbid SUD. For example, n-acetylcysteine (NAC) has been increasingly investigated as a pharmacologic agent for several different psychiatric disorders, including addictive disorders. A recent study[63] explored the efficacy of NAC in the treatment of PTSD and SUD, with encouraging results. The participants treated with NAC, in combination with psychotherapy, reported significant reduction in PTSD symptoms, craving and depression. The study is limited by its small sample size (N = 35), but is being investigated in a larger trial (see Table 13.1).

Ketamine, an NMDA receptor antagonist, is used as an anesthetic agent. In low doses which are subanesthetic, it produces a rapid reduction of depressive symptoms in individuals with depression and is currently used clinically particularly in treatment refractory depression.[64,65] An interesting finding was documented in a study of OEF/OIF service members who suffered serious burn injuries and who received ketamine during their surgeries; these individuals also reported a reduction in their PTSD symptoms.[66] This finding was replicated in a study by Feder et al.[67] in which ketamine infusion in 41 individuals was associated with a significant and rapid reduction in PTSD symptoms. Its use in comorbidity is unknown and should be considered carefully given the fact that ketamine has abuse liability.[68]

Guanfacine, the alpha-2 agonist, in a study of patients with cocaine use disorder by Fox et al., reduced substance-related anxiety, stress and cue-induced craving and arousal. While two studies of guanfacine for treatment of PTSD alone have been negative,[69,70] there is a possibility of a more beneficial effect for patients with comorbid PTSD and SUD.[71]

Another medication that is being investigated for the treatment of comorbid SUD and PTSD is an anticonvulsant zonisamide, which has shown some promise in the treatment of AUD. A study is currently underway to investigate zonisamide as an adjunctive treatment to Enhanced Cognitive Processing Therapy in veterans with comorbid PTSD and AUD (see clinicaltrials.gov). The noradrenergic agent doxazosin (which has a mechanism of action similar to prazosin, but longer-acting) has also been investigated (see clinicaltrials.gov).

CONCLUSIONS/CLINICAL IMPLICATIONS

Although currently there are no medications that are proven to treat both PTSD and SUD, there are several effective medications for the treatment of PTSD and SUD when occurring alone which have also shown some promise in the treatment of this comorbidity. Because there is no one medication that has been shown to treat both disorders, one clinical approach would be to treat both disorders with medications approved for that indication. For example, while SSRI

are used to treat PTSD, they do not seem to improve AUD. Since there is evidence that naltrexone can improve outcomes in AUD, combination may be clinically appropriate. Further studies may find that some of the newer compounds (e.g., n-acetylcysteine, or anticonvulsants similar to topiramate) may improve symptoms in both disorders.

It is also possible to address co-occurring SUD and PTSD using behavioral treatments perhaps in combination with medication. Clinically, acute symptom control can usually best be achieved with medications, but behavioral/cognitive treatments have been shown to be associated with longer term changes. The selection of medication should be guided by symptom presentation (PTSD symptoms vs. severe craving) and severity. Early initiation of PTSD treatment is important, especially keeping in mind the findings that PTSD severity reduction is likely to result in substance use improvement.[72] These findings make sense especially in the clinical settings where there is evidence of PTSD symptoms (e.g., sleep difficulties, distress with reminders) precipitating substance use relapse.

REFERENCES

1. Breslau N, Kessler RC, Chilcoat HD, Schultz LR, Davis GC, Andreski P. Trauma and posttraumatic stress disorder in the community: the 1996 Detroit Area Survey of Trauma. *Arch Gen Psychiatry.* 1998;55(7):626–632.
2. Benjet C, Bromet E, Karam EG, et al. The epidemiology of traumatic event exposure worldwide: results from the World Mental Health Survey Consortium. *Psychol Med.* 2016;46(2):327–343.
3. Kessler RC, Sonnega A, Bromet E, Hughes M, Nelson CB. Posttraumatic stress disorder in the National Comorbidity Survey. *Archives Gen Psychiatry.* 1995;52(12):1048–1060.
4. Karam EG, Friedman MJ, Hill ED, et al. Cumulative traumas and risk thresholds: 12-month PTSD in the World Mental Health (WMH) surveys. *Depress Anxiety.* 2014; 31(2):130–142.
5. Breslau N, Davis GC, Andreski P, Peterson E. Traumatic events and posttraumatic stress disorder in an urban population of young adults. *Arch Gen Psychiatry.* 1991;48(3): 216–222.
6. Kulka RA, Schlenger WE, Fairbank JA, et al. *Trauma and the Vietnam War Generation: Report of Findings from the National Vietnam Veterans Readjustment Study.* New York: Brunner/Mazel; 1990.
7. Pietrzak RH, Goldstein RB, Southwick SM, Grant BF. Prevalence and axis I comorbidity of full and partial posttraumatic stress disorder in the United States: results from Wave 2 of the National Epidemiologic Survey on Alcohol and Related Conditions. *J Anxiety Disord.* 2011;25(3): 456–465.

8. Seal KH, Cohen G, Bertenthal D, Cohen BE, Maguen S, Daley A. Reducing barriers to mental health and social services for Iraq and Afghanistan veterans: outcomes of an integrated primary care clinic. *J Gen Intern Med.* 2011; 26(10):1160−1167.

9. Tate SR, Norman SB, McQuaid JR, Brown SA. Health problems of substance-dependent veterans with and those without trauma history. *J Subst Abuse Treat.* 2007;33(1): 25−32.

10. McDevitt-Murphy ME, Williams JL, Bracken KL, Fields JA, Monahan CJ, Murphy JG. PTSD symptoms, hazardous drinking, and health functioning among U.S.OEF and OIF veterans presenting to primary care. *J Trauma Stress.* 2010;23(1):108−111.

11. Blanco C, Xu Y, Brady K, Perez-Fuentes G, Okuda M, Wang S. Comorbidity of posttraumatic stress disorder with alcohol dependence among US adults: results from National Epidemiological Survey on Alcohol and Related Conditions. *Drug Alcohol Depend.* 2013;132(3):630−638.

12. Saladin ME, Brady KT, Dansky BS, Kilpatrick DG. Understanding comorbidity between PTSD and substance use disorders: two preliminary investigations. *Addict Behav.* 1995;20(5):643−655.

13. Saladin ME, Back SE, Payne RA. *Posttraumatic Stress Disorder and Substance Use Disorder Comorbitidy.* Baltimore, MD: Lippincot Williams & Wilkins; 2009.

14. Blanchard EB, Jones-Alexander J, Buckley TC, Forneris CA. Psychometric properties of the PTSD checklist (PCL). *Behav Res Ther.* 1996;34(8):669−673.

15. Mayfield D, McLeod G, Hall P. The CAGE questionnaire: validation of a new alcoholism screening instrument. *Am J Psychiatry.* 1974;131(10):1121−1123.

16. Bush K, Kivlahan DR, McDonell MB, Fihn SD, Bradley KA. The AUDIT alcohol consumption questions (AUDIT-C): an effective brief screening test for problem drinking. Ambulatory Care Quality Improvement Project (ACQUIP). Alcohol Use Disorders Identification Test. *Arch Intern Med.* 1998;158(16):1789−1795.

17. McCarthy E, Petrakis I. Epidemiology and management of alcohol dependence in individuals with post-traumatic stress disorder. *CNS Drugs.* 2010;24(12):997−1007.

18. Norman SB, Myers US, Wilkins KC, et al. Review of biological mechanisms and pharmacological treatments of comorbid PTSD and substance use disorder. *Neuropharmacology.* 2012;62(2):542−551.

19. Ralevski E, Olivera-Figueroa LA, Petrakis I. PTSD and co-morbid AUD: a review of pharmacological and alternative treatment options. *Subst Abuse Rehabil.* 2014;5:25−36.

20. Sofuoglu M, Rosenheck R, Petrakis I. Pharmacological treatment of comorbid PTSD and substance use disorder: recent progress. *Addict Behav.* 2014;39(2):428−433.

21. Petrakis IL, Simpson TL. Posttraumatic stress disorder and alcohol use disorder: a critical review of pharmacologic treatments. *Alcohol Clin Exp Res.* 2017;41(2):226−237.

22. Taylor M, Petrakis I, Ralevski E. Treatment of alcohol use disorder and co-occurring PTSD. *Am J Drug Alcohol Abuse.* 2017;43(4):1−11.

23. Simpson TL, Lehavot K, Petrakis IL. No wrong doors: findings from a critical review of behavioral randomized clinical trials for individuals with co-occurring alcohol/drug problems and posttraumatic stress disorder. *Alcohol Clin Exp Res.* 2017;41(4):681−702.

24. Jonas DE, Amick HR, Feltner C, et al. Pharmacotherapy for adults with alcohol use disorders in outpatient settings: a systematic review and meta-analysis. *JAMA.* 2014; 311(18):1889−1900.

25. Petrakis IL, Poling J, Levinson C, et al. Naltrexone and disulfiram in patients with alcohol dependence and comorbid post-traumatic stress disorder. *Biol Psychiatry.* 2006;60(7):777−783.

26. Petrakis IL, Ralevski E, Desai N, et al. Noradrenergic vs serotonergic antidepressant with or without naltrexone for veterans with PTSD and comorbid alcohol dependence. *Neuropsychopharmacology.* 2012;37(4):996−1004.

27. Foa EB, Yusko DA, McLean CP, et al. Concurrent naltrexone and prolonged exposure therapy for patients with comorbid alcohol dependence and PTSD: a randomized clinical trial. *JAMA.* 2013;310(5):488−495.

28. Johnson B, Ait-Daoud N, Bowden C, et al. Oral topiramate for treatment of alcohol dependence: a randomised controlled trial. *Lancet.* 2003;361:1677−1685.

29. Johnson BA, Rosenthal N, Capece JA, et al. Topiramate for treating alcohol dependence: a randomized controlled trial. *JAMA.* 2007;298(14):1641−1651.

30. Alderman CP, McCarthy LC, Condon JT, Marwood AC, Fuller JR. Topiramate in combat-related posttraumatic stress disorder. *Ann Pharmacother.* 2009;43(4):635−641.

31. Batki SL, Pennington DL, Lasher B, et al. Topiramate treatment of alcohol use disorder in veterans with posttraumatic stress disorder: a randomized controlled pilot trial. *Alcohol Clin Exp Res.* 2014;38(8):2169−2177.

32. Tucker P, Trautman RP, Wyatt DB, et al. Efficacy and safety of topiramate monotherapy in civilian posttraumatic stress disorder: a randomized, double-blind, placebo-controlled study. *J Clin Psychiatry.* 2007;68(2):201−206.

33. Yeh MS, Mari JJ, Costa MC, Andreoli SB, Bressan RA, Mello MF. A double-blind randomized controlled trial to study the efficacy of topiramate in a civilian sample of PTSD. *CNS Neurosci Ther.* 2011;17(5):305−310.

34. Marshall RD, Beebe KL, Oldham M, Zaninelli R. Efficacy and safety of paroxetine treatment for chronic PTSD: a fixed-dose, placebo-controlled study. *Am J Psychiatry.* 2001;158(12):1982−1988.

35. Brady K, Pearlstein T, Asnis GM, et al. Efficacy and safety of sertraline treatment of posttraumatic stress disorder: a randomized controlled trial. *JAMA.* 2000;283(14): 1837−1844.

36. Davidson JR, Rothbaum BO, van der Kolk BA, Sikes CR, Farfel GM. Multicenter, double-blind comparison of sertraline and placebo in the treatment of posttraumatic stress disorder. *Arch Gen Psychiatry.* 2001;58(5):485−492.

37. van der Kolk BA, Dreyfuss D, Michaels M, et al. Fluoxetine in posttraumatic stress disorder. *J Clin Psychiatry.* 1994; 55(12):517−522.

38. Martenyi F, Brown EB, Zhang H, Prakash A, Koke SC. Fluoxetine versus placebo in posttraumatic stress disorder. *J Clin Psychiatry*. 2002;63(3):199–206.

39. Davidson J, Rothbaum BO, Tucker P, Asnis G, Benattia I, Musgnung JJ. Venlafaxine extended release in posttraumatic stress disorder: a sertraline- and placebo-controlled study. *J Clin Psychopharmacol*. 2006;26(3):259–267.

40. Hertzberg MA, Feldman ME, Beckham JC, Kudler HS, Davidson JR. Lack of efficacy for fluoxetine in PTSD: a placebo controlled trial in combat veterans. *Ann Clin Psychiatry*. 2000;12(2):101–105.

41. Friedman MJ, Marmar CR, Baker DG, Sikes CR, Farfel GM. Randomized, double-blind comparison of sertraline and placebo for posttraumatic stress disorder in a Department of Veterans Affairs setting. *J Clin Psychiatry*. 2007;68(5): 711–720.

42. Brady K, Sonne S, Roberts J. Sertraline treatment of comorbid post traumatic stress disorder and alcohol dependence. *J Clin Psychiatry*. 1995;56:502–505.

43. Brady KT, Sonne S, Anton RF, Randall CL, Back SE, Simpson K. Sertraline in the treatment of co-occurring alcohol dependence and posttraumatic stress disorder. *Alcohol Clin Exp Res*. 2005;29(3):395–401.

44. Hien DA, Levin FR, Ruglass LM, et al. Combining seeking safety with sertraline for PTSD and alcohol use disorders: a randomized controlled trial. *J Consult Clin Psychol*. 2015;83(2):359–369.

45. Raskind MA, Peskind ER, Hoff DJ, et al. A parallel group placebo controlled study of prazosin for trauma nightmares and sleep disturbance in combat veterans with post-traumatic stress disorder. *Biol Psychiatry*. 2007;61(8): 928–934.

46. Taylor FB, Martin P, Thompson C, et al. Prazosin effects on objective sleep measures and clinical symptoms in civilian trauma posttraumatic stress disorder: a placebo-controlled study. *Biol Psychiatry*. 2008;63(6):629–632.

47. Germain A, Richardson R, Moul DE, et al. Placebo-controlled comparison of prazosin and cognitive-behavioral treatments for sleep disturbances in US Military Veterans. *J Psychosom Res*. 2012;72(2):89–96.

48. Raskind MA, Peterson K, Williams T, et al. A trial of prazosin for combat trauma PTSD with nightmares in active-duty soldiers returned from Iraq and Afghanistan. *Am J Psychiatry*. 2013;170(9):1003–1010.

49. Raskind MA, Peskind ER, Chow B, et al. Trial of prazosin for post-traumatic stress disorder in military veterans. *N Engl J Med*. 2018;378(6):507–517.

50. Rasmussen DD, Alexander LL, Raskind MA, Froehlich JC. The alpha1-adrenergic receptor antagonist, prazosin, reduces alcohol drinking in alcohol-preferring (P) rats. *Alcohol Clin Exp Res*. 2009;33(2):264–272.

51. Le AD, Funk D, Juzytsch W, et al. Effect of prazosin and guanfacine on stress-induced reinstatement of alcohol and food seeking in rats. *Psychopharmacol Berl*. 2011; 218(1):89–99.

52. Simpson TL, Malte CA, Dietel B, et al. A pilot trial of prazosin, an alpha-1 adrenergic antagonist, for comorbid alcohol dependence and posttraumatic stress disorder. *Alcohol Clin Exp Res*. 2015;39(5):808–817.

53. Petrakis IL, Desai N, Gueorguieva R, et al. Prazosin for veterans with posttraumatic stress disorder and comorbid alcohol dependence: a clinical trial. *Alcohol Clin Exp Res*. 2016;40(1):178–186.

54. Wilkinson ST, Stefanovics E, Rosenheck RA. Marijuana use is associated with worse outcomes in symptom severity and violent behavior in patients with posttraumatic stress disorder. *J Clin Psychiatry*. 2015;76(9):1174–1180.

55. Wilkinson ST, Radhakrishnan R, D'Souza DC. A systematic review of the evidence for medical marijuana in psychiatric indications. *J Clin Psychiatry*. 2016;77(8):1050–1064.

56. Fraser GA. The use of a synthetic cannabinoid in the management of treatment-resistant nightmares in posttraumatic stress disorder (PTSD). *CNS Neurosci Ther*. 2009; 15(1):84–88.

57. Cameron C, Watson D, Robinson J. Use of a synthetic cannabinoid in a correctional population for posttraumatic stress disorder-related insomnia and nightmares, chronic pain, harm reduction, and other indications: a retrospective evaluation. *J Clin Psychopharmacol*. 2014;34(5):559–564.

58. Roitman P, Mechoulam R, Cooper-Kazaz R, Shalev A. Preliminary, open-label, pilot study of add-on oral Delta9-tetrahydrocannabinol in chronic post-traumatic stress disorder. *Clin Drug Investig*. 2014;34(8):587–591.

59. Meier MH, Caspi A, Ambler A, et al. Persistent cannabis users show neuropsychological decline from childhood to midlife. *Proc Natl Acad Sci U S A*. 2012;109(40): E2657–E2664.

60. Large M, Sharma S, Compton MT, Slade T, Nielssen O. Cannabis use and earlier onset of psychosis: a systematic meta-analysis. *Arch Gen Psychiatry*. 2011;68(6):555–561.

61. Moreira FA, Wotjak CT. Cannabinoids and anxiety. *Curr Top Behav Neurosci*. 2010;2:429–450.

62. Haney M, Evins AE. Does cannabis cause, exacerbate or ameliorate psychiatric disorders? An oversimplified debate discussed. *Neuropsychopharmacology*. 2016;41(2):393–401.

63. Back SE, McCauley JL, Korte KJ, et al. A double-blind, randomized, controlled pilot trial of N-Acetylcysteine in veterans with posttraumatic stress disorder and substance use disorders. *J Clin Psychiatry*. 2016;77(11):e1439–e1446.

64. Berman RM, Cappiello A, Anand A, et al. Antidepressant effects of ketamine in depressed patients. *Biol Psychiatry*. 2000;47(4):351–354.

65. Murrough JW, Iosifescu DV, Chang LC, et al. Antidepressant efficacy of ketamine in treatment-resistant major depression: a two-site randomized controlled trial. *Am J Psychiatry*. 2013;170(10):1134–1142.

66. McGhee LL, Maani CV, Garza TH, Gaylord KM, Black IH. The correlation between ketamine and posttraumatic stress disorder in burned service members. *J Trauma*. 2008;64(suppl 2):S195–S198; discussion S197–S198.

67. Feder A, Parides MK, Murrough JW, et al. Efficacy of intravenous ketamine for treatment of chronic posttraumatic stress disorder: a randomized clinical trial. *JAMA Psychiatry*. 2014;71(6):681–688.

68. Liu Y, Lin D, Wu B, Zhou W. Ketamine abuse potential and use disorder. *Brain Res Bull.* 2016;126(pt 1):68–73.

69. Neylan TC, Lenoci M, Samuelson KW, et al. No improvement of posttraumatic stress disorder symptoms with guanfacine treatment. *Am J Psychiatry.* 2006;163(12):2186–2188.

70. Davis LL, Ward C, Rasmusson A, Newell JM, Frazier E, Southwick SM. A placebo-controlled trial of guanfacine for the treatment of posttraumatic stress disorder in veterans. *Psychopharmacol Bull.* 2008;41(1):8–18.

71. Bernardy NC, Friedman MJ. Psychopharmacological strategies in the management of posttraumatic stress disorder (PTSD): what have we learned? *Curr Psychiatry Rep.* 2015;17(4):564.

72. Hien DA, Jiang H, Campbell AN, et al. Do treatment improvements in PTSD severity affect substance use outcomes? A secondary analysis from a randomized clinical trial in NIDA's Clinical Trials Network. *Am J Psychiatry.* 2010;167(1):95–101.

CHAPTER 14

When Food Is an Addiction

A. BENJAMIN SRIVASTAVA, MD • MARK S. GOLD, MD

INTRODUCTION

Over 1/3 of adults in the United States are considered obese, defined as body mass index (BMI) ≥30, and an additional 1/3 are considered overweight, defined as BMI ≥25.[1] Obesity is one of the leading public health problems in the United States, contributing to significant morbidity, mortality, and public health cost. Obesity-related illnesses, including cardiovascular disease, stroke, and certain types of cancer are some of the leading causes of preventable deaths.[2] Medical costs of managing obesity and obesity-related illnesses accounts for nearly over 20% of healthcare spending, over $190 billion in 2005,[3] which, if unchecked, could exceed $66 billion by 2030.[4]

Certainly, environmental factors have important implications in obesity. High calorie, palatable foods, which are staples of the so-called "Western" diet, and increasingly sedentary lifestyles have contributed to the obesity epidemic.[5,6] Traditionally, primary care physicians will recommend diet and exercise for obese patients; however, nonadherence is high, and even when some patients adhere to strict diet and exercise regimens, they are unable to lose weight, possibly due to genetic and epigenetic factors.[5,7] Similarly, not all individuals who eat high calorie diets and/or engage in sedentary lifestyles become obese, providing further evidence that endogenous factors may be relevant to the pathophysiology of obesity.[5,7] Given the enormous public health burden associated with obesity, substantial efforts and resources have been directed toward further understanding mechanisms and pathophysiology of obesity in order to develop a more sophisticated understanding of the illness as well as more effective management and treatment strategies.[5]

Increasingly, because investigation into "peripheral" causes (e.g., lipid dysregulation, insulin sensitivity) has failed to make an impression on the problem of obesity as a whole, conceptualization of obesity and treatment developments has shifted to more central causes. While neuroendocrine influences on appetite and satiety are well characterized, neuroscientists are increasingly investigating brain systems involving reward, motivation, and hedonic experiences as they relate to hedonic eating.[8] Through much preclinical and clinical research based on dopaminergic function, two parallel models of obesity have emerged, the reward deficit model and the reward surfeit model.[9] In the former model, striatal dopamine is increased in response to food, suggesting a positive-reinforcement schedule of reward, whereas the latter model suggests that affected individuals have a genetically determined baseline blunted DA release, resulting in cravings and search for rewarding stimuli (including food).[9]

An abundance of evidence exists for both of these models, and a discussion of the competing hypotheses is beyond the scope of this chapter. However, this dichotomy raises an important point. Obesity is a syndrome, principally defined by an epidemiologically based cutoff on weight, a continuous metric.[10] However, in 1972, John Feighner, Eli Robbins, and Sam Guze of the Department of Psychiatry at Washington University in St. Louis School of Medicine, inspired by the practice in other disciplines in medicine, implored clinicians and researchers to define psychiatric illness by longitudinal history, family history, pathophysiology, and delimitation from other illness in addition to the clinical picture.[11] This tradition has continued in every iteration of the Diagnostic and Statistical Manual for Psychiatric Disorders (DSM) since DSM III was published in 1980.[12] Thus, that obesity, which in a strict sense is a cross-sectional clinical description, should have multiple, valid and replicable evidence bases for pathophysiology is a foregone conclusion, and thus one must focus on both "top down" (i.e., phenotypically driven) as well as bottom-up (neuroscience informed) components when classifying obesity in terms of its psychiatric components.

In this chapter, we will largely focus on the reward-deficit model, which as described by Blum et al., is a well-validated model of drug and alcohol addiction (called the "Reward Deficiency Syndrome) and extend

The Assessment and Treatment of Addiction. https://doi.org/10.1016/B978-0-323-54856-4.00014-6

this idea that in some individuals, obesity may be the manifestation of food addiction.[9,13] We will discuss historical concepts, advances in fundamental neuroscience, clinical descriptions, relationship to substance use disorders, other behavioral addictions, and eating disorders, and ultimately treatment.

PRECLINICAL EVIDENCE

Behavioral Pharmacology

The idea that certain, highly palatable foods containing sugar and/or fat could have addictive properties was inspired by the behavioral (i.e., DSM) criteria for substance use disorders, specifically tolerance, withdrawal, and loss of control.[14–16] In a series of classic experiments in Bartley Hoebel's laboratory at Princeton University, rodents were given 12-h access to both lab chow and glucose/sucrose solutions and then subsequently deprived of food for 12 hours. This cycle was repeated for 3 weeks, which induces a state of spontaneous binge eating when exposed to food. Compared to control rodents offered ad libitum access to a sucrose solution and/or lab chow, the rats in the 12-h access/restriction group show binge usage (increased intake during the first hour of food exposure), spontaneous binge periods during the time when food is offered, increased lever presses for sugar, and opioid-like withdrawal symptoms either following either sugar/chow removal or naloxone administration.[14,15] Additionally, rats on a maintenance/restricted intake paradigm demonstrate locomotor cross-sensitization to amphetamine and increased alcohol intake.[17,18] A critical observation from these experiments is that simply having unlimited access to food or sugar does not produce an addiction-like phenotype; the restricted access paradigm appears absolutely necessary for the behavioral change to occur.[14]

Interestingly, when rats binge on sugar alone, they do not gain weight, yet when rats are offered sugar and fat, they tend to binge and gain weight.[19] Rats that binge on fat alone do not show evidence of opioid-like withdrawal when naloxone is administered,[20] yet binge-prone rats will tolerate high levels of shock when it is paired with a high sugar/high fat food available for consumption.[21] Additionally, Bocarsley et al. found that rats with access to solutions containing high fructose corn syrup, one of the commonest additives in food today,[22] experienced increased abdominal adiposity, weight gain, and hypertriglyceridemia.[23] Collectively, these preclinical findings indicate that individual macronutrients may selectively modulate addictive-like behaviors through both convergent and divergent mechanisms.[19,20,24] As humans typically consume food consisting of a multifarious array of nutrients, we can envisage a model in which high sugar, high fat foods consumed in the so-called "western diet" interact with underlying genetic and environmental factors, resulting in the food addiction-obesity syndrome.[24]

Neurotransmitter Systems: Dopamine

Many decades of research have implicated the neurotransmitter dopamine (DA) as central to drug addiction in terms of binge intoxication (acute surge in striatal dopamine release in the nucleus accumbens [NAc] with substance use), withdrawal negative affect (depletion of dopamine following cessation), and preoccupation/anticipation (dopamine release in the presence of anticipating use or experiencing use-associated salience).[25] Emerging evidence suggests that parallel changes in dopamine release, receptor density, and receptor gene expression characteristic of drug addiction may underlie the behavioral manifestations of rats who display addictive behaviors regarding food.[19,26] Food intake results in striatal dopamine release, and in rats exposed to food ad libitum after satiety is achieved, the novelty of the food, even highly palatable food, wears off and dopamine release is blunted.[19,26] However, in rats who *binge* on highly palatable food, dopamine release in the nucleus accumbens (NAc) surges as occurs in the binge-intoxication of drugs of abuse.[27] Additionally, obese rats have been found to have a downregulation of D2 receptors, a consistent phenomenon found in addiction, and D2R knockout rats demonstrate compulsive like food seeking behavior when exposed to highly palatable foods.[26]

Neurotransmitter Systems: Opioids

The endogenous opioid system also appears to have important implications for overconsumption of highly palatable foods and food addiction. In murine models, binge-like consumption of highly palatable foods is associated with increased expression of the mu-opioid receptor (MOR) in the cingulate cortex, hippocampus, locus coeruleus, and shell of the nucleus accumbens, key areas involved in emotion, memory, and stress response that have similarly been implicated in addiction.[8] As such, a variety of MOR agonists have been shown to increase intake of highly palatable foods, particularly in binge-eating animals, and MOR antagonists such as naltrexone have been shown to decrease binge consumption of highly palatable foods.[8,14] As mentioned previously, administration of MOR antagonist naloxone produces symptoms similar to opioid withdrawal in rats with a history of sugar binging.[14,15]

Other Neurotransmitter Systems: Endocannabinoids, Orexin (CASA), Ghrelin, and Leptin

The endocannabinoids comprise a complex neurotransmitter system that plays a key role in addiction to substances such as cannabis and alcohol, and cannabis itself binds to the CB1 receptor.[28] Additionally, the endocannabinoids are thought to modulate key neurotransmitters that affect appetite and satiety.[29] The CB1 receptor inverse agonist rimonabant was indeed shown to be efficacious for weight reduction in obese patients; however, adverse psychiatric side effects (including suicidal ideation) led to withdrawal from the worldwide market.[30,31] Orexin (or hypocretin) is a neuropeptide that regulates arousal, appetitive, and feeding behavior that has also been implicated in cue-induced drug seeking.[32] Ghrelin, an orexigenic hormone, and leptin, and antiorexigenic hormone, are important regulators of appetite and are thought to play key roles in the reward valuation of food.[8]

The Dark Side of Addiction: Revisited

George Koob has described the "Dark Side of Addiction" in which negative reinforcement mechanisms influence drug-taking behavior. Briefly, the drug taking initiates as an *impulsive* behavior (pleasure seeking) mediated by striatal dopamine release; however, over time, drug taking becomes *compulsive* (distress avoidance) mediated by the extended amygdala and enhanced corticotrophin releasing hormone (CRH) signalling.[25,33] Thus, the primary motivation is mediated through a negative reinforcement system in which the drug is taken to relieve a withdrawal/negative affect state, a process called allostasis.[25,33] Animal models support the idea of a similar process vis-a-vis hedonic eating. When food is withdrawn from binge eating rats that previously had been selected from binge eating, depressive and anxiety-like symptomatology is observed, and when these rats are allowed access to food, a compulsive pattern of binge eating is observed with a concurrent reduction in anxiety and depressive behaviors.[15,34,35]

CLINICAL EVIDENCE FROM NEUROIMAGING

There is an abundance of literature on neurobiology of obesity as it relates to addiction implicating a variety of brain regions including the ventral striatum, medial prefrontal cortex, habenula, and insula.[36] An in-depth review of said literature is beyond the scope of this chapter, but we wish to highlight major findings to further illustrate how the reward deficit syndrome, a

useful heuristic for understanding drug and alcohol addictions may be likewise useful for understanding food addiction. In healthy (nonobese) individuals, ingestion of palatable foods results in striatal dopamine release in an amount proportional to the subjective rating of the food.[37] However, just as ingestion of substances of abuse results in a blunted activation of reward circuitry in the addicted individual, ingestion of highly palatable food results in blunted activation of reward circuitry in obese individuals.[25,38] Additionally, exposure to highly palatable food (high fat/high sugar diets) is associated with striatal D2R downregulation, decreased dopamine transporter (DAT) expression and function, and decreased DA concentration in the nucleus accumbens.[9] Collectively, these data support the "reward deficit" heuristics of both substance and food addictions: changes in reward circuitry (a "less responsive system") underlie parallel behavior changes in both drug taking and binge eating (from "impulsive" to "compulsive" use/eating).[9,13]

FOOD ADDICTION: A CLINICAL SYNDROME

As we have described above, current standards dictate that psychiatric diagnoses be formulated through clinical symptomatology, longitudinal course of the illness, delimitation from other illnesses, family history, and biomarkers.[11] The final criterion, despite numerous attempts and decades of research, has not fully materialized for clinical purposes. The advent of the National Institute of Mental Health's Research Domain Criteria (RDoc), an emphasis toward a classification system that incorporates more "biologically" driven data, appears to be on the horizon; however, one of the problems that has arisen is attempts at characterizing psychopathology based on the valences of given categories in a the RDocs matrix.[39] Simply put, illnesses cannot be reliably defined based on arbitrary "cutoff points" on continuous metrics, and this is especially true for obesity.[39] Translational research on obese subjects has yielded inconsistent, though important findings. Similarly, efforts to characterize levels of "reward valuation" or "cognitive control" without a more definitive clinical syndrome other than a BMI-based indication of obesity would likely prove fruitless. Thus, a valid, clinical ("top down") model of food addiction is indispensable.[30]

The putative instrument for evaluating and diagnosing food addiction is the Yale Food Addiction Scale (YFAS) developed by Gearhardt, Corbin, and Brownwell at Yale in 2009 inspired by the phenomenological overlap between hedonic consumption of food and drug/alcohol addiction and corresponding neurobiological underpinnings discovered elucidated in the preclinical models described earlier in this chapter.[40,41] Gearhardt and colleagues developed and validated criteria based on the DSM-IV-TR criteria for substance use disorders, emphasizing features such as tolerance, withdrawal, loss of control, and clinically significant impairment in functioning.[40,41] The YFAS also has convergent validity with other measures that gauge problematic eating as well as discriminant validity against a measure for alcoholism.[40] Gearhardt and colleagues further added construct validity to the YFAS using functional magnetic resonance imaging, demonstrating that in both healthy and obese subjects, YFAS scores correlated with increased BOLD signaling in the anterior cingulate cortex (ACC), amygdala, and medial orbitofrontal cortex (mOFC), areas that have been shown consistently to have implications in both drug addiction and feeding/appetitive motivation.[42] The YFAS has since been updated to reflect DSM-5 criteria (YFAS 2.0)[43] and a version for children has been developed (YFAS-C).[44]

FOOD ADDICTION EPIDEMIOLOGY AND RELATION TO OBESITY

Evidence regarding the prevalence of YFAS defined food addiction is still somewhat preliminary[30]; however, in surveying over 130,000 women enrolled in the Nurses' Health Study, Flint and colleagues found that nearly 6% of women met YFAS defined criteria for food addiction, with a positive association between higher BMI and food addiction diagnoses.[45] Using much smaller, general population-based samples, the prevalence of food addiction in overweight/obese subjects, one study found the prevalence of food addiction to be approximately 7%, while another found the prevalence of food addiction to be approximately 15%.[46,47] In a clinical sample of obese patients seeking bariatric weight loss surgery, nearly 54% met criteria for food addiction.

RELATIONSHIP WITH OTHER EATING DISORDERS

Epidemiologic data suggest that patients with DSM-defined eating disorders (ED),[48] namely Anorexia Nervosa (AN), Bulimia Nervosa (BN), and Binge Eating Disorder (BED), are affected by comorbid substance use disorders at a prevalence five times greater than the general population.[30,49] BED is characterized by periods of persistent and uncontrolled intake of food without compensatory (i.e., weight reducing) behaviors.[50] Individuals with BED will typically beyond

satiety, which generates feelings of dysphoria and guilt, which drives further binge eating as a compensatory mechanism.[50] Patients with BED are at high risk for medical complications including and stemming from obesity,[50] and as many as 27% have comorbid substance use disorders.[51] BN is characterized by cycles of binge eating followed by compensatory or purging behavior (e.g., self-induced vomiting, exercise, etc.).[50] Similar to BED, patients with BN often have co-morbid substance use disorders (approximately 37%).[51] Finally, AN is characterized by either severe food restriction or restriction with binges and purges to maintain an abnormally low body weight.[50] As is the case with BED and BN, prevalence of comorbid substance use is high (27%).[51]

Eating disorders and substance use disorders share phenomenological similarities including loss of control continued behavior despite negative consequences, cravings, and impulsivity.[52,53] In eating disorders, however, the pathologic and diagnostic focus is on the thought processes and self-evaluation of the patient rather than the food; whereas in substance use disorders, the substance itself is considered of capital importance.[30] This distinction represents the key delimitation between the two diagnostic categories, and food addiction represents a bridge between the two constructs: certain genetic vulnerabilities and neuro-adaptive changes may represent an endophenotype of the food-addicted person, and certain characteristics of a given food (palatability, sugar content) may increase its addiction liability relative to other foods.[30]

Studies have demonstrated that patients who meet criteria for BN and BED frequently meet YFAS criteria for food addiction.[30] Compared to individuals without BED, individuals with BED tend to meet criteria for food addiction, and conversely individuals with food addiction tend to also meet criteria for BED compared to those who do not meet criteria for food addiction.[30] Preliminary work shows that an even higher percentage of patients with BN meet YFAS criteria for comorbid food addiction than do patients with BED.[54] Additionally, a bulk of evidence suggests that individuals with BED or BN who meet criteria for food addiction appear to exhibit more severe food and eating-related pathology than individuals with BED or BN without comorbid food addiction.[30] See Fig. 14.1 for a comparison between the symptomatology between food addiction, BED, and BN. Though AN and food addiction have overlapping symptomatology, research has not yet examined the prevalence of YFAS diagnosed food addiction in subjects with AN.[30]

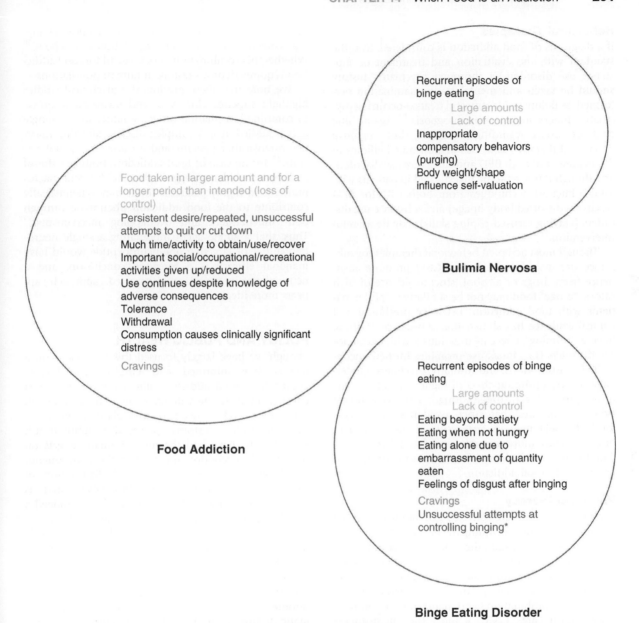

Bulimia Nervosa

Recurrent episodes of
binge eating
Large amounts
Lack of control
Inappropriate
compensatory behaviors
(purging)
Body weight/shape
influence self-valuation

Food Addiction

Food taken in larger amount and for a
longer period than intended (loss of
control)
Persistent desire/repeated, unsuccessful
attempts to quit or cut down
Much time/activity to obtain/use/recover
Important social/occupational/recreational
activities given up/reduced
Use continues despite knowledge of
adverse consequences
Tolerance
Withdrawal
Consumption causes clinically significant
distress
Cravings

Binge Eating Disorder

Recurrent episodes of binge
eating
Large amounts
Lack of control
Eating beyond satiety
Eating when not hungry
Eating alone due to
embarrassment of quantity
eaten
Feelings of disgust after binging
Cravings
Unsuccessful attempts at
controlling binging*

FIG. 14.1 Symptom overlap between food addiction, bulimia nervosa, and binge eating disorder.

EVALUATION AND TREATMENT

Limited literature and guidelines exist on the evaluation
and treatment of food addiction. Though the actual prevalence of food addiction is unknown, given that over
50% of obese patients may meet YFAS criteria for food
addiction, screening for food addiction in the obese patient in primary care, psychiatric, and other settings
may be prudent.[30] Additionally, given the comorbidity
between substance use disorders, eating disorders, and
food addiction, we recommend that patients who undergo evaluations for eating disorders undergo evaluation for addictive disorders and vice versa.[30] Further,
both of these groups of patients should be screened for
food addiction.[30] Monitoring of weight is standard practice in the treatment of eating disorders, and we have suggested the same for patients in substance treatment.[50,55]

Behavioral Therapies

If a diagnosis of food addiction is considered, as is the standard with the evaluation and treatment of substance use disorders, a thorough psychiatric history should be taken and mental status examination performed, as failure to identify and treat co-occurring psychiatric illness may worsen prognosis.[30] Again, little evidence exists regarding treatment, but cognitive behavioral therapy (CBT) has demonstrated efficacy in the treatment of both BED and substance use disorders, and though it has yet to be investigated in patients with food addiction, techniques from both CBT for BED (focus on distorted body image) and substance use disorders (craving-focused coping skills) may be a useful intervention.[56]

Though most accepted behavioral therapies for substance use disorders (including CBT) promote abstinence from drugs or alcohol, strict avoidance of high caloric "binge" food may not be similarly helpful in patients with food addiction. Extensive preclinical and clinical evidence has shown that substances of abuse have a "priming" effect in individuals with substance use disorders (i.e., index use promotes further, uncontrolled consumption), and similarly, preclinical models have shown a priming effect of highly palatable foods in the promotion of binge eating.[56] However, clinical evidence indicates that strict avoidance of "trigger" foods in BED may in fact result in more frequent binges.[56] Thus, more research is needed to better elucidate the role of abstinence versus controlled eating in patients with food addiction.[30]

Pharmacotherapy

Several medications are currently FDA approved for the treatment of obesity including the pancreatic and gastric lipase inhibitor orlistat, the selective $5HT_{2C}$ agonist Lorcaserin, GLP-1 agonist Liraglutide, a phenteramine—topiramate combination, and a naltrexone—bupropion combination.[5] Of these, Lorcaserin, phenteramine—topiramate combination, and naltrexone—bupropion combination are CNS acting. The naltrexone—bupropion combination might target pathways involved in the reward deficit (i.e., food addiction) model of obesity including a bupropion-mediated attenuated hypothalamic response to food cues and enhanced activation in areas associated with inhibitory control (anterior cingulate cortex), internal awareness (superior frontal gyrus, insular cortex, superior parietal lobe), and memory (hippocampus) regions.[57] Additionally, preclinical work has shown that a high-dose baclofen—naltrexone combination significantly decreases (compared to either drug alone or vehicle)

consumption of highly palatable foods without changing consumption of standard, laboratory chow.[58] Whether this combination, too, is useful for food addiction requires rigorous testing in human populations.

We note that these preclinical and clinical studies highlight superior efficacy of and increased response to combination pharmacotherapy rather than a single agent. Addiction is a complex disease, affecting many neurotransmitter systems and an array of neural circuits.[25] In the case of food addiction, both preclinical and clinical evidence suggests that the different macronutrients in highly palatable foods may synergistically contribute to the food addiction phenotype through both independent and overlapping mechanisms.[59] Thus, that a single agent modulating a single neurotransmitter or targeting one neuropeptide would have marginal efficacy is a foregone conclusion, and a neuroscience-informed, multitargeted approach appears more ideal.

POLICY AND PUBLIC HEALTH

Though we have largely focused this discussion on a neuroscience informed and empirically validated approach to food addiction and treatment, the most effective interventions will likely come on public health and policy levels. Indeed, when looking at addiction treatment from a historical perspective, public health interventions have had the most dramatic effects on outcomes in every domain. Though the 18th amendment, which banned the sale and distribution of alcohol ("Prohibition"), was short lived and is frequently taught as political mishap, it was indeed a significant public health success. During its 13-year existence, rates of alcohol-related deaths and cirrhosis plummeted, as did admissions to institutions for alcohol-related psychosis.[60] Additionally, the raising of the drinking age to 21 and implementation of drunk driving laws have also resulted in many lives saved.[60] Another great addiction-public health success is the dramatic decline in smoking. The prevalence of cigarette smoking has declined from over 42% of American adults in 1965% to 15.1% in 2015.[61,62] Though many factors are contributory to this successful outcome (with still more work to do), clean air laws including smoke-free restaurant mandates and tobacco taxes have truly been the driving force behind this success.[61]

Similar approaches are being implemented to target obesity. Beginning in 2006, under the leadership of then Mayor Michael Bloomberg, New York City implemented a number of policies directed toward reducing sugar consumption including caloric and drink size restrictions that, along with an aggressive media campaign, has effectively reduced sugar consumption in New York.[63] Additionally, a number of municipalities and countries have instituted taxes on sodas and other sugary drinks, which have the potential of significantly reducing obesity through net caloric consumption reduction as well as more funding for obesity prevention programs generated from the taxes themselves.[64] Though data on health outcomes specifically has not been gathered, when such taxes were introduced in Mexico, taxed sweetened beverage purchases decreased substantially. Thus, public health interventions implemented from a food addiction conceptual framework (explicitly, interventions targeting access to and consumption of highly palatable foods) can have large-scale implications in addressing the obesity epidemic.

FUTURE DIRECTIONS

In defining psychiatric illness, we are tasked with "carving nature at its joints,"[65] and we have argued that food addiction represents a theory cut from a "natural kind."[66] We have reviewed preclinical and clinical work that strongly supports the hypothesis of food addiction as a distinct syndrome, yet, as is the case with other psychiatric illness, determining the most refined, neuroscience informed, and defining features of the illness require much more research.[67] Additionally, the addiction liability of specific foods and whether certain combinations of foods may be necessary for the food addiction syndrome to manifest remains to be determined.[68,69] Further, the impact from industry cannot be understated. Recent work using fMRI has shown that food advertisements can impact food consumption and weight gain, possible through a differential effect on activity in the ventral striatum.[70] Dr. Ashley Gearhardt is currently leading the Food and Addiction Science and Treatment Lab at the University of Michigan (http://fastlab.psych.lsa.umich.edu/), a state-of-the-art translational research center with current investigations focused the effect environment and context has on the development of hedonic eating and food addiction.

These unanswered questions notwithstanding, given the social, economic, and public health burden of the obesity epidemic, dismissing the idea of food addiction is not on a conceptual, but also a practical error.[67] Though available treatments are indeed limited, progress is being made, and a number of researchers have taken cues from discoveries from translational neuroscience research in obesity and have investigated using neuromodulation interventions such as transcranial magnetic stimulation (TMS), transcranial direct-current stimulation (tDCS), vagus nerve stimulation (VNS), and deep brain stimulation (DBS) to target regions involved in addiction in obese patients, with some positive, preliminary findings.[71] Identifying obese individuals who meet criteria for food addiction allows for a more empathic understanding of the patient in terms of illness and a more personalized approach to treatment, including psychotherapy, psychopharmacology, and neuromodulation, and embracing the concept as a whole may yield more fruitful public policy.

REFERENCES

1. Ogden CL, Carroll MD, Fryar CD, Flegal KM. *Prevalence of Obesity Among Adults and Youth: United States, 2011–2014.* Hyattsville, MD: National Center for Health Statistics; 2015.
2. National Institutes of Health, National Heart Lung, Blood Institute. Clinical guidelines on the identification, evaluation, and treatment of overweight and obesity in adults: the evidence report. US Department of Health and Human Services. *Obes Res.* 1998.
3. Cawley J, Meyerhoefer C. The medical care costs of obesity: an instrumental variables approach. *J Health Econ.* 2012; 31(1):219–230.
4. Wang YC, McPherson K, Marsh T, Gortmaker SL, Brown M. Health and economic burden of the projected obesity trends in the USA and the UK. *Lancet.* 2011;378(9793): 815–825.
5. Heymsfield SB, Wadden TA. Mechanisms, pathophysiology, and management of obesity. *N Engl J Med.* 2017; 376(3):254–266.
6. Fung TT, Rimm EB, Spiegelman D, et al. Association between dietary patterns and plasma biomarkers of obesity and cardiovascular disease risk. *Am J Clin Nutr.* 2001; 73(1):61–67.
7. Ochner CN, Tsai AG, Kushner RF, Wadden TA. Treating obesity seriously: when recommendations for lifestyle change confront biological adaptations. *Lancet Diabetes Endocrinol.* 2015;3(4):232–234.
8. Murray S, Tulloch A, Gold MS, Avena NM. Hormonal and neural mechanisms of food reward, eating behaviour and obesity. *Nat Rev Endocrinol.* 2014;10(9):540–552.
9. Blum K, Thanos PK, Gold MS. Dopamine and glucose, obesity, and reward deficiency syndrome. *Front Psychol.* 2014;5:919.
10. Centers for Disease Control, Prevention. *Defining Adult Overweight and Obesity;* 2016. https://www.cdc.gov/obesity/adult/defining.html.
11. Feighner JP, Robins E, Guze SB, Woodruff Jr RA, Winokur G, Munoz R. Diagnostic criteria for use in psychiatric research. *Arch Gen Psychiatry.* 1972;26(1):57–63.

12. Kendler KS, Munoz RA, Murphy G. The development of the Feighner criteria: a historical perspective. *Am J Psychiatry*. 2010;167(2):134—142.

13. Blum K, Thanos PK, Oscar-Berman M, et al. Dopamine in the brain: hypothesizing surfeit or deficit links to reward and addiction. *J Reward Defic Syndr*. 2015;1(3):95—104.

14. Avena NM, Bocarsly ME, Hoebel BG, Gold MS. Overlaps in the nosology of substance abuse and overeating: the translational implications of "food addiction". *Curr Drug Abuse Rev*. 2011;4(3):133—139.

15. Avena NM, Rada P, Hoebel BG. Evidence for sugar addiction: behavioral and neurochemical effects of intermittent, excessive sugar intake. *Neurosci Biobehav Rev*. 2008;32(1):20—39.

16. Gold MS. From bedside to bench and back again: a 30-year saga. *Physiol Behav*. 2011;104(1):157—161.

17. Avena NM, Carrillo CA, Needham L, Leibowitz SF, Hoebel BG. Sugar-dependent rats show enhanced intake of unsweetened ethanol. *Alcohol*. 2004;34(2—3):203—209.

18. Avena NM, Hoebel BG. A diet promoting sugar dependency causes behavioral cross-sensitization to a low dose of amphetamine. *Neuroscience*. 2003;122(1):17—20.

19. Avena NM. The study of food addiction using animal models of binge eating. *Appetite*. 2010;55(3):734—737.

20. Bocarsly ME, Berner LA, Hoebel BG, Avena NM. Rats that binge eat fat-rich food do not show somatic signs or anxiety associated with opiate-like withdrawal: implications for nutrient-specific food addiction behaviors. *Physiol Behav*. 2011;104(5):865—872.

21. Oswald KD, Murdaugh DL, King VL, Boggiano MM. Motivation for palatable food despite consequences in an animal model of binge eating. *Int J Eat Disord*. 2011;44(3):203—211.

22. Bray GA. Fructose: pure, white, and deadly? Fructose, by any other name, is a health hazard. *J Diabetes Sci Technol*. 2010;4(4):1003—1007.

23. Bocarsly ME, Powell ES, Avena NM, Hoebel BG. High-fructose corn syrup causes characteristics of obesity in rats: increased body weight, body fat and triglyceride levels. *Pharmacol Biochem Behav*. 2010;97(1):101—106.

24. Avena NM, Gold JA, Kroll C, Gold MS. Further developments in the neurobiology of food and addiction: update on the state of the science. *Nutrition*. 2012;28(4):341—343.

25. Koob GF, Volkow ND. Neurobiology of addiction: a neurocircuitry analysis. *Lancet Psychiatry*. 2016;3(8):760—773.

26. Johnson PM, Kenny PJ. Dopamine D2 receptors in addiction-like reward dysfunction and compulsive eating in obese rats. *Nat Neurosci*. 2010;13(5):635—641.

27. Rada P, Avena NM, Hoebel BG. Daily bingeing on sugar repeatedly releases dopamine in the accumbens shell. *Neuroscience*. 2005;134(3):737—744.

28. Maldonado R, Valverde O, Berrendero F. Involvement of the endocannabinoid system in drug addiction. *Trends Neurosci*. 2006;29(4):225—232.

29. Berridge KC. 'Liking' and 'wanting' food rewards: brain substrates and roles in eating disorders. *Physiol Behav*. 2009;97(5):537—550.

30. The National Center on Addiction, Substance Abuse (CASA) at Columbia University. *Understanding and Addressing Food Addiction: A Science Based Approach to Policy, Practice, and Research*. 2016. New York.

31. Christensen R, Kristensen PK, Bartels EM, Bliddal H, Astrup A. Efficacy and safety of the weight-loss drug rimonabant: a meta-analysis of randomised trials. *Lancet*. 2007;370(9600):1706—1713.

32. Sakurai T. The role of orexin in motivated behaviours. *Nat Rev Neurosci*. 2014;15(11):719—731.

33. Koob GF. The dark side of addiction: the Horsley Gantt to Joseph Brady connection. *J Nerv Ment Dis*. 2017;205(4):270—272.

34. Cottone P, Sabino V, Roberto M, et al. CRF system recruitment mediates dark side of compulsive eating. *Proc Natl Acad Sci U S A*. 2009;106(47):20016—20020.

35. Moore CF, Sabino V, Koob GF, Cottone P. Neuroscience of compulsive eating behavior. *Front Neurosci*. 2017;11:469.

36. Volkow ND, Wang GJ, Tomasi D, Baler RD. The addictive dimensionality of obesity. *Biol Psychiatry*. 2013;73(9):811—818.

37. Small DM, Jones-Gotman M, Dagher A. Feeding-induced dopamine release in dorsal striatum correlates with meal pleasantness ratings in healthy human volunteers. *NeuroImage*. 2003;19(4):1709—1715.

38. Stice E, Spoor S, Bohon C, Veldhuizen MG, Small DM. Relation of reward from food intake and anticipated food intake to obesity: a functional magnetic resonance imaging study. *J Abnorm Psychol*. 2008;117(4):924—935.

39. Weinberger DR, Glick ID, Klein DF. Whither research domain criteria (RDoC)?: the good, the bad, and the ugly. *JAMA Psychiatry*. 2015;72(12):1161—1162.

40. Gearhardt AN, Corbin WR, Brownell KD. Preliminary validation of the Yale food addiction scale. *Appetite*. 2009;52(2):430—436.

41. Gearhardt AN, Corbin WR, Brownell KD. Food addiction: an examination of the diagnostic criteria for dependence. *J Addict Med*. 2009;3(1):1—7.

42. Gearhardt AN, Yokum S, Orr PT, Stice E, Corbin WR, Brownell KD. Neural correlates of food addiction. *Arch Gen Psychiatry*. 2011;68(8):808—816.

43. Gearhardt AN, Corbin WR, Brownell KD. Development of the Yale food addiction scale Version 2.0. *Psychol Addict Behav*. 2016;30(1):113—121.

44. Gearhardt AN, Roberto CA, Seamans MJ, Corbin WR, Brownell KD. Preliminary validation of the Yale food addiction scale for children. *Eat Behaviors*. 2013;14(4):508—512.

45. Flint AJ, Gearhardt AN, Corbin WR, Brownell KD, Field AE, Rimm EB. Food-addiction scale measurement in 2 cohorts of middle-aged and older women. *Am J Clin Nutr*. 2014;99(3):578—586.

46. Eichen DM, Lent MR, Goldbacher E, Foster GD. Exploration of "food addiction" in overweight and obese treatment-seeking adults. *Appetite*. 2013;67:22—24.

47. Pedram P, Wadden D, Amini P, et al. Food addiction: its prevalence and significant association with obesity in the general population. *PLoS One*. 2013;8(9):e74832.

48. American Psychiatric Association. *Diagnostic and Statistical Manual of Mental Disorders.* 5th ed. 2013. Washington, DC.

49. The National Center on Addiction, Substance Abuse (CASA) at Columbia University. *Food for Thought: Substance Abuse and Eating Disorders.* 2003. New York.

50. Mehler PS, Andersen AE. *Eating Disorders: A Guide to Medical Care and Complications.* Baltimore, MD: The Johns Hopkins University Press; 2009.

51. Hudson JI, Hiripi E, Pope Jr HG, Kessler RC. The prevalence and correlates of eating disorders in the National Comorbidity Survey Replication. *Biol Psychiatry.* 2007;61(3): 348–358.

52. Compan V, Walsh BT, Kaye W, Geliebter A. How does the brain implement adaptive decision making to eat? *J Neurosci.* 2015;35(41):13868–13878.

53. Kaye WH, Wierenga CE, Bailer UF, Simmons AN, Wagner A, Bischoff-Grethe A. Does a shared neurobiology for foods and drugs of abuse contribute to extremes of food ingestion in anorexia and bulimia nervosa? *Biol Psychiatry.* 2013;73(9):836–842.

54. Gearhardt AN, Boswell RG, White MA. The association of "food addiction" with disordered eating and body mass index. *Eat Behaviors.* 2014;15(3):427–433.

55. Hodgkins C, Frost-Pineda K, Gold MS. Weight gain during substance abuse treatment: the dual problem of addiction and overeating in an adolescent population. *J Addict Dis.* 2007;26(suppl 1):41–50.

56. Gearhardt AN, White MA, Potenza MN. Binge eating disorder and food addiction. *Curr Drug Abuse Rev.* 2011;4(3): 201–207.

57. Wang GJ, Tomasi D, Volkow ND, et al. Effect of combined naltrexone and bupropion therapy on the brain's reactivity to food cues. *Int J Obes.* 2014;38(5):682–688.

58. Avena NM, Bocarsly ME, Murray S, Gold MS. Effects of baclofen and naltrexone, alone and in combination, on the consumption of palatable food in male rats. *Exp Clinical Psychopharmacol.* 2014;22(5):460–467.

59. Schulte EM, Smeal JK, Gearhardt AN. Foods are differentially associated with subjective effect report questions of abuse liability. *PLoS One.* 2017;12(8):e0184220.

60. Gold MS, Adamec C. *The Encyclopedia of Alcoholism and Alcohol Abuse.* New York, NY: Infobase Publishing, Inc.; 2010.

61. National Center for Chronic Disease and Prevention, Health Promotion Office on Smoking and Health. *Reports of the Surgeon General. The Health Consequences of Smoking-50 Years of Progress: A Report of the Surgeon General.* Atlanta, GA: Centers for Disease Control and Prevention (US); 2014.

62. Jamal A, King BA, Neff LJ, Whitmill J, Babb SD, Graffunder CM. Current cigarette smoking among adults - United States, 2005-2015. *MMWR Morb Mortal Wkly Rep.* 2016;65(44):1205–1211.

63. Kansagra SM, Kennelly MO, Nonas CA, et al. Reducing sugary drink consumption: New York City's approach. *Am J Public Health.* 2015;105(4):e61–e64.

64. Andreyeva T, Chaloupka FJ, Brownell KD. Estimating the potential of taxes on sugar-sweetened beverages to reduce consumption and generate revenue. *Prev Med.* 2011;52(6): 413–416.

65. Kendler KS, Parnas J. *Philosophical Issues in Psychiatry IV: Psychiatric Nosology.* Oxford University Press; 2017.

66. Campbell J, O'Rourke M, Slater ME. *Carving Nature at Its Joints: Natural Kinds in Metaphysics and Science.* The MIT Press; 2011.

67. Avena NM, Gearhardt AN, Gold MS, Wang GJ, Potenza MN. Tossing the baby out with the bathwater after a brief rinse? The potential downside of dismissing food addiction based on limited data. *Nat Rev Neurosci.* 2012; 13(7):514; author reply 514.

68. Hebebrand J, Albayrak Ö AR, Adan R. "Eating addiction", rather than "food addiction", better captures addictive-like eating behavior. *Neurosci Biobehav Rev.* 2014;47(suppl C): 295–306.

69. Schulte EM, Potenza MN, Gearhardt AN. A commentary on the "eating addiction" versus "food addiction" perspectives on addictive-like food consumption. *Appetite.* 2017; 115:9–15.

70. Yokum S, Gearhardt AN, Harris JL, Brownell KD, Stice E. Individual differences in striatum activity to food commercials predict weight gain in adolescents. *Obesity (Silver Spring).* 2014;22(12):2544–2551.

71. Val-Laillet D, Aarts E, Weber B, et al. Neuroimaging and neuromodulation approaches to study eating behavior and prevent and treat eating disorders and obesity. *Neuro-Image Clin.* 2015;8:1–31.

CHAPTER 15

Quality, Accountability, and Effectiveness in Addiction Treatment: The Measurement-Based Practice Model

JOHN F. KELLY, PHD • DAVID MEE-LEE, MD

If you can't measure it, you can't improve it
LORD KELVIN (WILLIAM THOMSON)

INTRODUCTION

Alcohol and other drug (AOD) use disorders and related conditions pose a major threat to public health and safety among middle and high-income countries globally.[1] These growing problems confer a prodigious burden of disease, disability, and premature mortality as well as an increasing economic toll related to lost productivity, criminal justice, and healthcare costs.[2] To address these endemic substance-related problems, many societies provide an array of formal prevention and treatment services (e.g., screening and brief intervention, medications, outpatient, inpatient, residential treatments, recovery housing) across a broad range of healthcare settings as well as informal services (e.g., community-based peer supports, mutual-help organizations such as Alcoholics Anonymous [AA]).[3] In the United States, there are approximately 14,000 treatment facilities focused on treating AOD problems with costs for treatment in the tens of billions annually. It is anticipated that spending on SUD treatment is predicted to grow from $24.3 billion in 2009 to $42.1 billion in 2020.[4]

While the cost of treating AOD disorders care may be increasing substantially, the quality and effectiveness of treatments remains largely unknown. This is due, in part, to an implicit assumption that implementing best practices will produce better outcomes than treatment as usual. Thus, the fiscal appropriation and provision of such services is presumed to be sufficient to

reduce the public health impact of AOD on the population. However, among clinicians who adopt science-based standards of care, adequate *adherence* to the evidence-based protocols and the clinical *competence* with which such protocols are delivered vary greatly.[5] Additionally, studies have found that patients receiving treatment using evidence-based standards of care delivered with a high degree of adherence and competence do not actually have better clinical outcomes as compared to treatment as usual.[6,7] The large variability in the quality and benefit of implementing presumed best practices has been compounded by some treatment programs making outrageous claims of fantastically high success rates (despite rarely, if ever, defining success) and guaranteed recovery (despite no verification of these claims).

In sum, immense variation in the uptake and implementation of evidence-based practices; large variability in the quality of the delivery of care—even when evidence-based practices are adopted; inadequate demonstration of improved patient outcomes when programs deliver evidence-based practices with high fidelity; and the overselling of AOD treatment by some sectors of the treatment field has led to calls for much greater accountability in the AOD treatment field.

One way of improving the standard model of care is to move from evidence-based practice to measurement-based practice (MBP).[8,9] MBP has the potential to enhance accountability among providers and programs while improving the quality and effectiveness of AOD care through longitudinal capture, scoring, summarization, and relational graphic and/or tabular representation of brief, psychometrically validated patient-reported

The Assessment and Treatment of Addiction. https://doi.org/10.1016/B978-0-323-54856-4.00015-8

outcomes at the point of care.[8] This chapter will provide the following: (1) The rationale for MBP; (2) The potential benefits of MBP for patients, providers, programs, and payors; (3) A brief review of scientific findings regarding the demonstrated impact of implementing MBP approaches on care; and (4) A discussion of the implications of the findings of an MBP approach for addiction health care.

RATIONALE FOR MEASUREMENT-BASED PRACTICE

Healthcare costs continue to rise in the United States without concomitant improvements in patients' clinical outcomes. While insurers, practitioners, and clinical programs do their best to reimburse for and provide best practices to maximize health outcomes, system-wide inefficiencies remain. Health services are often based in clinical science; more specifically, they consist ideally of practices that have been proven under rigorous research conditions to provide an added benefit in patients' clinical outcomes and quality of life. Consequently, these are known as evidence-based practices (EBPs). One of the major problems faced in addiction health care, however, is determining what type and how much service to provide, as there is a lack of data on the observed degree of benefit accrued once the EBPs are implemented.

This lack of detailed data on patient outcomes is pervasive across health care and is particularly absent among the highly stigmatized addiction disorders. This has meant more recently that addiction treatment programs have come under increasing pressure to demonstrate effectiveness and be more accountable to justify their costs. If, for example, a family has $30,000 in life savings that they are willing and able to contribute toward care for a loved-one's addiction, should they spend it all on 28 days in "rehab"? If so, which program? Or, should they spend their money on a few years of outpatient treatment? Or, perhaps a combination of residential and outpatient treatment? Where is the evidence that can truly guide such decisions?

Research to Practice Gap and Barriers to Research Implementation

Evidence-based and evidence-informed practices have been buzz words for the past 20 years. The emergence of these concepts and terminology stemmed from calls from the Institute of Medicine of the National Academy of Sciences to help bridge the observed chasm in quality between the clinical science base and actual clinical

care—the so-called "research to practice gap".[10] This was an effort that mobilized a generation of researchers to develop new behavioral and pharmacological treatments and to conduct rigorous studies of their potential benefit. In turn, this brought widespread attempts to adopt and implement EBPs based on the results from these randomized clinical trials.[11] However, several challenges exist that hinder the timely acquisition of systematic clinical knowledge in the behavioral health and addiction fields, as well as science-based clinical practice dissemination and implementation in an attempt to improve patients' outcomes. These challenges include the following: (1) The long time lag between recognizing the need to answer a specific clinical question through research and being able to answer it; (2) The wide variability among addiction providers and programs in the adoption and implementation of EBPs; (3) The poor fidelity with which EBPs actually may be delivered in clinical care; and (4) The lack of convincing evidence that patients' outcomes are improved when EBPs are adopted and implemented with high fidelity.

The Long Time Lag Between Posing the Clinical Research Question and Finding Out Its Answer Through Standard Clinical Research Protocols

One of the challenges in devising and conducting clinical trials is the expense and sheer length of time they take to complete. A clinical researcher, for instance, may pose an important research question that needs to be answered. If motivated, the researcher then will conceive of a testable study design and spend several months writing a grant application to obtain the money needed to run the study. Once the grant is submitted to a funding institution (e.g., the United States National Institutes of Health), it might take four to five months for the institution to review the grant, assign a score, and provide feedback. Even if the response is favorable, grant funding institutions commonly ask grant writers to submit a revised application. It typically takes another year to submit a revised application and have it reviewed. If the funding institution approves the study, it may take several months thereafter to obtain the money. Finally, the researcher can *begin* the study. Clinical studies often last several years due to the need to recruit participants and follow clinical cases longitudinally over time. Thus, it may take five years of study recruitment and follow-up, statistical analyses, and writing of the study's results before the findings begin to be published. Even then, it can take another few years for the findings to be disseminated and discovered by treatment agencies and clinicians before the results are implemented in frontline practice settings. Therefore, while the clinical researcher needed that question answered at the time he or she first thought of it and decided to study it more systematically, it may be 10 years before any semblance of an answer will come to light. By that time, intervening changes (e.g., in clinical practices or funding/reimbursement structures) may render that question irrelevant. Additionally, the effects of using exclusion criteria add to the frustratingly long timeline of such studies. If relative improvements *are* found in a study under rigorously controlled experimental conditions, the benefits may not always be transferred to real-world clinical settings because certain types of more severe and medically and psychiatrically complex patients—the type seen in day to day real-world clinical practice settings—may have been excluded from those studies. Furthermore, there may be other unintended therapeutic artifacts operating under ideal controlled research conditions, such as the additional clinical researcher attention and support (which can have additional therapeutic benefit) and assessment reactivity,[12] which can enhance outcomes in clinical trials—therapeutic elements that are typically absent in frontline clinical care.

The Wide Variability Among Addiction Practitioners and Programs in the Adoption and Implementation of EBPs

It has long been known that there is wide variation in the degree to which clinical providers and programs adopt and implement EBPs. One reason for this is a simple lack of knowledge about new practices or innovations (e.g., "I didn't know about it"). Most practitioners and programs do not read academic journals and are therefore not exposed to the latest innovations in clinical science, leaving them unperturbed in continuing to implement existing practices. A further barrier is a presumed (or actual) lack of incremental benefit of a sufficient magnitude to justify the effort and expense of implementation (i.e., "it won't be worth the hassle"). Unless clinicians and programs perceive that the expense and effort needed to change practices is worth it, they are unlikely to adopt new practices or innovations. A study of clinicians conducted by Miller et al.[13] found that clinicians would only be willing to adopt a new addiction care practice if it resulted in at least a 10% benefit in patients' outcomes. Another obstacle is structural barriers including insufficient time, financial resources, and system support to teach and train practitioners in the new practices or to supervise them over time to ensure maintenance of the new

practices. Many programs and providers are required to maximize the amount of time spent in face-to-face clinical treatment delivery to maximize reimbursement and pay for overhead costs. Adopting and learning to deliver new practices can be an expensive disruption to healthcare systems. Finally, ideological barriers may cause providers and programs to object to the adoption and implementation of a particular approach even if evidence is strong (e.g., methadone/buprenorphine for the treatment of opioid use disorders) because they "don't believe in it" or believe "it's unethical."

The Poor Fidelity With Which EBPs May Be Actually Delivered in Standard Clinical Care

Another challenge in delivering high-quality addiction treatment is that while the implementation of an evidence-based practice is shown to result in better outcomes, it is difficult to ensure that clinicians and programs are using it with acceptable degrees of competence and adherence. It has been found, for example, that clinicians and programs who believe and report that they are using evidence-based practices may not actually be doing so. Examination of videotaped sessions from programs reporting that they are implementing evidence-based practices shows that the sessions have little to no resemblance to the actual evidence-based practice.[14] Given the disconnect between the apparent belief in adherence to proper implementation of evidence-based practices and the lack of actual resemblance to them, a question lingers around how to enforce or ensure proper use of evidence-based practices. MBP can allow for variability in EBP implementation by focusing more on the evaluation of outcomes. This eliminates the challenge of policing the competent deployment of evidence-based practices. Given the enormous burden of disease, disability, premature mortality, and economic costs (approaching $700 billion annually) attributed to alcohol and other drug use disorders in the United States, poorly implemented evidence-based practices and the lack of meaningful real-world benefit, even if they are implemented well, are of urgent concern.

The Lack of Convincing Evidence that Even When EBPs Are Adopted and Implemented With High Fidelity, Patients' Outcomes Are Improved

A further challenge is the striking finding that even when clinicians are trained and supervised to implement EBPs in addiction care (e.g., cognitive-behavioral therapy) and the new treatment is delivered, patients' clinical outcomes are not better than existing practices.[6,7]

While it is alluring to believe that the technical aspects of a particular therapy are responsible for conveying its therapeutic effects (e.g., teaching cognitive and behavioral coping skills in CBT), it has been observed that any rational, active, behavioral addiction treatment mobilizes the same underlying therapeutic factors, thus producing similar outcome benefits.[15] A noteworthy example of this is the findings from the largest multisite clinical trial of psychosocial treatment for alcohol use disorder known as Project MATCH.[16,17] In this trial, 1724 men and women with alcohol use disorder (AUD) were randomly assigned to receive one of three individually delivered treatments: (1) twelve sessions of cognitive-behavioral therapy (CBT); (2) four sessions of motivational enhancement therapy (MET), based on the principles of motivational interviewing; or (3) twelve sessions of Twelve-Step Facilitation (TSF) therapy intended simply to get patients engaged with community Alcoholics Anonymous meetings. Despite strong a priori predictions that CBT—given its strong existing empirical and theoretical base—would be a standout winner, all treatments did equally well on the main outcomes (i.e., on the average number of alcoholic drinks consumed per drinking day and the percentage of days in which patients were abstinence in the past 90 days across the 3-year follow-up period), with a slight advantage for TSF. Such findings are important as they suggest that several different well-articulated approaches, although differing in theory and conceptual language, produce similar benefits. Such findings are common.[18,8] Given the challenges and barriers to the standard care model of EBP implementation, we believe a more productive paradigm is to switch emphasis from evidence-based practice to measurement-based practice (MBP). Not only does MBP help to overcome these challenges, it also possesses a number of distinct advantages that can supplement EBP implementation. In the next section, we describe what MBP is and its potential advantages.

MBP AND ITS POTENTIAL BENEFITS FOR PATIENTS, PROVIDERS, PROGRAMS, AND PAYORS

We define MBP as the systematic capture, aggregation, summarization, and representation (e.g., graphic) of brief nonproprietary psychometrically validated clinically meaningful outcomes, captured at the point of care, and intended to enhance the quality, effectiveness, and accountability of addiction and behavioral healthcare organizations. It achieves this through providing clinically useful and easy to understand and interpret feedback to providers and patients, helping providers have instant access to data summarization capabilities regarding each patient or patient caseload and enabling them to monitor their own clinical effectiveness and improvement. It provides programs and systems with data summarization capabilities to monitor improvements in such things as patients' engagement, retention, and progress on targeted clinical outcomes and to compare such improvements within as well as across programs and systems.

More specifically, clinicians, programs, treatment systems, and insurers can be armed with vital clinical information that can help direct, and instantly and constantly, evaluate the provision of clinical care by using brief, nonproprietary, standardized and validated measures commonly used in clinical research, which can be captured easily in a few minutes using electronic tablet devices in the waiting room prior to each visit (e.g., on iPad-like devices) and then automatically and instantly aggregated, summarized, related to prior scores, and archived. These results can be fed back to patients to increase or maintain motivation and can alert clinicians to risky trends that could signify a high probability of treatment dropout or symptom exacerbation and relapse. At the program level and at the healthcare system level, it also helps to identify under- and over-performing clinicians and clinical programs that may be doing particularly well, as well as help identify patient subgroups for whom current best practices are not helping. This readily available information, in turn, can signal the need for clinical innovations that can be developed, implemented, and evaluated rapidly in a matter of months instead of years, because outcomes are continuously measured using the same standardized metrics used in clinical trials. This facilitates the immediate ability to test whether novel practice innovations can help particularly vulnerable patient subgroups in the actual specific contexts in which they are being treated. This shifts the emphasis from evidence-based practice to practice-based evidence driven by measurement-based practice.

We believe investment in and systematic use of MBP has the potential to revolutionize addiction and mental health care. MBP provides immediate clinical metrics regarding real-world impacts on the frontline where it has most meaning and relevance, reducing the need to wait years for results from long-term and expensive research studies that may ultimately have little real-world relevance and impact.

In many areas of medicine, a version of MBP is already in use to help inform and direct care. Blood pressure readings are always taken during hypertensive visits and blood sugar/A1c readings at diabetes care visits.

These provide the basis for monitoring and directing care and formulating recommendations and a treatment plan. Like these medical vital signs used for decades in medical care, the MBP approach assesses addiction/mental health vital signs to measure the outcomes and responses to treatment from mental health and addiction patients. Because we do not currently have biologically based vital signs (biomarkers) to examine response to addiction care, addiction vital signs are typically things like subjective reports of craving, and the number of days in the past week or month in which patients maintained abstinence from substances, the number of days in which they were intoxicated, the longest periods of continuous abstinence, and the number of days that alcohol/drug use interfered with functioning. Measures of psychiatric symptoms (e.g., depression, anxiety) can also be assessed and monitored as they commonly co-occur in the context of substance use and can undermine addiction recovery efforts if left unattended.

Patients and Providers

The beneficiaries of such an approach will be patients, providers, programs, payors, and treatment systems (Table 15.1). Patients will have immediate knowledge of, and access to, their own data-based clinical response to treatment that can be presented graphically for easy interpretation. This type of concrete visual feedback can empower and motivate patients to make necessary changes or maintain current behavioral management strategies. Clinicians will know concretely how well each individual patient in their case load is doing and will be able to see how well all their patients are doing overall; they will be able to monitor and evaluate whether they are improving in quality and effectiveness in the delivery of their own care over time. When set up appropriately, MBP approaches also allow for comparisons of effectiveness across providers within or across treatment programs, as well as across programs in systems.

TABLE 15.1

Benefits of Measurement-Based Practice (MBP) Models At Different Levels of Analysis and Examples of Common Clinical Questions That Can Be Answered Using It

Level	Benefits	Specific Questions Answered
Patient	Enhances patient engagement, interest, satisfaction, and clinical outcomes.	How am I doing in treatment? Am I getting worse, stabilizing, getting better?
Provider	Enhances provider awareness and empowerment through aggregation and visible summarization of validated clinically informative metrics.	How are my patients doing in treatment? What are my dropout/retention rates? Am I improving in the delivery of my care over time?
Program	Increases knowledge of program performance and quality of care; enhances identification of patient subgroups who are not responding to standard "best practice" approaches; facilitates rapid development and implementation of innovative practices in real-world setting, with built in evaluation of that innovation.	Which clinicians are under- and over-performing in my clinic? How is my program doing in treating addiction? Are there particular patient subgroups in my program that are falling through the cracks and not responding to standard best practice implementation? Are there some patient subgroups who are doing particularly well?
Payor	Provides psychometrically validated clinical evidence of provider/program performance leading to greater efficiency in health care insurance reimbursement, funding, and appropriations.	Which services should we pay for? What is the optimal configuration and implementation of successful practices? What is the best value model?
System	Identifies under- and over-performing clinical programs and uncovers new effective clinical paradigms leading to dissemination and wider spread clinical enhancements with immediate ecological validity.	Which programs are under- or over-performing? What factors are responsible for these differences?

Programs and Systems

Because of the aggregation of data using the same standardized validated outcome metrics used in clinical trials, programs can determine how well their patients are performing relative to those in clinical trials through comparing standardized effect sizes. Obviously, these need to be adjusted for differences in patient case-mix (i.e., demographic and clinical differences across samples), but even within programs, it is possible to determine whether a particular clinical program is continuing to improving outcomes year after year.

Continuous Quality Improvement

Because it is accruing and aggregating its own psychometrically validated clinical data over time, MBP also allows for easy identification of patient subgroups who are not responding as well to the standard of care being implemented. This can lead to immediate development and testing of novel clinical strategies to help determine if these outcomes can be improved. Importantly, because outcomes are being continuously measured, those vulnerable patient subgroups' responses to new clinical strategies can be assessed immediately and in a matter of months, rather than years. The quick turnaround in assessing the effectiveness of clinical indices is an important advantage compared to the standard research paradigm, which takes years of clinical trials for data to emerge only to then be met with skepticism as to if the results will apply in a specific clinical context or population.

From the broader treatment system standpoint, MBP will help identify under- and over-performing programs (after adjusting for patient case-mix variation allowing for "apples to apples" comparisons). Programs performing well can be identified and informed of such, as they not otherwise be aware of their success relative to other programs. This method will help uncover progressive new teams and new innovations that can be adopted and implemented elsewhere to positively affect more patients. Under-performing programs can also become of their shortcomings, prompting them to begin identifying weak links in the treatment process and ultimately innovate and improve their practices.

A major problem with the research to practice paradigm is that rather than driving progress through innovation clinicians often feel forced to deliver an external "evidence-base" that seems to undervalue and override their clinical experience, expertise and judgement, which leads to passivity, perceived impotence, even resentment. Alternatively, MBP empowers clinicians through providing data-based feedback and aggregation that allows for trend and subgroup analyses to identify

improvements as well as patients in need of greater attention.

The ability to identify over-performing providers and programs is a particular benefit of MBP that is not always immediately apparent. The continuous systematic monitoring of patient outcomes makes it possible to identify programs within a treatment system, region or country, who may have hit upon an optimal configuration of services or are doing something innovative that is producing particularly positive outcomes. This type of approach has been shown helpful in other areas of medicine such as the Cystic Fibrosis Foundation (CFF), which has collected detailed data from all of its affiliated clinics ($k = 117$) nationally for more than 50 years. In the 1960s, a physician named LeRoy Matthews of Cleveland, Ohio was claiming an extraordinarily low 2% mortality rate while the national mortality rate at the time was at least 20%, with most affected individuals deceased are 3-year olds. To test Matthews' claim, CFF in 1964 gave University of Minnesota (UMN) pediatrician Warren Warwick $10,000 to collect reports on every patient treated at the 31 Cystic Fibrosis (CF) care centers in the United States. The median age at death for patients in Matthews's center was 21 years—seven times older than patients treated elsewhere. Upon further investigation, Warwick found that Matthews' team was trying new procedures based on practices learned in other countries, providing more assertive patient disease management and monitoring. Matthews' model soon became the national standard and by the 1970s 95% of patients with CF were living past their 18th birthday.

As MBP begins to provide valid data for cost-effectiveness analyses, federal, state, and private insurers can begin to see the effectiveness and efficiency of healthcare provision and expenditure. However, because there could be potential challenges with programs only taking in "good prognosis" patients ("creaming") or otherwise reporting certain data and not others (biased reporting), programs will need to ensure proper adherence to an MBP approach by agreeing to independent random auditing much like healthcare quality accreditation agencies do (e.g., the Joint Commission on Accreditation of Healthcare Organizations [JCAHO], the Commission on Accreditation of Rehabilitation Facilities [CARF]). An added benefit is the ability to compare similar programs in a healthcare system or region or nationally depending on the degree of adoption of the MBP system around the country. The MBP approach provides continuous measurement that advances quality, accountability, and effectiveness.

We anticipate that this type of model will lead to greater patient engagement, retention, clinical response, and outcomes (Table 15.2). It will lead to greater clinical provider satisfaction, program awareness, and accountability to insurers and to the general public. These are important factors when addressing highly stigmatized conditions like addiction. Payors will know which programs/clinicians are good, better, and best. Best practices can be identified where it really matters—in the actual real-world healthcare delivery context with real, complex, patients. Excellent programs can be identified and informed that they have hit upon a winning formula. These winning formulae, in turn, can be shared to the benefit of more patients.

MBP approaches allow questions such as: What is my clinic's no-show rate this year? Last year? Last month? How has this changed over the past year or 5 years? What is my clinic's dropout rate within the first month that patients are in care? Are men or women more likely to drop out of treatment early? Are individuals with greater clinical severity more or less likely to drop out of treatment? Are individuals with opioid addiction compared to alcohol or other drug use disorders more or less likely to drop out of my treatment program? How is my program doing in terms of the proportion of patients achieving abstinence and remission in the first 3 months of care? Does this differ by gender, diagnosis, severity? These highly relevant clinical questions can be answered **easily and instantly** with a few clicks of a mouse through MBP software systems and the answers can subsequently be presented in easy to read tables and graphs. These data can be shared with staff, insurers and other stakeholders, without waiting for weeks for queries to be run on electronic medical record systems that do not possess the detailed levels of clinical outcome data.

SUMMARY

One of the significant benefits of the implementation of measurement-based practice models is that it can provide contextually specific outcome data and allow for continuous quality improvement through the ongoing accrual of psychometrically validated outcomes. This has two major benefits: (1) It helps to eliminate the substantial time lags between the discovery of clinical treatment innovations from efficacy research and clinical trials and the translation and implementation of those findings in front-line clinical practice settings (i.e., the "research to practice" gap); and (2) It removes the patient case-mix differences that often occur between efficacy research trials (which often have numerous exclusion criteria) and the more complex and diverse patient caseloads seen in real-world community-based addiction treatment programs. Furthermore, due to the continuous aggregation of data on patient

TABLE 15.2
Specific Features and Benefits of Measurement-Based Practice Domains

Measurement-based Practices Domains	Specific Features and Benefits
Assessment Type	Standardized, psychometrically validated patent-reported clinical outcome measures that have clinical utility and concurrent and predictive validity.
Assessment Frequency	Regular point of care (e.g., weekly) repeated measures assessment.
Assessment Scoring, Presentation, and Report Generation	Instant computerized scoring algorithms, summarization, and relational graphic/tabular presentation. Ability to generate instant reports of queries regarding patients' enrolment, engagement, retention, and clinical outcomes.
Level of analysis	Allows for data collection, scoring, summarization, and relational representation at the patient-, provider-, program-, and systems-level.
Quality Improvement	Allows for continuous quality improvement as well as uncovering and identification of vulnerable patient subgroups who are not responding to best practice implementation.
Clinical Innovation	Allows for quick frontline contextually specific clinical innovation to develop and test novel practices to help vulnerable patient subgroups and improve clinical outcomes.

characteristics, patient engagement and retention, and patients' clinical outcomes, MBP makes it possible for programs and treatment systems themselves to identify moderators of treatment response; it identifies which patients may or may not be responding to standard care. The increase of data aggregation over time allows for the simultaneous testing of multiple factors, which can help identify patient subgroups who may be "falling through the cracks." Clinical trials, on the other hand, cannot generally answer the important clinical question as to which patients are best suited to this specific intervention (i.e., personalized medicine), as they are typically powered statistically to detect main effects and not interactions (and when they are, they are usually only powered to detect one moderator variable, such as sex/gender or high/low severity effects). By implementing MBP, an investigator can move past simply asking "Do men and women do equally well in my treatment program?" and can act on clinical observations made at the clinic to ask a more complex question such as, "Do young women with opioid use disorder do as well on average, as all other patients treated in my program?". Here, it is not only sex/gender that is being considered, but age (young women) as well as primary substance (opioids). In this way, common clinical anecdotal observations regarding specific vulnerable patient subgroups can be examined more formally using the large accrued dataset that employs the same kinds of validated metrics utilized in clinical trials (e.g., percent days abstinent, number of days substance use interfered with functioning, etc.). This methodology allows for comparison with the published scientific literature, while noting any demographic or clinical differences between samples.

Providing insufficient timely and specific feedback to patients leads to a lack of awareness of their own progress and in what ways they are or are not progressing during SUD treatment. This is a disservice to patients. Feedback is often provided in the care of other medical disorders such as hypertension and diabetes where blood pressure and blood sugar markers are collected at the point of care and fed back to patients. Moreover, these indices serve as the basis for treatment plan evaluation and change when needed. Another challenge stemming from a lack of MBP is the absence of clinician awareness of patients' specific status, trends, and patterns on important clinical variables. Furthermore, programs feel disempowered to make changes or defend themselves to criticisms regarding their services if they are unaware of their own clinical effectiveness (e.g., rates of engagement, retention/dropout, response, success rates) (Box 15.1).

BOX 15.1
Advantages of MBP

Enhanced patient awareness of current status, trends, and patterns, on clinically relevant intermediate/ultimate outcomes (e.g., craving, days of use, pain).

Enhanced clinician awareness of patients' status, trends, and patterns, etc., that can highlight off-course cases early and raise consciousness and allow adjustments to course and intensify of treatment.

Enhanced program awareness of program's effectiveness in engagement, retention, clinical response to delivered care through continuous data aggregation.

Enhanced ability to detect patient subgroups failing to respond to standard of care lowering overall program effectiveness.

Enhanced awareness of poor patient response for patient subgroups facilitates immediate development, testing, and evaluation of clinical innovations NOW to meet needs of vulnerable populations (i.e., constant QI).

Clinic/program-level data comparison across collaborating centers and systems can allow identification of over-performing programs (as well as under-performing programs).

System-wide MBP can allow for continual identification of the most effective programs/practices and clinical innovations that have real-world ecological validity removing barriers of "research to practice" lags and translation.

Identify where exactly in the treatment causal therapeutic chain the treatment fails and thus enhance theories of SUD-related behavior change identifying the mobilizers, mechanisms, and moderators of such change.

WHAT IS CURRENTLY KNOWN EMPIRICALLY ABOUT THE EFFECTIVENESS OF MBP APPROACHES IN CLINICAL CARE?

Most, if not all, clinicians would likely agree with the assertion that it is vital to measure patients' responses to the care they are receiving. Any conscientious clinician will likely check in at every visit regarding goals and progress. This, however, is typically done informally through verbal means without the aid of standardized validated metrics. One of the challenges with this informal approach is that clinicians often have difficulty predicting patients' deterioration or impending treatment dropout.[19,20] Variations in more formal and systematic measurement-based systems have been around for many years,[21] but it is only more recently that sophisticated studies, including randomized controlled trials, have been conducted that show real-world benefits from implementation of MBP models.[22] The vast majority of this work has been conducted in general psychotherapy samples with an array of presenting problems and pathology.[23–26] Typically, these types of MBP have taken the form of systematic capture of patient-reported outcome measures that are scored, aggregated, and related to prior scores to mark symptom improvements or deterioration, other kinds of behavioral outcomes and functioning (e.g., number of days using alcohol or other drugs in the past week; urine toxicology screens), or treatment engagement (e.g., days attending treatment or number of sessions attended). These scores are then used by clinicians to monitor and guide treatment in an ongoing fashion. Data are sometimes directly fed back to patients to enhance interest, personal engagement, retention, and outcomes. Michael Lambert[27] and Scott Miller[22] are pioneers of implementation and evaluation of MBP. The available findings suggest that the routine implementation of some kind of outcome monitoring is likely to result in one or more of the following: (1) Double the treatment effect size and increase the proportion of patients with reliable and clinically significant change; (2) Reduce treatment dropout rates by half; (3) Reduce the risk of clinical deterioration by a third; (4) Shorten the length of treatment by two-thirds; and (5) Reduce the economic costs associated with treatment.[22] As in many interventions, however, feedback may not always enhance outcomes and may only do so under certain conditions. A randomized clinical trial by De Jong et al.[28] found that feedback was only effective for deteriorating, not-on-track clinical cases and among therapists who used the feedback. This highlights that therapist factors may also be important to consider in evaluating the magnitude of the effects of these approaches in some psychiatric populations.

Studies have also shown that treatment engagement, retention, and clinical outcomes can be enhanced in substance use disorder and addiction specific applications of MBP protocols. A randomized clinical trial by Raes et al.[29,30] found that compared to patients receiving treatment as usual without measurement-based feedback, patients receiving direct measurement-based feedback had increased adherence to treatment at and beyond eight sessions (53% vs. 34%) as well as at and beyond 12 sessions (34% vs. 21%). Another addiction specific multisite trial in three outpatient substance use disorder treatment clinics found that providing measurement-based feedback significantly reduced alcohol and drug use as well as

improved psychosocial functioning and symptoms[29] compared to treatment as usual.

While existing data are promising, more studies are needed to understand and pinpoint the nature, frequency, and scope of MBP and patient and clinician variable moderators of impact, as well as the healthcare cost necessary for its adoption and systematic use. That said, conservatively, it can be concluded from existing data from mental health and addiction populations that in most cases, MBP has the potential to improve and enhance patients' treatment engagement, retention, and outcomes. Furthermore, it does this in and of itself, without explicitly addressing any theoretically relevant variable as far as pathogenesis or maintaining factors are concerned. It merely raises consciousness of the change process by frequently highlighting the impact of any given intervention on relevant target outcome variables (e.g., abstinence motivation or self-efficacy, number of days abstinent, psychiatric distress) using standardized, psychometrically validated measures of high clinical utility. Thus, MBP models can be considered an additive beneficial component to whatever kind of theoretically driven treatment is being delivered.

IMPLICATIONS OF MBP APPROACHES FOR THE FUTURE OF ADDICTION HEALTH CARE

In the modern era, a great deal of focus and expenditure has been targeted at the adoption, implementation, and maintenance of evidence-based practice with the ultimate, worthy, goal of improving patients' clinical outcomes and quality of life. An implicit assumption of such efforts is that clinicians and healthcare systems would readily adopt and implement such practices, deliver them with close adherence to the original protocols and with high clinical competence, and that patients would subsequently be better off. Evidence accumulated during the past 20 years, however, has revealed that in addiction health care, voluntary uptake of such practices has been slow or delivered with low fidelity when adopted. Evidence-based practices have largely failed to enhance patients' outcomes in real-world settings despite being delivered with high fidelity and close adherence to the protocols that have shown to be beneficial under tightly controlled clinical research conditions. Furthermore, the development and testing of new clinical research protocols can take up to 10 years from research conception to study findings when trying to answer an important clinical research question—a question that had clinical relevance at the time it was posed but unknown relevance at the time the answer is finally revealed 10 years later. In addition, the applicability of the findings obtained under tightly controlled conditions with circumscribed and narrowly defined clinical populations often presents difficulties in translation to community settings, which cater to a broader mix of individuals with a more diverse range of severity, greater complexity, and comorbidity. This time lag from the conception of a clinical research question to obtaining the study results, coupled with the challenges of translation, adoption, and implementation of such findings to real-world care, substantially diminishes the efficiency of our models of clinical care. For these reasons, we argue that the addiction field move away from the narrow concept of evidence-based practice to the broader and more inclusive concept of measurement-based practice, consisting of reliable, valid, regular measurement of clinical and functional outcomes obtained as addiction vital signs at each point-of-care. These are analogous to physical vital signs that are assessed to both appraise and direct treatment planning in other chronic illness (e.g., obtaining blood pressure readings at each clinic visit in the treatment of hypertension). Use of standardized metrics in other fields of medical care, such as hypertension and diabetes, not only empowers clinicians to understand more reliably how a patient is responding to treatment, but allows them, their health systems, and insurance payers, to appraise clinical effectiveness and response to the current standard of care. Feedback to patients based on these metrics also can help patients more accurately assess how they are responding to care. This can motivate them to initiate, strengthen, or maintain salutary behavior changes. Evidence from the implementation of such measurement-based practice models suggests that such a paradigm increases patients' engagement with treatment as well as their clinical outcomes. Although not yet evaluated, these MBP models are likely to be highly cost-effective too, as greater treatment response means less relapse and less use of related expensive acute care medical services.

At the system level, this allows for evaluation of programs and detection of both under-performing and, equally important, over-performing programs—programs that have struck on a new approach or combination of approaches producing much better clinical outcomes. Such clinical system monitoring and surveillance has been adopted in other areas of medicine (e.g., cystic fibrosis) with the result that the quality, accountability, and effectiveness of clinical care have dramatically improved with many more lives saved.

Another important aspect of MBP is the aggregation of clinical data with high clinical utility, as such data are gathered with meaningful and valid metrics and are contextually relevant, stemming from and thus having direct applicability to the population at hand. Over time, this allows for the identification of patient subgroups for whom the standard of care is not working as well. In clinical research, these are known as statistical interactions or moderator effects. The difference with the MBP approach is the ability to examine high-order interactions with the larger and ever expanding datasets. Thus, instead of only evaluating whether a specific program or approach works as well for women as it does for men, one can evaluate whether women who are young and have a primary opioid addiction do as well as the rest of the clinical population. In other words, it allows for identification of more complex and vulnerable clinical profiles involving multiple characteristics instead of just one. Due to continuous outcomes measurement, clinical innovators using the MBP system can feel more empowered to act to remedy any shortfall in improvement that is observed in more vulnerable patient subgroups, while simultaneously evaluating the impact of these innovations in real-time.

CONCLUSION

In most middle- and high-income countries around the world, alcohol- and other drug-related conditions are among the greatest contributors to disease, disability, and premature mortality, conferring an immense economic burden on the bottom line of these nations. Healthcare service provision varies widely in cost across these different countries, but invariably absorbs a large chunk of these nations' gross domestic product (GDP). Addiction healthcare systems adopting MBP as a part of routine operations are likely to enhance patients' outcomes, empower clinicians, increase job satisfaction, and lead to more efficient use of resources. This MBP approach does not replace the evidence-based practice paradigm. Rather, measurement-based practice is the very essence of evidence-based practice, but with the evidence coming directly from the clinical population of relevance. The ready availability of data with high clinical utility and applicability means quicker identification and remediation of vulnerable and nonresponsive patient subgroups leading to enhanced overall outcomes and greater clinical efficiency. In turn, this can lead to greater accountability, quality, and effectiveness in addiction health care.

REFERENCES

1. *Global Status Report on Alcohol and Health*. Geneva, Switzerland: World Health Organization; 2014.
2. Facing addiction in America. *The Surgeon General's Report on Alcohol, Drugs, and Health: Executive Summary*. Washington, D.C.: US Department of Health and Human Services, Office of the Surgeon General; 2016.
3. Kelly JF, White WL. *Addiction Recovery Management: Theory, Research, and Practice*. New York: Humana Press/Springer Science Media LLC; 2011.
4. Substance Abuse, Mental Health Services Administration. *Projections of National Expenditures for Treatment of Mental and Substance Use Disorder, 2010-2020*. Rockville, MD.: HSS Publication No. SMA-14–4883; 2014.
5. Carroll KM, Kiluk BD, Nich C, et al. Toward empirical identification of a clinically meaningful Indicator of treatment outcome: features of Candidate Indicators and evaluation of Sensitivity to treatment effects and relationship to one Year follow up Cocaine Use outcomes. *Drug Alcohol Dependence*. 2014;137:3–19.
6. Morgenstern J, Blanchard KA, Morgan TJ, Labouvie E, Hayaki J. Testing the effectiveness of cognitive-behavioral treatment for substance abuse in a community setting: within treatment and posttreatment findings. *J Consult Clin Psychol*. 2001;69(6):1007–1017. https://doi.org/10.1037/0022-006x.69.6.1007.
7. Smedslund G, Berg RC, Hammerstrom KT, et al. Motivational interviewing for substance abuse. *Cochrane Database Syst Rev*. 2011;(5).
8. Kelly JF, Bergman BG, O'Connor C. Evidence-based Treatment of Addictive Disorders. An overview. In: McKillop J, McKenna G, Ray L, eds. *Integrating Psychological and Pharmacological Treatments for Addictive Disorders: An Evidence-based Guide*. New York: Taylor and Francis; 2016.
9. Miller SD, Mee-Lee D, Plum W, Hubble MA, Lebow J, eds. *Making Treatment Count: Client-directed, Outcome-informed Clinical Work with Problem Drinkers*. Hoboken, NJ: John Wiley & Sons; 2005:281–308.
10. Olsen L, McGinnis JM, eds. *Redesigning the Clinical Effectiveness Research Paradigm*. Washington, DC: Institute of Medicine; 2010.
11. Mittman BS. Creating the evidence base for quality improvement collaborative. *Ann Intern Med*. 2004;140(11):897.
12. Clifford PR, Maisto SA, David CM. Alcohol treatment research assessment exposure subject reactivity effects: part I. Alcohol use and related consequences. *J Studied Alcohol Drugs*. 2007;68(4):519–528.
13. Miller WR. *Enhancing Motivation for Change in Substance Abuse Treatment*. Rockville, MD: Center for Substance Abuse Treatment; 1999.
14. Sholomskas DE, Syracuse-Siewert G, Rounsaville BJ, Ball SA, Nuro KF, Carroll KM. We don't train in vain: a dissemination trial of three strategies of training clinicians in cognitive-behavioral therapy. *J Consult Clin Psychol*. 2005;73(1):106–115.
15. Mee-Lee D, McLellan AT, Miller SD. What works in substance abuse and dependence treatment, in the Heart and Soul of change. 2nd ed. Washington, DC. *Am Psychol Assoc*. 2010:393–417.
16. Project MATCH Research Group. Project MATCH: rationale and methods for a multisite clinical trial matching patients to alcoholism treatment. *Alcohol Clin Exp Res*. 1993;17:1130–1145.
17. Project MATCH Research Group. Matching alcoholism treatments to client heterogeneity: Project MATCH posttreatment drinking outcomes. *J Stud Alcohol*. 1997;58:7–29.
18. Longabaugh R, Donovan DM, Karno MP, McCrady BS, Morgenstern J, Tonigan JS. Active ingredients: how and why evidence-based alcohol behavioral treatment interventions work. *Alcohol Clin Exp Res*. 2005;29(2):235–247.
19. Hannan C, Lambert MJ, Harmon C, et al. A lab test and algorithms for identifying clients at risk for treatment failure. *J Clin Psychol*. 2005;61(2):155–163.
20. Hartfield D, McCullough L, Frantz SHB, Krieger K. Do we know when our clients get worse? An investigation of therapists' ability to detect negative client change. *Clin Psychol Psychotherapy*. 2009;17(1):24–32.
21. Howard KI, Moras K, Brill PL, et al. Evaluation of psychotherapy: efficacy, effectiveness, and patient progress. *Am Psychol*. 1996;51:1059–1064.
22. Miller SD, Hubble MA, Chow D, Seidel J. Beyond measures and monitoring: realizing the potential of feedback-informed treatment. *Psychotherapy*. 2015;52(4):449–457.
23. Amble I, Gude T, Stubdal S, Anderson BJ, Wampold BE. The effect of implementing the Outcome Questionnaire-45.2 feedback system in Norway: a multisite randomized clinical trial in a naturalistic setting. *Psychotherapy Res*. 2014;25(6):669–677.
24. Bickman L, Kelley SD, et al. Effects of routine feedback to clinicians on mental health outcomes of youths: results of a randomized trial. *Pschiatr Serv*. 2011;62(12):1423–1429.
25. Knaup C, Koesters M, et al. Effects of feedback of treatment outcome in specialist mental healthcare: meta-analysis. *Br J Psychiatry*. 2009;195(01):15–22.
26. Probst T, Lambert MJ, et al. Feedback on patient progress and clinical support tools for therapists: improved outcome for patients at risk of treatment failure in psychosomatic in-patient therapy under the conditions of routine practice. *J Psychosomatic Res*. 2013;75(3):255–261.
27. Lambert MJ, Shimokawa K. Collecting client feedback. *Psychother Relationships That Work*. 2011:203–223.
28. De Jong K, Sluis PV, Nugter MA, Heiser WJ, Spinhoven P. Understanding the differential impact of outcome monitoring. Therapist variables that moderate feedback effects in a randomized clinical trial. *Psychotherapy Res*. 2012;22(4):464–474.
29. Crits-Christoph P, Ring-Kurtz S, Hamilton JL, et al. A preliminary study of the effects of individual patient-level feedback in outpatient substance abuse treatment programs. *J Subst Abuse Treat*. 2012;42(3):301–309.
30. Raes V, De Jong CA, Bacquer DD, Broekaert E, Maeseneer JD. The effect of using assessment instruments on substance-abuse outpatients adherence to treatment: a multi-centre randomised controlled trial. *BMC Health Serv Res*. 2011;(1):11.

CHAPTER 16

Functional Assessment and Treatment of Alcohol Use Disorders

JEFFREY BECKER, MD, ABIHM • ITAI DANOVITCH, MD, MBA, DFASAM, FAPA

INTRODUCTION

Alcohol use disorders (AUD) are a major preventable cause of morbidity and mortality. Effective interventions exist[1]; however, there are many barriers to optimal outcomes. Well-established psychosocial and pharmacological interventions for AUD can be limited by disengagement, tolerability, nonadherence, and high relapse rates.[2] There is a need for additional interventions that are safe, well tolerated, acceptable to patients, and effective. Natural molecular treatments—or functional treatments, such as high-dose vitamins, minerals, amino acids and other metabolites—are supported by several lines of evidence and may engage patients who are reluctant to accept pharmaceutical medications. Such interventions are not a replacement for effective pharmacotherapy or psychosocial interventions, but they may have salutary benefits, support recovery, and engage patients in fostering nutritional health. This chapter explores the rationale supporting functional treatments in AUD and clinical considerations in assessment and treatment. After describing functional medicine in general, we characterize four natural interventions for which there is evidence of efficacy, followed by a series of less well-established interventions that warrant consideration.

FUNCTIONAL TREATMENT DEFINED

Functional Medicine (FM) is not a separate branch of medicine, such as Ayurveda, acupuncture, or energy healing, disciplines that are sometimes referred to as complimentary, holistic, or alternative medicine. FM approaches disease in a manner consistent with Western medical paradigms, addressing pathophysiologic mechanisms in disease to reduce pathology and support restoration of health. However, FM prioritizes use of commonly available nutritional entities to address imbalances with perceived incremental negative effect over time. Typical interventions include vitamins, minerals, and nutrients.

WHY ARE FUNCTIONAL TREATMENTS IMPORTANT IN AUD

Alcohol is one of the oldest known intoxicating substances used by humans. Excessive alcohol use can have both acute and chronic toxic effects.[3] Gastrointestinal enterocytes may become degraded, impairing barrier function and leading to absorption of inflammatory bacterial cell-wall components (e.g., lipopolysaccharide). Hepatic toxicity, as well as innate immune system hyperstimulation, may contribute to the development of cirrhosis. Gut-related toxicity inhibits absorption of numerous vitamins, minerals and nutrients, leading to deficiencies not easily corrected through low-dose oral repletion strategies. Renal toxicity may decrease reabsorption or increase excretion of necessary nutrients, compounding the effect of impaired intestinal absorption. Thus, alcohol may both cause and magnify nutritional deficiencies in drinkers. Excessive alcohol use can deplete vitamin and mineral cofactors, leading to deficiencies and degradation of antioxidant systems, leaving tissues vulnerable to free-radical and inflammatory assault. Recognizing patterns of AUD toxicity and understanding the role of nutritional depletion sets the stage for functional treatment.

THIAMINE

Thiamine, also known as Vitamin B1, is a coenzyme required by several enzymes critical to energy metabolism. Thiamine is found in whole grains, yeast, and legumes and is absorbed in the small intestine via active transport and passive diffusion. Thiamine has a half-life of 10−20 days, and its metabolites are excreted via urine and bile. Thiamine storage is limited,

The Assessment and Treatment of Addiction. https://doi.org/10.1016/B978-0-323-54856-4.00016-X

necessitating continuous dietary consumption to maintain adequate levels. Deficiency may result from inborn errors of metabolism, poor absorption, or inadequate nutrition.

The best-known complication of severe thiamine deficiency in persons with AUD is Wernicke's encephalopathy, an acute neurological syndrome characterized by progressive encephalopathy, oculomotor dysfunction, and gait ataxia; unaddressed, this can lead to long-term complications such as Korsakoff's dementia.[4] However, subclinical thiamine deficiency is much more common in AUD and may still have significant neurological consequences.[5]

Thiamine is poorly phosphorylated to its active diphosphate form in the context of inadequate nutrition and hepatic insufficiency, reducing its activity as an essential cofactor for a number of enzymes in the tricarboxylic acid cycle. Deficiency reduces dependent enzymatic activity, but it also reduces overall concentrations of both thiamine-dependent and thiamine-independent enzymes in the murine tricarboxylic acid cycle.[6] Thiamine deficiency degrades ATP productive capacity, which contributes to neuronal injury, particularly in the mammillary bodies, impairs cardiac function, and compromises other vulnerable tissues and organ systems. Direct toxic effects of thiamine deficiency are further compounded by indirect effects that increase oxidative stress.[7]

Most commercial laboratories offer serum thiamine testing, with a normal range of 70–180 nmol/L (3.0–7.7 µg/dL). Thiamine deficiency can be detected through an inadequate erythrocyte thiamine transketolase[8] response to a thiamine pyrophosphate challenge test.[9] However, the sensitivity and specificity of this test is not well characterized, nor is it readily available at point of care. Cerebral spinal fluid thiamine monophosphate levels are potentially more sensitive and specific for thiamine deficiency[10]; however, these too are impractical in general practice when a clinical determination is sufficient to justify supplementation.

Thiamine is readily available over the counter for oral intake and by prescription for parenteral administration. It is low cost, well tolerated, and indicated in the treatment of acute alcohol detoxification. Normal dietary requirements are 1–2 mg daily; however, in the setting of insufficiency, significantly higher levels of repletion are required. A recent systematic review concluded there is insufficient evidence to dictate specific recommendations for dose, frequency, or route of thiamine administration.[11] However, the Royal College of Physicians published a rigorous guideline for treatment and prevention of Wernicke's encephalopathy, recommending parenteral thiamine dosing of 500–750 mg three times per day for a minimum of 5 days, and to continue for as long as improvement occurs. They also recommend parenteral administration of riboflavin, pyridoxine, nicotinamide, vitamin C, and magnesium.[12] Other recommendations suggest 500 mg thiamine parenterally three times per day for 2 days, followed by 250 mg parenterally for 5 days.[13] Supplementation of thiamine should precede glucose administration, as glucose metabolism depletes thiamine and can exacerbate deficiency.

Oral thiamine is poorly absorbed, such that treatment of AUD in outpatient settings should include high-dose oral thiamine supplementation or use of highly absorbed thiamin congeners, such as benfotiamine. Benfotiamine (S-benzoylthiamine-O-monophosphate) is a high-potency thiamine analog found within the allium family (e.g., garlic, onions, leeks). It is the most studied and most potent of the alli-thiamines, a class of natural thiamine congeners with enhanced absorption and blood–brain barrier penetration (e.g., benfotiamine, sulbutiamine, fursultiamin).[14] These thiamine analogs are of particular interest in AUD because they offer increased absorption in compromised individuals. A study of 120 nontreatment seeking, actively drinking, alcohol-dependent adults found that 600 mg daily oral benfotiamine was well tolerated and was associated with a significant reduction in total mean alcohol intake over 6 months (−611 drinks vs. −159 drinks) in women, but not in men.[15] A study at a teaching hospital found that inadequate thiamine repletion was documented in 97.6% of high-risk inpatients, resulting from inappropriate dosing, frequency and route of delivery.[16] Given the favorable risk-benefit profile of thiamine, supplementation should be considered for all patients with moderate to severe alcohol use disorder.

N-ACETYLCYSTEINE

N-acetylcysteine (NAC) is a low-cost, well-tolerated dietary supplement, available both over-the-counter and by prescription. NAC is a prodrug to L-cysteine, the limiting amino acid precursor to the endogenous antioxidant glutathione. NAC is FDA approved to prevent hepatic injury after acetaminophen overdose and is believed to exert its protective effects through restoration of glutathione levels depleted by the toxic acetaminophen metabolite N-acetyl-p-benzoquinoneimine. NAC has shown promise in several psychiatric conditions and substance use disorders.[17]

Both cysteine and glutathione can become depleted in AUD.[18] Low consumption of protein or poor digestive function can limit absorption. In addition, hepatic insufficiency can impair transsulfuration, which is required to recover cysteine from homocysteine.[19] One marker of depletion is gamma-glutamyl transferase (GGT), which is used as a marker of excessive drinking because GGT increases as the body attempts to restore alcohol-related depletion of cysteine and glutathione. Glutathione also plays a direct and essential role in NMDA receptor activity through regulation of many redox sensitive processes, such as receptor activation and signal transduction.[20] NMDA receptor hyperactivity may mediate acute and postacute alcohol withdrawal symptoms and influence long-term mood regulation and risk of relapse.

To date, most research on NAC in AUD has focused on alcoholic hepatitis. One study evaluated 5 days of IV NAC versus placebo given with prednisolone in 174 human subjects with severe alcoholic hepatitis, reporting a notable decrease in 1-month all-cause mortality (hazard ratio, 0.58; 95% CI, 0.14 to 0.76; $P = .006$) though their primary outcome measurement at 6 months fell short of significance (hazard ratio, 0.62; 95% CI, 0.37 to 1.06; $P = .07$).[21] However, given that functional interventions are unlikely to continue working for 6 months after only 5 days of treatment, the duration of administration may not have been adequate. In future research, transition to oral NAC dosing might be considered.

Typical dosing for NAC is 1200 mg orally twice daily; however, doses as high as 8000 mg/day have been administered safely and without adverse effects.[22] A double-blinded randomized controlled study of NAC at 2400 mg/day in veterans with post-traumatic stress disorder and SUD (over 80% had AUD) demonstrated improvements in clinical scores for depression, PTSD and drug craving (alcohol, cocaine and opiate; $P < .05$), though craving was a secondary outcome.[23]

At this point in time, there is not much direct evidence to support the use of NAC for AUD. However, as the preceding discussion indicates, there are several reasons why NAC may be therapeutic, and additional studies are warranted to examine its efficacy. Clinicians may consider using NAC on a case by case basis, weighing the positive safety profile against the potential, but as of yet unproven, benefits.

MAGNESIUM

Magnesium is an alkaline metal with wide ranging physiological activity, supporting over 300 enzymatic reactions throughout the human body.[24] Magnesium ions are predominantly stored intracellularly, such that depletion is not readily apparent from serum tests. Hypomagnesemia can cause neuromuscular hyperexcitability, cardiac arrhythmias, and abnormalities in calcium metabolism. In addition, hypokalemia occurs in 40%–60% of patients with hypomagnesemia.[25]

Hypomagnesemia is common in AUD, occurring in up to one-third of patients presenting to hospitals, 37% of those with cirrhosis and 86% of those with delirium tremens.[26] Deficiency occurs due to reduced intake and absorption, and sharply increased urinary loses within minutes of alcohol ingestion[27–29] due to impaired renal tubular reabsorption, or as a side effect of hypophosphatemia or increased lactate.[29] Hypomagnesemia has been associated with osteoporosis and cardiovascular disease in alcoholism,[28,30] stroke, sarcopenia, cardiomyopathy, steatohepatitis, cirrhosis,[31] and angina.[32] A study of ICU patients with AUD linked severe magnesium deficiency with mortality risk.[33] Severe and rapid negative effects of magnesium depletion may be an issue in binge drinking as well.

In early sobriety, lingering low magnesium levels may contribute to common psychiatric symptoms including depression, anxiety, memory problems, and insomnia given its role as a natural intracellular NMDA receptor antagonist. In a massive "Triple-Hit," chronic alcohol intake simultaneously induces hypomagnesemia, NMDA receptor hypersensitivity and GABA-B receptor hyposensitivity,[34] a powerfully negative combination that may make early abstinence emotionally difficult and fraught with insomnia and physical activation. Magnesium supplementation has shown safety and efficacy in anxiety disorders,[35] depression,[36] and insomnia associated with subacute alcohol withdrawal.[37]

Assessment of magnesium status through serum values is likely to underestimate the prevalence and severity of magnesium deficiency. Serum-ionized magnesium failed to identify severely deficient cirrhotic patients identified with magnesium loading tests.[38] Magnesium is predominantly stored intracellularly, and if magnesium load testing is unavailable, RBC levels may help rule-in deficiency; however, in patients with chronic magnesium-wasting tubulopathies, RBC levels may not be helpful.[39] Given the difficulty of ruling-out magnesium deficiency, empiric supplementation of magnesium to patients with moderate to severe AUD may be considered. Labs can be drawn but inherently poor sensitivity must be acknowledged in translation to treatment.

Supplement formulation is important, with poorly absorbed forms of magnesium commonly prescribed for osmotic laxative effects. While IV magnesium treatments are sometimes offered in inpatient settings, oral dosing of magnesium sufficient to achieve whole-body repletion requires higher doses and longer periods of time than is commonly prescribed. Magnesium citrate can be the right choice in individuals with constipation, while magnesium hydroxide is generally only appropriate for constipation. Magnesium glycinate may be the most easily tolerated and absorbed. A study confirming that transcutaneous permeation of magnesium can occur primarily through hair follicles[40] implies possible benefits from high concentration magnesium sulfate (i.e., Epsom salt) baths. Magnesium repletion in AUD may require significant doses for extended periods. In a study of 49 persons with AUD, 15 mmol of magnesium as mixed lactate and citrate salts (dose split TID) for 6 weeks significantly reduced AST, ALT and GGT levels, and improved numerous electrolytes (Na, K, P, Mg, Ca) and muscle strength compared to placebo.[41] In recently abstinent persons with AUD, eight weeks of 500 mg of magnesium (in split dose as magnesium carbonate, acetate and hydroxide) was associated with improved mean serum AST scores compared to placebo.[42]

ZINC

Zinc is an essential trace element incorporated into hundreds of specific enzymes that perform numerous essential metabolic functions. It is vital to DNA transcription and supports antioxidant function, immune function, wound healing, protein synthesis, and sense of taste and smell. Sufficient daily intake is required because no zinc storage system exists in the human body. Zinc deficiency leads to growth impairment, mental lethargy, anorexia, alopecia, diarrhea, and skin lesions.[43]

Multiple mechanisms conspire to cause severe zinc deficiency in alcoholism, including increased urinary losses, decreased intake, reduced intestinal absorption, and impaired albumin-related carrying capacity. Serum Zinc levels were reported to be critically low in patients with cirrhosis compared to controls (0.82 vs. 11.22 μmol/L; $P < .001$), and levels were worse still in patients with encephalopathy and ascites ($P = .002$).[44] Severity of zinc deficiency was correlated to Child-Pugh groups,[44] implying that deficiency may play a large and direct role in cirrhosis mortality. However, it should be noted that liver biopsy revealed severe zinc depletion in alcoholics both with cirrhosis (−55%) and without (−30%)[45]; thus, deficiency should be evaluated at all stages of treatment. Zinc deficiency can influence metabolism of other essential nutrients such

as niacin, which is implicated in alcoholic pellagra[46] and may be involved in many conditions commonly comorbid with AUD including anorexia, skin lesions, hypogonadism, retinal dysfunction, congenital malformations, immune dysfunction, cancer,[47] anosmia, poor sense of taste, brain fog, hair loss, weight loss, poor wound healing, night blindness, and diarrhea.[48]

Laboratory assessment of zinc status, while potentially useful, must be interpreted with caution, as zinc is primarily an intracellular ion that easily buffers to plasma, normalizing serum levels even in circumstances of severe intracellular depletion. As such, serum testing can provide false reassurance, leading to inadequate prescriptive supplementation. For instance, in healthy subjects with AUD, alveolar macrophages were zinc deficient despite normal serum levels, and this was correlated to poor phagocytic functioning.[49] In patients with alcoholic cirrhosis, zinc sulfate at 600 mg/day corrected serum zinc levels in 10 days, but it took 60 days to normalize levels in liver tissue.[50] The limitations of laboratory testing necessitate close clinical assessment of signs and symptoms of zinc deficiency.

Zinc repletion can be achieved through oral supplementation; however, some formulations of zinc are poorly absorbed and/or tolerated and research into optimal forms is needed.[51] It is important to note that high-dose zinc supplementation can drive down copper levels[52]; however, this can be managed through serial laboratory assessment (i.e., serum ceruloplasmin or copper), allowing clinicians to prescribe doses of zinc that achieve repletion goals. Patients exhibit variable tolerance for different zinc formulations and thus it is reasonable to suggest a number of different products to identify one that is tolerable. Generally, chelated forms of zinc (e.g., orotate, picolinate, and glycinate) are better tolerated and they may have some absorption advantages, though they can be harder to find and more expensive per milligram.

While 1 month of repletion at 400 mg/day of zinc sulfate improved visual capacity in subjects with AUD and visual neuropathy,[53] 3 days of zinc at 40 mg/day did not affect parameters of acute withdrawal.[54] In patients with alcoholic cirrhosis, 200 mg of zinc sulfate for 2 months produced significant improvement in immune function.[55] And, despite starting with normal serum levels, high-dose zinc sulfate (200 mg TID for 6 weeks) restored taste function, raised prothrombin and alkaline phosphatase levels, and lowered levels of bilirubin and carotene in patients with cirrhosis.[56]

In summary, zinc repletion is likely to be a critical leverage point in AUD recovery, especially in severe cases. Low-dose supplementation is unlikely to meet the needs of many patients with AUD and mere dietary improvement during recovery may be inadequate to replete zinc deficiency. For example, after 30 days, rehab patients still exhibited significantly lower zinc levels compared to controls in one study,[57] and after 21 days, serum zinc and selenium levels did not improve without supplementation in another.[58] Clinicians working with AUD should perform clinical and laboratory assessment of zinc and copper status and prescribe supplementary zinc in doses sufficient to achieve meaningful clinical and laboratory outcomes. High copper levels commonly associated with AUD can be corrected through zinc repletion, but if copper levels are normal or low then a copper supplement at 1 or 2 mg/day should be included to avoid inducing copper deficiency. Even high copper levels can eventually become depleted by high-dose zinc supplementation, so serial serum copper or ceruloplasmin levels can be warranted.

OTHER FUNCTIONAL SUPPORT

The interventions that follow are organized in terms of generalized support or specific clinically relevant symptomatic support.

General Vitamin and Mineral Support

In AUD, it would be easier to ask which vitamins and minerals are not depleted. Documented deficiencies can be severe and include: Thiamine/B1,[16,59] Niacin/B3,[46,60] Folate/B9,[61] Cobalamin/B12,[62−65] Zinc,[44,46,47,66−68] Magnesium,[28,64,65,67,69] Phosphate,[64,70] Vitamin D,[28,64,65,67,68,70,71] Vitamin A,[66,68,72,73] Iron,[65] CoQ10,[74,75] Carnitine,[76] Vitamin C,[59,68,77,78] and Vitamin E.[68,73,79] Given the general safety of supplements and the broad potential for progressive damage should deficiencies go unaddressed, prescriptions for comprehensive, even aggressive, nutrient repletion can be justified.

Prescribing an effective supplement regimen can require attention to several different factors including the following:

- **Pricing and Quality**—The supplement industry produces products that vary greatly in quality and price, two factors that are not necessarily correlated. The independent quality testing and pricing analysis produced by the online resource Consumer Lab (www.consumerlab.com) is a helpful clinical resource.
- **Convenience and Compliance**—There are a number of quality supplement manufacturers producing well-designed synergistic nutrient combinations.

Formulas combining commonly coprescribed nutrients (e.g., CoQ10 & Acetyl-L-Carnitine, or zinc & magnesium) can reduce cost and filler content, and increase convenience and compliance.

- **Absorption and Tolerability**—Nutrient formulation can affect absorption and tolerance (e.g., magnesium oxide vs. magnesium glycinate, or ferrous sulfate vs. ferrous succinate). While there are many places to turn for information in this regard, clinicians may find the online monographs found at Examine (www.examine.com) helpful (Table 16.1).

Mood, Anxiety and Stress Support

AUD has been associated with states of low mood and impaired hedonic drive.[80] One strategy to support recovery is to supplement precursors involved in mood regulation. While this chapter does not permit a thoroughly detailed exploration of this arena, the following natural treatments may have some utility and theoretical basis for use in AUD. The evidence for efficacy in humans is admittedly thin, but consideration of these interventions may be warranted by the combination of a favorable safety profile, and at least some theoretical basis or preliminary experimental findings.

Rhodiola rosea is frequently used in complementary and alternative medicine for antistress and mood-elevating effects. It is considered an adaptogen (a natural substance thought to promote homeostasis or support physiological adaptation to stress) and has been shown to modulate catecholaminergic neurotransmitters,[81] perhaps in part through monoamine oxidase inhibition.[28,82]

Hypericum perforatum, also known as St. John's Wort (SJW), has been used as a mood tonic for 2000 years and may have benefits for depressive symptoms associated with AUD. Attention to CYP effects is warranted given pharmacokinetic interaction with several commonly prescribed medications. While no human studies have been reported, alcohol-preferring rats significantly reduced intake when placed on a high-dose extract alone and when lower doses were used in conjunction with naltrexone.[83] The mechanism of action may involve effects upon serotonin and norepinephrine reuptake, and/or extracellular GABA and acetylcholine.[84]

Cognitive and Cholinergic Support

In addition to long-term effects on the GABAergic system, AUD appears to induce alterations in the cholinergic system.[85] Alterations in cholinergic transmission may underlie a broad set of symptoms in recovery

TABLE 16.1
Key Vitamin, Mineral and Nutrient Categories With Dosing Range and Clinical Issues

Class Effect	Specific Nutrient	Forms	Low Dosing	High Dosing	Notes
Vitamin Support	General Multi-vitamin and Stress B Complex	Various	One daily	Three/day	Choose products with active B-vitamin forms such as methylcobalamin, methylfolate, pyridoxal 5'-phosphate. Comprehensive products with other antioxidants (e.g., CoQ10, carnitine, resveratrol) may improve cost and compliance. Almost all vitamins and minerals can be depleted in AUD, so choose a comprehensive formula.
	Thiamine	Thiamine Oral	100 mg	300 mg	High doses are often needed.
		Thiamine IM	100 mg	1500 mg	May be only effective form in early recovery. Requires prescription and teaching injection procedure to patient.
		Benfotiamine	100 mg	300 mg	More easily absorbed at gut and maybe at blood–brain barrier. Best researched.
		Sulbutaimine	100 mg	200 mg	Less researched.
	Vitamin D	D_3 or cholecalciferol	1,000 IU	10,000 IU	Use initial and follow-up blood levels to guide dosing strategy. Prescription strength may be warranted. Consider repeat labs if product or formulation changes. Long-term supplementation ≤2,000 IU/day generally does not require monitoring.
Mineral Support	Zinc	Zinc Orotate, Zinc Citrate, Zinc Picolinate	30 mg	300 mg	Offer a few products to patients to help them determine which is most tolerable. Split daily dose in BID or TID fashion and take with food if possible. Dosing is likely to be higher than expected. Check copper or ceruloplasmin before and periodically to avoid copper depletion and include a copper supplement as needed.
	Magnesium	Magnesium Glycinate, Magnesium Citrate, Magnesium Taurinate	400 mg	1,200 mg	Intake can be limited by laxative effects. Split dose and use chelated forms. May have immediate benefits after binging.
	Multimineral	Molybdenum, Chromium, Manganese, Selenium, Copper (see zinc note)			Covers wide range of micromineral needs. May already be incorporated in a comprehensive multiple. Copper is often high in AUDs so keep dosing of this low if labs confirm. Watch for copper depletion over months if high doses of zinc are prescribed.

Category	Compound	Form	Low dose	High dose	Notes
Mitochondrial support	CoQ10	Ubiquinone, Ubiquinol	100 mg	400 mg	Best absorbed if taken with fat. Can be combined with Omega-3 supplements.
	Carnitine	Acetyl-L–Carnitine & L-Carnitine	500 mg	2,000 mg	Acetyl group may allow better absorption.
Antioxidant & antiinflammatory	Cysteine	N-Acetylcysteine	600 mg	2,000 mg	Easy to supplement orally. Do not trade for glutathione supplements which are probably just an expensive source of L-cysteine.
	Resveratrol	Resveratrol	100 mg	400 mg	Antioxidant component of grapes, wine and other plants sources. May be particularly well suited to addressing innate immune system hyperstimulation.
		Pterostilbene	25 mg	100 mg	A more potent version of resveratrol.
	Curcumin	Curcuminoids	100 mg	500 mg	Combine with piperine to enhance absorption. Other proprietary versions exist. Raw and dried turmeric are potential options
	Omega-3 Fatty Acids	Triglycerides Ethyl Esters	1,000 mg	8,000 mg	Variety of strengths and various ratios of EPA and DHA exist. Consider esterified or prescription strength versions for their potency.
Neurotransmitter & amino acid support	Acetylcholine	CDP choline	200 mg	2,000 mg	AKA Citicoline
		L-Alpha glyceryl-phosphorylcholine	400 mg	1,200 mg	AKA Alpha-GPC. 40% choline.
		Choline Bitartrate	300 mg	1,000 mg	May be less capable of crossing BBB
	Dopamine and Norepinephrine	L-Tyrosine	500 mg	2,000 mg	May help with anhedonia and brain fog in early and sustained recovery.
	Taurine	Taurine	2,000 mg	6,000 mg	Natural analog of acamprosate.
GI Support	L-glutamine	L-glutamine powder	2 g	8 g	May reduce withdrawal symptoms. Is a precursor for glutamate and GABA and improves GI barrier function.
Stress Support	Rhodiola rosea	Standardized Extract	250 mg	500 mg	Complex pharmacology, but generally standardized for 3% rosavins and 1% salidroside.
	Hypericum perforatum	Standardized Extract	600 mg	1,200 mg	AKA St. John's Wort. Ideally in thrice daily dosing. Some propriety extracts have research support. Can inhibit CYP enzymes and reduce oral birth control efficacy.

(e.g., brain fog and cognitive deficits, emotional dysregulation, depression).[86] Furthermore, cholinergic transmission is involved in growth hormone (GH) regulation, and impairments may adversely influence GH release.[87]

Transdermal administration of the cholinergic medication galantamine to AUD subjects who had completed detoxification shortened time to severe relapse by 28%, but reduced mean grams of alcohol consumed on drinking days after relapse by 24%.[88] Cytidine diphosphate-choline, also known as citicoline or CDP-choline, is a substrate for production of acetylcholine and phosphatidylcholine. A review of nine studies in cocaine use disorder reported promising results,[89] and a study investigating effects on heavy alcohol consumption is currently underway.[90] It is possible that other cholinergic supplemental support (e.g., DMAE, centrophenoxine, choline, phosphatidylcholine) would be helpful in AUD but research is lacking.

Mitochondrial Support

The mitochondrion is an organelle involved in metabolism, aerobic respiration, and energy production. Mitochondrial ALDH is involved in conversion of acetaldehyde to acetate, one of the key steps in the metabolism of alcohol. Excessive alcohol degrades mitochondrial function,[91] resulting in impaired respiration, reduced ATP levels, and increased production of reactive oxygen species implicated in several alcohol-related pathological pathways, including cardiac and liver toxicity.[92] It induces reductions in carnitine palmitoyltransferase and mitochondrial complexes I and V, negatively affecting ATP production.[93] Many vitamin and mineral deficiencies already discussed have a negative impact on mitochondrial function, but two natural molecules warrant specific mention.

Acetyl-L-Carnitine (ALC) is a natural and well-tolerated over-the-counter supplemental form of carnitine. In vivo, carnitine transports fatty acids from the cytoplasm across mitochondrial membranes to provide fuel for oxidative respiration. It also contributes to acetylcholine production through donation of acetyl groups. Approximately 25% of daily carnitine need is synthesized de novo from methionine and lysine and requires niacin, B6, iron and ascorbic acid as cofactors, all of which are commonly depleted in AUD. The rest is acquired from an adequate diet through GI absorption, both of which are also commonly compromised. In addition, the biochemical compromise in cirrhosis directly impairs de novo synthesis.

Carnitine availability may play a role in alcohol-related morbidity, though the mechanisms are not clear

and conflicting findings have been reported, with some studies finding high[94] and others low plasma levels.[76] It is possible that chronic alcohol use leads to low levels, whereas decompensated liver function can result in elevations.[95]

Acute administration of L-carnitine with alcohol had no effect on blood alcohol level but decreased mean plasma acetate AUC by 23% and increased urinary acetylcarnitine levels, implying that supplemental L-carnitine was trapping excess acetyl groups produced in ethanol metabolism.[96] Acetyl-L-carnitine successfully reversed alcohol-induced increases in superoxide and hydroxyl in human brain endothelial cells in vitro,[97] and coadministration with alcohol reduced frontal cortical oxidative damage and neuronal loss, and restored LTP-related neurotransmission in male mice.[98]

A multicenter double-blinded randomized trial evaluated the effects of ALC 2 g per day in patients with AUD and cognitive deficits who were abstinent for 1 month, showing improved performance in several cognitive domains.[99] A more recent study of ALC 2 g twice per day improved a broad spectrum of parameters assessing mental status, cognition, and liver function.[100]

Ubiquinone or CoQ10 is a vitamin-like coenzyme involved with Complex I, II and III in the electron transport chain, a series of reactions involved in mitochondrial energy production. CoQ10 is readily available over the counter as a supplement, is well tolerated, and relatively low cost. Oxidative respiration is responsible for up to 95% of human energy production and insufficient concentrations of CoQ10 can adversely impact tissues with high energy demand (e.g., cardiac, brain, liver). CoQ10 depletion can also increase chances of electron escape from the electron transport chain and increase levels of superoxide, a powerful free radical.

CoQ10 levels are negatively affected by oxidative stress, reduced endogenous synthesis in the liver, and poor dietary intake. Any or all of these mechanisms can occur in AUD and CoQ10 levels were reported to be only 27% of controls in cirrhotic alcoholics and 53% in noncirrhotic alcoholics.[74] Deficiency in this critically important molecule is likely to affect the health of many individuals with AUD.

In rats, CoQ10 dose dependently reduced alcohol induced neuropathy and hyperalgesia[101] and protected gastric mucosal tissues from alcohol-induced damage.[102] While there are no human studies supporting the use of CoQ10 in AUD, supplemental CoQ10 is already a reasonably well-accepted treatment in heart disease and further research is warranted to evaluate putative benefits in AUD.

Amino Acid Support

Poor nutritional status in AUD may lead to inadequate stores of essential amino acids (AAs). A study of patients with AUD and niacin deficiency found that essential and conditionally essential amino acids (e.g., tryptophan, methionine, phenylalanine, arginine and tyrosine) were reduced by 40% or more, while nonessential AAs and neuroexcitatory glutamic acid were increased.[103] Low levels of essential AAs can deplete several critical neurotransmitters and functional support may include L-type amino acids to facilitate synthesis (e.g., 5HTP in depression, L-Tyrosine in attention deficit).

A food supplement containing D-phenylalanine, L-glutamine, and L-5-hydroxytriptophan reportedly reduced some psychiatric symptoms compared to placebo in 20 AUD patients undergoing alcohol detoxification, though several laboratory measures were unchanged.[104] Taken on an empty stomach, supplemental L-type AAs flood transporters at the blood—brain barrier and may increase brain levels beyond that seen with improved diet alone. In combination with key vitamins and minerals (e.g., B6, C, folate, B12, zinc, magnesium and iron), AA supplementation may help provide symptomatic improvement in early recovery.

Taurine is a sulfonic acid derivative of the amino acid cysteine. It is essential for cardiac function and acts as an endogenous antioxidant. Within the central nervous system, it protects against glutamate excitotoxicity through inhibitory effects on neurotransmission.[105] Taurine has notable natural overlap in its receptor effects with those of alcohol, including a potentiation of GABA and glycine receptors and inhibition of excitatory amino acid receptors and calcium channels.[106] The FDA has approved acamprosate, a homotaurine derivative, for use in AUD. Taurine at 2 g three times daily, administered over a period of 3 months, significantly reduced liver enzyme levels, improved B-vitamin status, reduced reactive oxygen species, and increased the activities of alcohol dehydrogenase and aldehyde dehydrogenase in subjects with AUD.[107]

Anti-inflammatory Support

Chronic alcohol use provokes inflammation that can persist well beyond periods of active drinking. High levels of TNF-α, IL-8, and malondialdehyde,[73] oxidative stress caused by depleted CoQ10 and degraded oxidative phosphorylation,[75] and damaged glutathione peroxidase (GPx), superoxide dismutase (SOD), and catalase[79] have all been described. Nuclear factor kappa beta (NFKβ) can stimulate the innate immune system and is upregulated by many factors increased by alcohol use including TNF-α,[108] oxidized glutathione,[109] ROS,[110] lipopolysaccharide,[111] and elevated glutaminergic neurotransmission.[112]

Resveratrol is a natural antioxidant and NFKβ-antagonist with a potential protective role in alcohol-induced inflammation. To date, there are no human studies. Animal studies suggest resveratrol may reverse alcohol-induced elevations in liver enzymes, TNF-α, IL-1 and lipid peroxides, and reverse deficiencies in the endogenous antioxidant enzymes SOD, catalase, and GPx.[113,114]

Similarly, curcumin is a constituent of turmeric with broad anti-inflammatory effects and indications of potential efficacy for depression.[115] Animal models suggest potential benefits from curcumin in the setting of pathology resulting from excessive alcohol[116—118]; however, human studies are lacking.

Gastrointestinal Support

While much of the inflammatory burden of alcohol is attributable to overt toxicity, increased gastrointestinal permeability may contribute indirect toxic effects.[119] Damage to enterocytes and tight-junction integrity by aldehyde and proliferation of gram-negative bacterial species may increase circulating endotoxin and pepdidoglycan, triggering innate inflammatory systems in the liver.[120] Endocrine peptides from the GI tract are known to influence corticostriatal-limbic circuitry[121]; thus, treatments oriented toward restoration of bowel ecology and physiology may be useful in recovery. Glutamine is an AA thought to have positive effects upon intestinal barrier function in parenteral nutrition,[122] but it has not been studied directly in AUDs. Though some animal studies with probiotics are encouraging, a human trial in patients with pancreatitis produced a twofold increased risk of mortality[123] and thus more study is necessary before this can be recommended. While alcohol-related GI tract vulnerability may make supplementation of exogenous strains of bacteria inadvisable, prebiotic supplements that support endogenous probiotic species are likely to be more safe. Lactulose is a prescription prebiotic sugar that has been shown to support probiotic species in the colon. It increased lactobacilli species in cirrhotic patients[124] and reduced endotoxin, TNF-α, IL-6 and IL-18 in cirrhotic patients with minimal encephalopathy.[125] Trials with natural prebiotics are lacking (e.g., inulin, fructooligosaccharides) but one review reports that L-glutamine, zinc, and oats may help improve intestinal function.[120]

CONCLUSIONS

Despite converging evidence and a favorable risk-benefit profile, functional treatments are rarely utilized in AUD. Several factors may inhibit adoption of functional treatments. The small effect sizes of natural treatments make it difficult to ascertain outcomes. Problems with absorption may limit the effectiveness of commonly used repletion strategies. Reliance on standard serum laboratory assays to determine metabolic and physiological health may fail to detect early markers. Clearly, more research is needed to determine what elements of AUD pathology are most appropriately targeted with FM interventions, what patient populations are most likely to benefit, what dose and duration of interventions are required, and what clinical or laboratory assays are effective in monitoring treatment outcomes.

This review sought to bring to together existing research and literature on FM interventions for AUD. The following is a summary of key points:

- There is ample evidence documenting multiple, severe, interacting vitamin, mineral and metabolic deficiencies at all disease stages.
- Nutrient deficiencies are associated with AUD morbidity, likely both resulting from and exacerbating alcohol-related pathophysiology.
- Research establishing efficacy of nutritional interventions is limited, and existing studies are beset with challenges related to adequacy of formulation and dosing, duration of treatment, and tissue-specific assessment of efficacy.
- There are studies with adequate nutrient dosages for sufficient time reporting notably positive outcomes.
- More research is needed to establish the role and relevance of functional treatments in AUD. There is also a need for research examining synergistic supplement combinations that address multiple arenas of pathophysiology simultaneously.

REFERENCES

1. Jonas DE, Amick HR, Feltner C, et al. Pharmacotherapy for adults with alcohol use disorders in outpatient settings: a systematic review and meta-analysis. *JAMA.* 2014;311(18):1889–1900. https://doi.org/10.1001/jama.2014.3628.
2. Rapp RC, Xu J, Carr CA, Lane DT, Wang J, Carlson R. Treatment barriers identified by substance abusers assessed at a centralized intake unit. *J Subst Abuse Treat.* 2006;30(3):227–235. https://doi.org/10.1016/j.jsat.2006.01.002.
3. Lieber CS. Relationships between nutrition, alcohol use, and liver disease. *Alcohol Res Health J Natl Inst Alcohol Abuse Alcohol.* 2003;27(3):220–231.
4. Latt N, Dore G. Thiamine in the treatment of Wernicke encephalopathy in patients with alcohol use disorders. *Intern Med J.* 2014;44(9):911–915. https://doi.org/10.1111/imj.12522.
5. Krishel S, SaFranek D, Clark RF. Intravenous vitamins for alcoholics in the emergency department: a review. *J Emerg Med.* 1998;16(3):419–424.
6. Bubber P, Ke Z-J, Gibson GE. Tricarboxylic acid cycle enzymes following thiamine deficiency. *Neurochem Int.* 2004;45(7):1021–1028. https://doi.org/10.1016/j.neuint.2004.05.007.
7. Hazell AS, Faim S, Wertheimer G, Silva VR, Marques CS. The impact of oxidative stress in thiamine deficiency: a multifactorial targeting issue. *Neurochem Int.* 2013;62(5):796–802. https://doi.org/10.1016/j.neuint.2013.01.009.
8. Leigh D, McBurney A, McIlwain H. Erythrocyte transketolase activity in the Wernicke-Korsakoff syndrome. *Br J Psychiatry J Ment Sci.* 1981;139:153–156.
9. Edwards KA, Tu-Maung N, Cheng K, Wang B, Baeumner AJ, Kraft CE. Thiamine assays-advances, challenges, and caveats. *ChemistryOpen.* 2017;6(2):178–191. https://doi.org/10.1002/open.201600160.
10. Tallaksen CM, Bøhmer T, Bell H. Concentrations of the water-soluble vitamins thiamin, ascorbic acid, and folic acid in serum and cerebrospinal fluid of healthy individuals. *Am J Clin Nutr.* 1992;56(3):559–564.
11. Day E, Bentham PW, Callaghan R, Kuruvilla T, George S. Thiamine for prevention and treatment of Wernicke-Korsakoff Syndrome in people who abuse alcohol. *Cochrane Database Syst Rev.* 2013;(7):CD004033. https://doi.org/10.1002/14651858.CD004033.pub3.
12. Thomson AD, Cook CCH, Touquet R, Henry JA, Royal College of Physicians, London. The Royal College of Physicians report on alcohol: guidelines for managing Wernicke's encephalopathy in the accident and Emergency Department. *Alcohol Alcohol.* 2002;37(6):513–521.
13. Cook CC, Hallwood PM, Thomson ADB. Vitamin deficiency and neuropsychiatric syndromes in alcohol misuse. *Alcohol Alcohol.* 1998;33(4):317–336.
14. Gibson GE, Hirsch JA, Cirio RT, Jordan BD, Fonzetti P, Elder J. Abnormal thiamine-dependent processes in Alzheimer's Disease. Lessons from diabetes. *Mol Cell Neurosci.* 2013;55:17–25. https://doi.org/10.1016/j.mcn.2012.09.001.
15. Manzardo AM, He J, Poje A, Penick EC, Campbell J, Butler MG. Double-blind, randomized placebo-controlled clinical trial of benfotiamine for severe alcohol dependence. *Drug Alcohol Depend.* 2013;133(2):562–570. https://doi.org/10.1016/j.drugalcdep.2013.07.035.
16. Isenberg-Grzeda E, Chabon B, Nicolson SE. Prescribing thiamine to inpatients with alcohol use disorders: how well are we doing? *J Addict Med.* 2014;8(1):1–5. https://doi.org/10.1097/01.ADM.0000435320.72857.c8.
17. McClure EA, Gipson CD, Malcolm RJ, Kalivas PW, Gray KM. Potential role of N-acetylcysteine in the management of substance use disorders. *CNS Drugs.* 2014;28(2):95–106. https://doi.org/10.1007/s40263-014-0142-x.

18. Kumar SM, Haridoss M, Swaminathan K, Gopal RK, Clemens D, Dey A. The effects of changes in glutathione levels through exogenous agents on intracellular cysteine content and protein adduct formation in chronic alcohol-treated VL17A cells. *Toxicol Mech Methods*. 2017;27(2):128−135. https://doi.org/10.1080/15376516.2016.1268229.

19. Lu SC. Regulation of glutathione synthesis. *Mol Aspects Med*. 2009;30(1−2):42−59. https://doi.org/10.1016/j.mam.2008.05.005.

20. Do KQ, Cabungcal JH, Frank A, Steullet P, Cuenod M. Redox dysregulation, neurodevelopment, and schizophrenia. *Curr Opin Neurobiol*. 2009;19(2):220−230. https://doi.org/10.1016/j.conb.2009.05.001.

21. Nguyen-Khac E, Thevenot T, Piquet M-A, et al. Glucocorticoids plus N-acetylcysteine in severe alcoholic hepatitis. *N Engl J Med*. 2011;365(19):1781−1789. https://doi.org/10.1056/NEJMoa1101214.

22. De Rosa SC, Zaretsky MD, Dubs JG, et al. N-acetylcysteine replenishes glutathione in HIV infection. *Eur J Clin Invest*. 2000;30(10):915−929.

23. Back SE, McCauley JL, Korte KJ, et al. A double-blind, randomized, controlled pilot trial of N-Acetylcysteine in veterans with posttraumatic stress disorder and substance use disorders. *J Clin Psychiatry*. 2016;77(11):e1439−e1446. https://doi.org/10.4088/JCP.15m10239.

24. Jahnen-Dechent W, Ketteler M. Magnesium basics. *Clin Kidney J*. 2012;5(suppl 1):i3−i14. https://doi.org/10.1093/ndtplus/sfr163.

25. Whang R, Ryder KW. Frequency of hypomagnesemia and hypermagnesemia. Requested vs routine. *JAMA*. 1990;263(22):3063−3064.

26. Sullivan JF, Wolpert PW, Williams R, Egan JD. Serum magnesium in chronic alcoholism. *Ann NY Acad Sci*. 1969;162(2):947−962. https://doi.org/10.1111/j.1749-6632.1969.tb13023.x.

27. Laitinen K, Lamberg-Allardt C, Tunninen R, et al. Transient hypoparathyroidism during acute alcohol intoxication. *N Engl J Med*. 1991;324(11):721−727. https://doi.org/10.1056/NEJM199103143241103.

28. Abbott L, Nadler J, Rude RK. Magnesium deficiency in alcoholism: possible contribution to osteoporosis and cardiovascular disease in alcoholics. *Alcohol Clin Exp Res*. 1994;18(5):1076−1082.

29. Elisaf M, Merkouropoulos M, Tsianos EV, Siamopoulos KC. Pathogenetic mechanisms of hypomagnesemia in alcoholic patients. *J Trace Elem Med Biol Organ Soc Miner Trace Elem GMS*. 1995;9(4):210−214. https://doi.org/10.1016/S0946-672X(11)80026-X.

30. Brown RA, Crawford M, Natavio M, Petrovski P, Ren J. Dietary magnesium supplementation attenuates ethanol-induced myocardial dysfunction. *Alcohol Clin Exp Res*. 1998;22(9):2062−2072.

31. Romani AMP. Magnesium homeostasis and alcohol consumption. *Magnes Res*. 2008;21(4):197−204.

32. Miwa K, Igawa A, Miyagi Y, Fujita M. Importance of magnesium deficiency in alcohol-induced variant angina. *Am J Cardiol*. 1994;73(11):813−816.

33. Chernow B, Bamberger S, Stoiko M, et al. Hypomagnesemia in patients in postoperative intensive care. *Chest*. 1989;95(2):391−397.

34. Knapp CM, Ciraulo DA, Datta S. Mechanisms underlying sleep-wake disturbances in alcoholism: focus on the cholinergic pedunculopontine tegmentum. *Behav Brain Res*. 2014;0:291−301. https://doi.org/10.1016/j.bbr.2014.08.029.

35. Boyle NB, Lawton C, Dye L. The effects of magnesium supplementation on subjective anxiety and stress—a systematic review. *Nutrients*. 2017;9(5). https://doi.org/10.3390/nu9050429.

36. Eby GA, Eby KL. Rapid recovery from major depression using magnesium treatment. *Med Hypotheses*. 2006;67(2):362−370. https://doi.org/10.1016/j.mehy.2006.01.047.

37. Hornyak M, Haas P, Veit J, Gann H, Riemann D. Magnesium treatment of primary alcohol-dependent patients during subacute withdrawal: an open pilot study with polysomnography. *Alcohol Clin Exp Res*. 2004;28(11):1702−1709.

38. Koivisto M, Valta P, Höckerstedt K, Lindgren L. Magnesium depletion in chronic terminal liver cirrhosis. *Clin Transpl*. 2002;16(5):325−328. https://doi.org/10.1034/j.1399-0012.2002.01141.x.

39. Elin RJ, Hosseini JM, Gill JR. Erythrocyte and mononuclear blood cell magnesium concentrations are normal in hypomagnesemic patients with chronic renal magnesium wasting. *J Am Coll Nutr*. 1994;13(5):463−466.

40. Chandrasekaran NC, Sanchez WY, Mohammed YH, Grice JE, Roberts MS, Barnard RT. Permeation of topically applied Magnesium ions through human skin is facilitated by hair follicles. *Magnes Res*. 2016;29(2):35−42. https://doi.org/10.1684/mrh.2016.0402.

41. Gullestad L, Dolva LO, Søyland E, Manger AT, Falch D, Kjekshus J. Oral magnesium supplementation improves metabolic variables and muscle strength in alcoholics. *Alcohol Clin Exp Res*. 1992;16(5):986−990.

42. Poikolainen K, Alho H. Magnesium treatment in alcoholics: a randomized clinical trial. *Subst Abuse Treat Prev Policy*. 2008;3:1. https://doi.org/10.1186/1747-597X-3-1.

43. Sandstead HH, Freeland-Graves JH. Dietary phytate, zinc and hidden zinc deficiency. *J Trace Elem Med Biol Organ Soc Miner Trace Elem GMS*. 2014;28(4):414−417. https://doi.org/10.1016/j.jtemb.2014.08.011.

44. Rahelić D, Kujundžić M, Romić Z, Brkić K, Petrovecki M. Serum concentration of zinc, copper, manganese and magnesium in patients with liver cirrhosis. *Coll Antropol*. 2006;30(3):523−528.

45. Rodriguez-Moreno F, González-Reimers E, Santolaria-Fernandez F, et al. Zinc, copper, manganese, and iron in chronic alcoholic liver disease. *Alcohol*. 1997;14(1):39−44. https://doi.org/10.1016/S0741-8329(96)00103-6.

46. Vannucchi H, Moreno FS. Interaction of niacin and zinc metabolism in patients with alcoholic pellagra. *Am J Clin Nutr*. 1989;50(2):364−369.

47. McClain CJ, Su LC. Zinc deficiency in the alcoholic: a review. *Alcohol Clin Exp Res*. 1983;7(1):5−10.

48. Zinc: fact sheet for health professionals. January 2018. https://ods.od.nih.gov/pdf/factsheets/Zinc-HealthProfessional.pdf.

49. Mehta AJ, Yeligar SM, Elon L, Brown LA, Guidot DM. Alcoholism causes alveolar macrophage zinc deficiency and immune dysfunction. *Am J Respir Crit Care Med.* 2013;188(6):716—723. https://doi.org/10.1164/rccm.201301-0061OC.

50. Zarski JP, Arnaud J, Labadie H, Beaugrand M, Favier A, Rachail M. Serum and tissue concentrations of zinc after oral supplementation in chronic alcoholics with or without cirrhosis. *Gastroenterol Clin Biol.* 1987;11(12):856—860.

51. McClain C, Vatsalya V, Cave M. Role of zinc in the development/progression of alcoholic liver disease. *Curr Treat Options Gastroenterol.* 2017;15(2):285—295. https://doi.org/10.1007/s11938-017-0132-4.

52. Fiske DN, McCoy HE, Kitchens CS. Zinc-induced sideroblastic anemia: report of a case, review of the literature, and description of the hematologic syndrome. *Am J Hematol.* 1994;46(2):147—150.

53. Béchetoille A, Ebran JM, Allain P, Mauras Y. Therapeutic affect of zinc sulfate on central scotoma due to optic neuropathy of alcohol and tobacco abuse. *J Fr Ophtalmol.* 1983;6(3):237—242.

54. Iber FL. Evaluation of an oral solution to accelerate alcoholism detoxification. *Alcohol Clin Exp Res.* 1987;11(3):305—308.

55. Labadie H, Verneau A, Trinchet JC, Beaugrand M. Does oral zinc improve the cellular immunity of patients with alcoholic cirrhosis? *Gastroentérologie Clin Biol.* 1986;10(12):799—803.

56. Weismann K, Christensen E, Dreyer V. Zinc supplementation in alcoholic cirrhosis. A double-blind clinical trial. *Acta Med Scand.* 1979;205(5):361—366.

57. De Vos N, Song C, Lin A h, et al. Lower serum zinc in relation to serum albumin and proinflammatory cytokines in detoxified alcohol-dependent patients without apparent liver disease. *Neuropsychobiology.* 1999;39(3):144—150. https://doi.org/26574.

58. Gueguen S, Pirollet P, Leroy P, et al. Changes in serum retinol, alpha-tocopherol, vitamin C, carotenoids, xinc and selenium after micronutrient supplementation during alcohol rehabilitation. *J Am Coll Nutr.* 2003;22(4):303—310.

59. Baines M. Detection and incidence of B and C vitamin deficiency in alcohol-related illness. *Ann Clin Biochem.* 1978;15(6):307—312.

60. Badawy AA-B. Pellagra and alcoholism: a biochemical perspective. *Alcohol Alcohol.* 2014;49(3):238—250. https://doi.org/10.1093/alcalc/agu010.

61. Blasco C, Caballería J, Deulofeu R, et al. Prevalence and mechanisms of hyperhomocysteinemia in chronic alcoholics. *Alcohol Clin Exp Res.* 2005;29(6):1044—1048.

62. Fragasso A, Mannarella C, Ciancio A, Sacco A. Functional vitamin B12 deficiency in alcoholics: an intriguing finding in a retrospective study of megaloblastic anemic patients. *Eur J Intern Med.* 2010;21(2):97—100. https://doi.org/10.1016/j.ejim.2009.11.012.

63. Cylwik B, Czygier M, Daniluk M, Chrostek L, Szmitkowski M. Vitamin B12 concentration in the blood of alcoholics. *Pol Merkur Lek Organ Pol Tow Lek.* 2010;28(164):122—125.

64. Wijnia JW, Wielders JPM, Lips P, van de Wiel A, Mulder CL, Nieuwenhuis KGA. Is vitamin D deficiency a confounder in alcoholic skeletal muscle myopathy? *Alcohol Clin Exp Res.* 2013;37(suppl 1):E209—E215. https://doi.org/10.1111/j.1530-0277.2012.01902.x.

65. Sobral-Oliveira MB, Faintuch J, Guarita DR, Oliveira CP, Carrilho FJ. Nutritional profile of asymptomatic alcoholic patients. *Arq Gastroenterol.* 2011;48(2):112—118.

66. Russell RM. Vitamin A and zinc metabolism in alcoholism. *Am J Clin Nutr.* 1980;33(12):2741—2749.

67. Wilkens Knudsen A, Jensen J-EB, Nordgaard-Lassen I, Almdal T, Kondrup J, Becker U. Nutritional intake and status in persons with alcohol dependency: data from an outpatient treatment programme. *Eur J Nutr.* 2014;53(7):1483—1492. https://doi.org/10.1007/s00394-014-0651-x.

68. Maillot F, Farad S, Lamisse F. Alcohol and nutrition. *Pathol Biol Paris.* 2001;49(9):683—688.

69. Turecky L, Kupcova V, Szantova M, Uhlikova E, Viktorinova A, Czirfusz A. Serum magnesium levels in patients with alcoholic and non-alcoholic fatty liver. *Bratisl Lekárske Listy.* 2006;107(3):58—61.

70. Vandemergel X, Simon F. Evolution of metabolic abnormalities in alcoholic patients during withdrawal. *J Addict.* 2015. https://doi.org/10.1155/2015/541536.

71. Neupane SP, Lien L, Hilberg T, Bramness JG. Vitamin D deficiency in alcohol-use disorders and its relationship to comorbid major depression: a cross-sectional study of inpatients in Nepal. *Drug Alcohol Depend.* 2013;133(2):480—485. https://doi.org/10.1016/j.drugalcdep.2013.07.006.

72. McClain CJ, Van Thiel DH, Parker S, Badzin LK, Gilbert H. Alterations in zinc, vitamin A, and retinol-binding protein in chronic alcoholics: a possible mechanism for night blindness and hypogonadism. *Alcohol Clin Exp Res.* 1979;3(2):135—141.

73. González-Reimers E, Fernández-Rodríguez CM, Candelaria Martín-González M, et al. Antioxidant vitamins and brain dysfunction in alcoholics. *Alcohol Alcohol.* 2014;49(1):45—50. https://doi.org/10.1093/alcalc/agt150.

74. Bianchi GP, Fiorella PL, Bargossi AM, Grossi G, Marchesini G. Reduced ubiquinone plasma levels in patients with liver cirrhosis and in chronic alcoholics. *Liver.* 1994;14(3):138—140.

75. Cunningham CC, Bailey SM. Ethanol consumption and liver mitochondria function. *Biol Signals Recept.* 2001;10(3—4):271—282. https://doi.org/46892.

76. Kępka A, Waszkiewicz N, Zalewska-Szajda B, et al. Plasma carnitine concentrations after chronic alcohol intoxication. *Postępy Hig Med Dośw Online.* 2013;67:548—552.

77. Ong J, Randhawa R. Scurvy in an alcoholic patient treated with intravenous vitamins. *BMJ Case Rep.* 2014;2014. https://doi.org/10.1136/bcr-2013-009479.

78. Shugalei IS. [Features of vitamin C metabolism and the functional status of the liver in alcoholism and alcoholic delirium in the stage of detoxification therapy]. *Zhurnal Nevropatol Psikhiatrii Im SS Korsakova Mosc Russ 1952.* 1987;87(2):240–243.

79. Zhou JF, Chen P. Studies on the oxidative stress in alcohol abusers in China. *Biomed Environ Sci BES.* 2001; 14(3):180–188.

80. Koob GF. The dark side of emotion: the addiction perspective. *Eur J Pharmacol.* 2015;753:73–87. https:// doi.org/10.1016/j.ejphar.2014.11.044.

81. *Rhodiola rosea.* Monograph. *Altern Med Rev J Clin Ther.* 2002;7(5):421–423.

82. van Diermen D, Marston A, Bravo J, Reist M, Carrupt P-A, Hostettmann K. Monoamine oxidase inhibition by *Rhodiola rosea* L. roots. *J Ethnopharmacol.* 2009;122(2): 397–401. https://doi.org/10.1016/j.jep.2009.01.007.

83. Perfumi M, Santoni M, Cippitelli A, Ciccocioppo R, Froldi R, Massi M. *Hypericum perforatum* CO_2 extract and opioid receptor antagonists act synergistically to reduce ethanol intake in alcohol-preferring rats. *Alcohol Clin Exp Res.* 2003;27(10):1554–1562. https://doi.org/ 10.1097/01.ALC.0000092062.60924.56.

84. Abenavoli L, Capasso F, Addolorato G. Phytotherapeutic approach to alcohol dependence: new old way? *Phytomedicine.* 2009;16(6–7):638–644. https://doi.org/ 10.1016/j.phymed.2008.12.013.

85. Arendt T. Impairment in memory function and neurodegenerative changes in the cholinergic basal forebrain system induced by chronic intake of ethanol. *J Neural Transm Suppl.* 1994;44:173–187.

86. Vescovi PP, Coiro V. Different control of GH secretion by gamma-amino- and gamma-hydroxy-butyric acid in 4-year abstinent alcoholics. *Drug Alcohol Depend.* 2001; 61(3):217–221.

87. Vescovi PP, Coiro V. Persistence of defective serotonergic and GABAergic controls of growth hormone secretion in long-term abstinent alcoholics. *Alcohol Alcohol.* 1997; 32(1):85–90.

88. Mann K, Ackermann K, Diehl A, et al. Galantamine: a cholinergic patch in the treatment of alcoholism: a randomized, placebo-controlled trial. *Psychopharmacol Berl.* 2006;184(1):115–121. https://doi.org/10.1007/ s00213-005-0243-9.

89. Wignall ND, Brown ES. Citicoline in addictive disorders: a review of the literature. *Am J Drug Alcohol Abuse.* 2014;40(4): 262–268. https://doi.org/10.3109/00952990.2014.925467.

90. Lyon J. More treatments on deck for alcohol use disorder. *JAMA.* 2017;317(22):2267–2269. https://doi.org/ 10.1001/jama.2017.4760.

91. Manzo-Avalos S, Saavedra-Molina A. Cellular and mitochondrial effects of alcohol consumption. *Int J Environ Res Public Health.* 2010;7(12):4281–4304. https:// doi.org/10.3390/ijerph7124281.

92. Cahill A, Cunningham CC, Adachi M, et al. Effects of alcohol and oxidative stress on liver pathology: the role of the mitochondrion. *Alcohol Clin Exp Res.* 2002;26(6): 907–915.

93. Haorah J, Rump TJ, Xiong H. Reduction of brain mitochondrial β-oxidation impairs complex I and V in chronic alcohol intake: the underlying mechanism for neurodegeneration. *PLoS One.* 2013;8(8):e70833. https://doi.org/10.1371/journal.pone.0070833.

94. Amodio P, Angeli P, Merkel C, Menon F, Gatta A. Plasma carnitine levels in liver cirrhosis: relationship with nutritional status and liver damage. *J Clin Chem Clin Biochem Z Klin Chem Klin Biochem.* 1990;28(9):619–626.

95. Alonso de la Peña C, Rozas I, Alvarez-Prechous A, Pardiñas MC, Paz JM, Rodriguez-Segade S. Free carnitine and acylcarnitine levels in sera of alcoholics. *Biochem Med Metab Biol.* 1990;44(1):77–83.

96. Adamo S, Siliprandi N, Dl Lisa F, et al. Effect of L-carnitine on ethanol and acetate plasma levels after oral administration of ethanol in humans. *Alcohol Clin Exp Res.* 1988;12(5):653–654.

97. Haorah J, Floreani NA, Knipe B, Persidsky Y. Stabilization of superoxide dismutase by acetyl-l-carnitine in human brain endothelium during alcohol exposure: novel protective approach. *Free Radic Biol Med.* 2011;51(8):1601–1609. https://doi.org/10.1016/j.freeradbiomed.2011.06.020.

98. Rump TJ, Abdul Muneer PM, Szlachetka AM, et al. Acetyl-L-carnitine protects neuronal function from alcohol-induced oxidative damage in the brain. *Free Radic Biol Med.* 2010;49(10):1494–1504. https://doi.org/ 10.1016/j.freeradbiomed.2010.08.011.

99. Tempesta E, Troncon R, Janiri L, et al. Role of acetyl-L-carnitine in the treatment of cognitive deficit in chronic alcoholism. *Int J Clin Pharmacol Res.* 1990;10(1–2): 101–107.

100. Malaguarnera M, Gargante MP, Cristaldi E, et al. Acetyl-L-carnitine treatment in minimal hepatic encephalopathy. *Dig Dis Sci.* 2008;53(11):3018–3025. https://doi.org/ 10.1007/s10620-008-0238-6.

101. Kandhare AD, Ghosh P, Ghule AE, Bodhankar SL. Elucidation of molecular mechanism involved in neuroprotective effect of Coenzyme Q10 in alcohol-induced neuropathic pain. *Fundam Clin Pharmacol.* 2013;27(6): 603–622. https://doi.org/10.1111/fcp.12003.

102. Karakaya K, Barut F, Hanci V, et al. Gastroprotective effects of CoQ10 on ethanol-induced acute gastric lesions. *Bratisl Lek Listy.* 2015;116(1):51–56.

103. Vannucchi H, Moreno FS, Amarante AR, de Oliveira JE, Marchini JS. Plasma amino acid patterns in alcoholic pellagra patients. *Alcohol Alcohol.* 1991;26(4):431–436.

104. Jukić T, Rojc B, Boben-Bardutzky D, Hafner M, Ihan A. The use of a food supplementation with D-phenylalanine, L-glutamine and L-5-hydroxytryptophan in the alleviation of alcohol withdrawal symptoms. *Coll Antropol.* 2011;35(4):1225–1230.

105. Leon R, Wu H, Jin Y, et al. Protective function of taurine in glutamate-induced apoptosis in cultured neurons. *J Neurosci Res.* 2009;87(5):1185–1194. https://doi.org/ 10.1002/jnr.21926.

106. Olive MF. Interactions between taurine and ethanol in the central nervous system. *Amino Acids.* 2002;23(4): 345–357. https://doi.org/10.1007/s00726-002-0203-1.

107. Hsieh Y-L, Yeh Y-H, Lee Y-T, Huang C-Y. Effect of taurine in chronic alcoholic patients. *Food Funct.* 2014;5(7): 1529–1535. https://doi.org/10.1039/c3fo60597c.

108. Fitzgerald DC, Meade KG, McEvoy AN, et al. Tumour necrosis factor-alpha (TNF-alpha) increases nuclear factor kappaB (NFkappaB) activity in and interleukin-8 (IL-8) release from bovine mammary epithelial cells. *Vet Immunol Immunopathol.* 2007;116(1–2):59–68. https://doi.org/10.1016/j.vetimm.2006.12.008.

109. Renard P, Zachary MD, Bougelet C, et al. Effects of antioxidant enzyme modulations on interleukin-1-induced nuclear factor kappa B activation. *Biochem Pharmacol.* 1997;53(2):149–160.

110. Chandel NS, Trzyna WC, McClintock DS, Schumacker PT. Role of oxidants in NF-kappa B activation and TNF-alpha gene transcription induced by hypoxia and endotoxin. *J Immunol Baltim Md 1950.* 2000;165(2):1013–1021.

111. Qin H, Wilson CA, Lee SJ, Zhao X, Benveniste EN. LPS induces CD40 gene expression through the activation of NF-kappaB and STAT-1alpha in macrophages and microglia. *Blood.* 2005;106(9):3114–3122. https://doi.org/10.1182/blood-2005-02-0759.

112. Meffert MK, Chang JM, Wiltgen BJ, Fanselow MS, Baltimore D. NF-kappa B functions in synaptic signaling and behavior. *Nat Neurosci.* 2003;6(10):1072–1078. https://doi.org/10.1038/nn1110.

113. Kasdallah-Grissa A, Mornagui B, Aouani E, et al. Resveratrol, a red wine polyphenol, attenuates ethanol-induced oxidative stress in rat liver. *Life Sci.* 2007;80(11): 1033–1039. https://doi.org/10.1016/j.lfs.2006.11.044.

114. Tiwari V, Chopra K. Resveratrol prevents alcohol-induced cognitive deficits and brain damage by blocking inflammatory signaling and cell death cascade in neonatal rat brain. *J Neurochem.* 2011;117(4):678–690. https://doi.org/10.1111/j.1471-4159.2011.07236.x.

115. Ng QX, Koh SSH, Chan HW, Ho CYX. Clinical use of curcumin in depression: a meta-analysis. *J Am Med Dir Assoc.* 2017;18(6):503–508. https://doi.org/10.1016/j.jamda.2016.12.071.

116. Rong S, Zhao Y, Bao W, et al. Curcumin prevents chronic alcohol-induced liver disease involving decreasing ROS generation and enhancing antioxidative capacity. *Phytomed Int J Phytother Phytopharm.* 2012;19(6):545–550. https://doi.org/10.1016/j.phymed.2011.12.006.

117. Zeng Y, Liu J, Huang Z, Pan X, Zhang L. Effect of curcumin on antioxidant function in the mice with acute alcoholic liver injury. *Wei Sheng Yan Jiu.* 2014;43(2): 282–285.

118. Samuhasaneeto S, Thong-Ngam D, Kulaputana O, Suyasunanont D, Klaikeaw N. Curcumin decreased oxidative stress, inhibited NF-kappaB activation, and improved liver pathology in ethanol-induced liver injury in rats. *J Biomed Biotechnol.* 2009;2009:981963. https://doi.org/10.1155/2009/981963.

119. Keshavarzian A, Holmes EW, Patel M, Iber F, Fields JZ, Pethkar S. Leaky gut in alcoholic cirrhosis: a possible mechanism for alcohol-induced liver damage. *Am J Gastroenterol.* 1999;94(1):200–207. https://doi.org/10.1111/j.1572-0241.1999.00797.x.

120. Purohit V, Bode JC, Bode C, et al. Alcohol, intestinal bacterial growth, intestinal permeability to endotoxin, and medical consequences: summary of a symposium. *Alcohol Fayettev N.* 2008;42(5):349–361. https://doi.org/10.1016/j.alcohol.2008.03.131.

121. Vadnie CA, Park JH, Abdel Gawad N, Ho AMC, Hinton DJ, Choi D-S. Gut-brain peptides in corticostriatal-limbic circuitry and alcohol use disorders. *Front Neurosci.* 2014;8. https://doi.org/10.3389/fnins.2014.00288.

122. van der Hulst RR, van Kreel BK, von Meyenfeldt MF, et al. Glutamine and the preservation of gut integrity. *Lancet Lond Engl.* 1993;341(8857):1363–1365.

123. Besselink MGH, van Santvoort HC, Buskens E, et al. Probiotic prophylaxis in patients with predicted severe acute pancreatitis: a randomised, double-blind, placebo-controlled trial. *Ned Tijdschr Geneeskd.* 2008;152(12): 685–696.

124. Riggio O, Varriale M, Testore GP, et al. Effect of lactitol and lactulose administration on the fecal flora in cirrhotic patients. *J Clin Gastroenterol.* 1990;12(4):433–436.

125. Jain L, Sharma BC, Srivastava S, Puri SK, Sharma P, Sarin S. Serum endotoxin, inflammatory mediators, and magnetic resonance spectroscopy before and after treatment in patients with minimal hepatic encephalopathy. *J Gastroenterol Hepatol.* 2013;28(7):1187–1193. https://doi.org/10.1111/jgh.12160.

Index

Note: Page numbers followed by "f" indicate figures, "t" indicate tables.

Printed and bound by CPI Group (UK) Ltd, Croydon, CR0 4YY

21/10/2024

01777198-0001